Teaching Students with Language and Communication Disabilities

Teaching Students with Language and Communication Disabilities

S. Jay Kuder
Rowan College

Allyn and Bacon
Boston • London • Toronto • Sydney • Tokyo • Singapore

Senior Editor: Ray Short
Editorial Assistant: Christine Svitila
Marketing Manager: Kris Farnsworth
Production Administrator: Annette Joseph
Production Coordinator: Susan Freese
Editorial-Production Service: WordCrafters Editorial Services, Inc.
Manufacturing Buyer: Megan Cochran
Composition Buyer: Linda Cox
Cover Administrator: Suzanne Harbison

Library of Congress Cataloging-in-Publication Data
Kuder, S. Jay.
    Teaching students with language and communication disabilities /
  S. Jay Kuder.
       p.   cm.
    Includes bibliographical references and index.
    ISBN 0-205-15694-0
      1. Handicapped children—United States—Language arts.
    2. Language disorders in children—United States.   3. Communicative
  disorders in children—United States.   I. Title.
    LC4028.K83   1997
    371.91′4—dc20   96-24905
                                                              CIP

Printed in the United States of America

10 9 8 7 6 5 4 3 2   01 00 99 98 97

Text Credits

Pages 112–113, case study about "Randy": from *Handbook of Autism and Pervasive Developmental Disorders*, edited by R. Paul, Copyright © 1987 John Wiley & Sons, Inc. Reprinted by permission of John Wiley & Sons, Inc. **Page 163**, case study about "Joey": Reprinted with permission from the March issue of *Learning*, 1991, Copyright The Education Center®, 1607 Battleground Ave., Greensboro, NC 27408. **Page 164**, case study about "Alfonso": From *Exceptional Children and Youths*, 6th ed., by Haring/McCormick, © 1982. Adapted by permission of Prentice-Hall, Inc., Upper Saddle River, NJ. **Page 165**, case study about "Ethan": From L. Michaud and A. Duhaime, "Traumatic Brain Injury," in *Children with Disabilities: A Medical Primer*, 3rd ed., edited by M. Batshaw and Y. Perret (Baltimore, MD: Brookes Publishing Co., 1992), pp. 541–542. Reprinted with permission of the authors and Brookes Publishing Co., P.O. Box 10624, Baltimore, MD 21285-0624. **Page 207**, case study about "Bob": From E. Wiig and E. Semel, *Language Assessment and Intervention for the Learning Disabled*. Copyright © 1984 by Allyn and Bacon. Reprinted by permission.

Brief Contents

Contents

List of Figures

List of Tables

Preface

What is it like to be a student who has difficulty understanding or using language? It may be a lot like the experience of being in a foreign country where you do not speak the language—at least not very well. If you have ever been in such a situation, you may recall your embarrassment when asking a simple question about directions, for instance. You may remember what it felt like to be laughed at by others or to fear being ridiculed because of your accent and grammatical errors. You may have been reluctant to order a meal or a taxi for fear of making a mistake, and you may have actually experienced physical sensations, such as sweating or nausea, before having to speak or participate in a conversation.

The problems experienced by students who have difficulties with language and communication may not be dissimilar from the feelings experienced by visitors to a foreign country. Students with communication difficulties may be reluctant to participate in class discussions because they fear being ridiculed by teachers or peers. They may misunderstand directions and fail to ask questions that would help them understand. Further, they may shy away from interaction with other students.

Sometimes students with language and communication difficulties are labeled as "special education students" and classified as "learning disabled," "communication handicapped," or even "mildly mentally retarded." Many of these children will not be labeled, but their problems may be no less serious.

The purpose of this book is to help teachers and other professionals who work with children identify, understand, and help those children with language difficulties. To achieve these goals, it is essential that all educators, special and regular, understand language—what it is *and* how to help children experiencing difficulty with it. Three current trends make this more imperative than ever.

The first trend is the present emphasis on the whole-language approach in educational practice. In order to be an effective user of the whole-language approach, the teacher must know about language and how it interrelates with the other language arts.

A second trend is toward delivery of speech and language services in the classroom, with the teacher acting as a partner in the intervention process. This approach relies heavily on the classroom teacher's ability to identify children with speech and language difficulties and to carry out classroom-based intervention strategies.

Finally, there is a trend toward including students with special needs in regular education classrooms. No longer can teachers rely on certain experts to remove from their classrooms children who are experiencing learning difficulties. Regular education teachers must develop skills in teaching *all* children—including those with language disorders. At the same time, it is essential that special education teachers develop skills—through collaboration and consultation with other teachers—that will enable them to support instruction in the regular education classroom.

If these three trends continue, all teachers can expect to work with children who have language difficulties. Moreover, additional responsibility for identifying and helping these children will be placed on the classroom teacher—both special and regular education.

This book is divided into three major units. Part I (Chapters 1–4) presents the components of speech, language, and communication and describes language development. Part II (Chapters 5–9) presents a description of the language abilities of students with a variety of disabilities. And Part III (Chapters 10–14) provides suggestions for assessment and intervention and discusses cultural factors and language.

I have tried to make this book one that will be useful to educators who do not have extensive backgrounds in linguistic and developmental theories. Therefore, I have tried to keep the use of technical language to a minimum, while retaining a solid base of research. My hope is that readers will feel better prepared to help their students develop those language and communication skills that are essential for success in school and the community.

Acknowledgments

A book such as this is more than the product of a few months or years; it is the result of a lifetime of learning and growth. Still, there are a few individuals to whom I am especially indebted. These include Dr. Diane Bryen of Temple University, who first sparked my interest in language and language disorders, and Dr. Paula Menyuk of Boston University, who helped refine my interest into a vocation. I also thank Dr. Hector Rios, for his suggestions regarding cultural and language differences, and Dr. Mary Ann Romski, for her most helpful comments on the subject of augmentative and alternative communication. In addition, I thank those individuals who reviewed earlier versions of this book for Allyn and Bacon: Barbara C. Gartin, University of Arkansas, and Steven F. Warren, Peabody at Vanderbilt.

Finally, I thank my wife—Lucy—and my children—Julia, Emily, and Suzanne—for giving me the courage to undertake this task and for their patience and understanding.

Part *I*

Understanding Language and Communication

The four chapters in this unit present background information about language and communication—their definitions, models of acquisition, and development. This information is essential for teachers and other professionals who want to identify, teach, and understand children with language and communication problems.

Language and communication are complex and fascinating processes. Defining them helps us better understand these processes and communicate with each other about them. Chapter 1 presents definitions of speech, language, and communication. Chapter 2 focuses on language and the various aspects that comprise it.

The mystery of language acquisition is described, but not entirely solved, in Chapter 3. Knowledge of language acquisition theories can be useful in understanding what may underlie the language and communication difficulties of some children. In addition, the theories provide models for language intervention.

The course of normal language development is described in Chapter 4. Understanding it can be helpful in the identification of deviations from the normal sequence. Although there is considerable variability in normal language development, there comes a point at which one may become concerned about children who are not keeping up with their peers.

After reading this unit you should have a better understanding of language and communication. You should be familiar with the major theories of language acquisition and have a general idea of the course of language development. This knowledge will help you identify and understand children with language problems.

C h a p t e r **1**

Language and Language Disorders

In this chapter we will explore the meaning of the terms speech, language, *and* communication. *It is important to understand the meaning of each of these terms since they will be used throughout the text. In addition, they are frequently used—and sometimes misused—to describe the difficulties experienced by some students.*

Once we are reasonably sure what we are talking about, it is possible to begin to identify children with language disorders. In this chapter we will also discuss the concept of language disorder *and consider some criteria for identifying students with language difficulties.*

After reading this chapter, you should be able to:

1. Differentiate among *speech, language,* and *communication.*
2. Explain the characteristics of a language.
3. Identify the components needed for successful communication.
4. Identify the characteristics of language disorder.

_____ **Kevin: A Case Study** _____

Kevin is a 9-year-old student in a regular fourth-grade classroom. Kevin seems bright and usually works hard, but he is a puzzle to his teacher. Sometimes it seems as though he's just not all there. He misunderstands directions—failing to complete all of the assignment or even working on the wrong pages. He is reluctant to answer questions in class. When he does answer, he stops and starts and seems confused. Kevin is a slow, hesitant reader. His teacher, Mrs. Ross, has noticed that his comprehension of text often seems to be ahead of his ability to read the words themselves. He is a poor speller. In his writing he tends to use short, choppy, sentences, and his output is often poorly organized. Although Kevin is good in math, he has difficulty with word problems. In addition to these problems with his schoolwork, Kevin often appears to be lost among his fellow students. He hangs behind the others when they go out to play and often eats by himself at lunch.

Mrs. Ross would like to help Kevin, but she is not sure what is wrong. Is he immature? Should he be referred for special education? Could there be some medical reason for Kevin's problems?

Kevin is typical of students who have problems with language and communication. He may be experiencing difficulty understanding incoming language and producing appropriate spoken responses of his own. He appears to lack some of the subtle communication skills that are critical to social acceptance by his peers. He is at risk for academic as well as social difficulties. If nothing is done, it is likely that Kevin's problems will get worse. As the pace of learning increases in middle and high school, he is likely to fall further behind. But what *should* be done? And just what *is* Kevin's problem?

In order to understand Kevin and children like him, it is first necessary to understand the nature of language and the related concepts of speech and communication. This may help in determining what kind of difficulty Kevin is experiencing. It may even help in the development of procedures to help Kevin and children like him to enhance their skills in language and communication.

Speech, Language, and Communication

Speech

Speech, language, and *communication*—all of these are words that are sometimes used in describing the language production and language difficulties of children. It may be that Kevin has a speech problem. Might he also have a language problem? Is this just another way of saying the same thing? He may well have some problems communicating with others. Does it make any difference what we call his problem, or is this just another tiresome academic debate?

One way to answer this question is to ask some other questions. Is it possible to have speech without language? Consider the 3-month-old baby as she begins to babble. Listen to the sounds she makes: "bah," "gah," "buh." Are these speech sounds? Linguists (people who study language) say that they *are* speech sounds, because they have characteristics that are identical to the same sounds produced by adults. What about people with echolalia? This is a condition prevalent in many children with autism and mental retardation in which they repeat back exactly what they hear. For example, I might say, "What did you have for dinner?" and a person with echolalia might respond, "What did you have for dinner?" Did this person use speech? Of course, the answer is yes.

In each of these examples it is clear that speech is being used, but most linguists would say that in neither case is true *language* being used. Although Mommy or Daddy may claim to understand what baby is saying, most outsiders would have a hard time interpreting the sounds being uttered. The baby's speech could hardly be said to be conforming to the rules of adult language. In the case of an individual with echolalia, although the speech output is certainly in the form of language, it is not being used in a meaningful way. It is not an appropriate response within the context of the conversation.

These observations can help us differentiate between speech and language. **Speech** can be defined as the neuromuscular act of producing sounds that are used in language. Not all sounds are speech sounds in a particular language. For example, I can make clicking sounds with my tongue. Although these may actually be speech sounds in some African languages, they are not speech sounds in English. Speech, then, is a physiological act in which the muscles involved in speech production are coordinated by the brain to produce the sounds of language.

Language

So, what *is* language? Before we can arrive at a definition, it is necessary to ask another question. Is it possible to have language without speech? The answer is yes. The best example is American Sign Language (ASL). ASL is, most linguists agree, a language. It is the primary mode of communication of many deaf persons. It is a gestural language that has its own unique grammatical structure. But why is it considered a language? What makes it so?

One feature may be obvious: A true language **communicates.** It communicates thoughts, ideas, and meaning. A second feature of language is that it is a **shared code.** That is, although not everyone may know ASL (just as not everyone knows Hungarian), those who know the language being used can communicate with each other. A third feature of language is that it consists of **arbitrary symbols.** That is, the symbols have meaning just because we say they do. There is no reason that a tree might not be called a "smook." There is nothing green and leafy about the word *tree.* Although a few ASL signs are iconic (they look like the things they represent), most are arbitrary symbols. Therefore, ASL has this feature of language. Another feature of language is that it is **generative.** Given a finite set of words and a finite number of rules, speakers can generate an infinite number of sentences. Although you are an educated person who has read widely, there are certainly sentences in this book that you have never encountered before. This is due to the generative property of language. Finally, language is **creative.** New words are constantly entering the language while existing words drop out of usage or change their meaning. Consider some of the new words that have entered the English language—*byte, teflon, laser.* How about words that have changed their meanings—*gay, cool, neat.*

Language is a complex phenomenon and, as such, is difficult to define (see Box 1.1). Although there are many definitions of language, none of them is completely adequate. In this book we will use a simple definition: **Language** is a rule-governed symbol system for communicating meaning through a shared code of arbitrary symbols. Although this may not be a perfect definition, it does convey the idea that language involves communication that is shared by a community. Which leads to our final definition, the definition of communication.

BOX 1.1   Do Animals Have Language?

This is a question that has long fascinated psychologists and linguists alike. Research has examined the so-called language abilities of many species. For example, studies by Karl Von Frisch (1967) and Konrad Lorenz (1971) revealed that bees possess an elaborate system of communication. Through a complex dance routine, bees can tell each other about the distance and direction from the hive to a source of nectar. Although this is a remarkable achievement, the communicative abilities of bees are very limited.

There is a long history of interest in the linguistic abilities of chimpanzees. Although early attempts by Winthrop and Luella Kellogg in the 1930s and Keith and Kathy Hayes in the 1940s to induce language in chimps by raising them just as they would a human infant were largely a failure, the interest in nonhuman primate language did not disappear. Beginning in the 1960s with research by Beatrice and Allan Gardner of the University of Nevada, interest in the potential language abilities of chimps and other nonhuman primates was revived. Using American Sign Language as the means of communication, the Gardners successfully trained a chimp named Washoe to use over 100 signs.

Even more exciting, they claimed that Washoe created *new* signs by combining signs she had already learned (Gardner & Gardner, 1969). Other research by David Premack (1972) and Duane Rumbaugh (1977) at the University of Georgia focused on the development of grammatical skills in chimps and produced interesting and controversial results.

Many of the claims put forward by the researchers on the language abilities of chimpanzees were challenged by Herbert Terrace of Columbia University (Terrace, 1980). His own research with a chimp named Nim and his review of the Gardners's earlier research caused him to conclude that many of the claims for evidence of chimps' language abilities were overblown and that the supposed uses of language were, in fact, merely instances of sophisticated imitation.

The debate on whether or not language is unique to humans will continue. Recent studies carried out with gorillas and with pygmy chimpanzees (Savage-Rumbaugh, 1990) has rekindled interest in the possible language abilities of nonhuman primates. These contemporary studies are exploring the possibility that animals may be able to understand more language than was previously thought.

Communication

Once again a question: Is it possible to have communication without language? If you have ever been in a noisy barroom, the answer should be obvious. A lot of communication can go on nonlinguistically. A smile, a shift in body position, a gesture, even the raise of an eyebrow can communicate a great deal. Sometimes these communicative attempts may be misinterpreted, causing problems. But, clearly, it is possible to communicate without spoken language.

Communication is the broadest of the three terms that we have attempted to define. **Communication** has been defined as "the process of exchanging information and ideas between participants" (Owens, 1992, p. 6). In order for communication to take place, there must be four elements:

1. A sender of the message
2. A receiver of the message

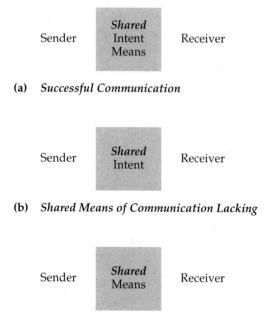

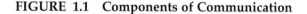

FIGURE 1.1   **Components of Communication**

3. A shared intent to communicate
4. A shared means of communication

When all of these elements are present, communication may occur (see Figure 1.1[a]). But when one or more of these elements is missing, there may be a breakdown in communication. Figure 1.1(b) shows what may happen if you meet someone in a foreign country. You may both want to communicate, but unless you share a common language, you may be unable to do so. Although you share the intent to communicate, you lack a shared means of communication. However, if you can get your messages across with gestures and facial expressions, you may be able to communicate with each other after all. Conversely, two speakers may share the means to communicate (i.e., a common language) but not share the same communicative intent (Figure 1.1[c]). For example, if I am teaching a class and suddenly feel hot, I may look at a student in the class who is seated near the window and say, "Gee, it's hot in here." If the student's response is to say, "Yes, it is," we have failed to communicate. My intent was for the student to open the window. The student's understanding of my message was that I was simply commenting on the room temperature. For communication to be successful, *all* of its elements must be in place: a speaker, a listener, a shared intent to communicate, and a shared means of communication.

We have seen that speech and language can be used for communication but are not essential for communication. Similarly, language can be either spoken or

FIGURE 1.2   Speech, Language, and Communication

Speech: The neuromuscular act of producing sounds that are used in language.

Language: A rule-governed symbol system for communicating meaning through a shared code of arbitrary symbols. Language:
- Communicates.
- Is a shared code.
- Consists of arbitrary symbols.
- Is generative.
- Is creative.

Communication: The process of exchanging information and ideas between participants (Owens, 1992). In order for communication to take place, there must be a:
- Sender of the message.
- Receiver of the message.
- Shared intent to communicate.
- Shared means of communication.

nonspoken (e.g., ASL). Speech can be used to express language or for nonlanguage utterances (e.g., babble or echolalia) (see Figure 1.2).

For our purposes it is important to understand the distinctions among speech, language, and communication because these distinctions can help us be more specific about the nature of the problems of a student such as Kevin. It could be that his difficulties are primarily the result of speech problems such as misarticulation. This could account for some of his reluctance to talk in class and for some of his difficulties in socializing with his peers. But a speech problem alone would not explain Kevin's difficulties in understanding language or his problems with reading and writing. Kevin clearly has some difficulties communicating with others. These could be caused by misunderstanding the communicative intentions of others or by deficiencies in the language skills that are necessary for communication. It is most likely that Kevin has a language disorder. His difficulties in using and interpreting language for learning and socialization support this conclusion.

Language Disorder

The American Speech-Language-Hearing Association (ASHA), the professional organization of speech-language specialists, has defined *language disorder* as follows:

> *A language disorder is impaired comprehension and/or use of spoken, written, and/or other symbol systems. This disorder may involve (1) the form of language (phonology, morphology, syntax), (2) the content of language (semantics), and/or (3) the function of language in communication (pragmatics) in any combination. (Ad Hoc Committee on Service Delivery in the Schools, 1993, p. 40)*

Let's take a look at this definition in more detail. The first major point highlighted by the ASHA definition is that language disorder includes both *comprehension* of language and language *production*. Children who have comprehension (receptive language) difficulties may have difficulty following directions and may appear to be inattentive. Students who have problems with language production (expressive language) may be reluctant to participate in activities that require the use of language. They may use more immature language than their peers. They may have difficulty relating personal experiences or retelling stories. Sometimes the productive language problems are more obvious, but difficulties in comprehension can be as much as or more of a problem in the classroom.

The second major point made by the definition is that the disorder can be identified in *either* spoken or written language. Usually we think of a language disorder as referring just to spoken language problems. But the definition points out that language is an essential part of writing as well. Sometimes problems in writing are caused by an underlying difficulty in using language.

The third major point is that language disorders can occur in one or more aspects of language. We will examine these elements of language in more detail in the next chapter, but the important point is that a language disorder can be pervasive or limited in scope.

It is important to distinguish language *disorders* from language *differences*. Many students come to school speaking a language other than English as their first language or a dialect that differs from standard English. These children must not be labeled "language disordered" merely because they talk differently from their teachers or from some societal standard. However, some children may talk differently *and* have a language disorder. Later in this book we will see how experts have devised ways to differentiate children with language differences from those with language disorders.

Language disorders can vary from very mild (e.g., problems in using metaphor in writing) to severe (e.g., no spoken language). There can be disorders in the rate or timing of language development and in specific aspects of language (syntax, semantics, etc.) (Leonard, 1990). The terms *delay* and *deviance* have also been used in relation to language disorders (de Villiers & de Villiers, 1978). *Delay* refers to the timing of language acquisition and includes late onset of development, a lagging rate of acquisition, and/or a final level of language proficiency significantly less than that of normal adult language. *Deviance* refers to differences in the sequence of language development or in the structures that are acquired.

Often children with language and communication disorders experience other problems as well. They may have difficulty interacting with their peers. They may be shy and reluctant to approach others. Other children may ignore them or, even worse, reject their attempts at friendship. Some children with language and communication disorders have difficulty with cognitive functioning. They may have difficulty organizing information for recall, may be less attentive than their peers, and may be generally slower to respond. Sometimes children with language and communication difficulties exhibit behavior problems. These problems may be the result of their own frustration with communication, or they may result from the response of others to their difficulties. Some children with language and communication disorders have physical disabilities that either cause or exacerbate their difficulty. For example, children with cleft palate often have difficulty with articulation, and children with mild, fluctuating hearing loss are at risk for a variety of language and communication disorders.

Language disorders are often associated with other disabilities such as autism and mental retardation. Children with language disorders may be called "dysphasic," "dyslexic," "dysnomic," "communication handicapped," "language-learning disabled," and so on. However, language disorders are not limited to children with classifications such as mental retardation and autism. Many students with mild language difficulties are never classified or are grouped under the general term *learning disabled*. In this book, I have chosen to organize the sections on specific language disorders by category of disability. This was no easy choice, and I recognize its potential for confusion. It may seem that the book is saying that all children with a particular disability (e.g., mental retardation) have language disorders when, in fact, this may not be the case. Alternatively, it may seem that a child has to be classified with a disability label to have a language disorder. This also is not true. However, special education tends to be organized on the basis of diagnostic categories, and much of the research on language disorders is related to diagnostic categories. So, while these categories may be misleading, they provide an organizing framework for understanding language disorders.

The key criterion in determining whether a language difficulty is serious enough to require intervention is the impact the problem has on the child and on others. Does the child appear to be concerned about the problem? Is the language difficulty interfering with the child's ability to learn and/or socialize? Do other children tease or reject the child because of difficulties the child may be experiencing with speech, language, or communication? If the answer to one or more of these questions is yes, the child may require some sort of intervention.

Because children with language and communication disorders are at risk for academic and social failure, it is important that their difficulties be identified as early as possible. In many cases it may be possible to correct or at least enhance their performance. Figure 1.3 provides a list of characteristics of children with language and communication difficulties that may be useful in identifying these children.

Recognizing the problem and determining the need for intervention is a necessary first step in helping children with language and communication difficulties. But it is only a first step. Knowing *what* the child should be able to do and how to help the child get to that point is the goal of the rest of this book.

Summary

Speech, language, and communication are related to each other yet also independent of each other. Communication is the broadest of these concepts, encompassing both verbal and nonverbal interaction. Speech refers to the neuromuscular act of sound production. Language is a complex phenomenon that involves the use of symbols that conform to rules that are used to express meaning.

FIGURE 1.3   Characteristics of Children with Language and Communication Disorders

Academic Performance
Reluctance to contribute to discussions
Difficulty organizing ideas
Difficulty recognizing phonemes
Difficulty producing sounds
Failure to follow directions
Difficulty finding the right word for things

Social Interaction
Reluctance to interact with other children
Exclusion or rejection by other children
Difficulty carrying on a conversation
Problems negotiating rules for games

Cognitive Functioning
Difficulty organizing information for recall
Slow responding
Inattentiveness

Behavior
High level of frustration
Frequent arguments
Fighting with peers
Withdrawing from interaction

Language disorders are deviations from the normal development and/or appropriate use of language. It is important to identify language disorders as early as possible, because such disorders can cause serious problems in learning and socialization. Moreover, with early identification it may be possible to help children make significant improvement in their language skills.

Review Questions

1. Is it possible to have speech without language? Why or why not? Give two examples that support your answer.

2. List and briefly explain three features that help define language.

3. When you are talking to yourself, are you communicating? Why or why not?

4. Describe the kinds of problems that a child with a language comprehension disorder might experience in a classroom situation.

5. A parent says to you, "Do you think Sharon (my 6-year-old child) should have speech therapy?" How would you respond?

6. One characteristic of human language is creativity. Give five examples of words that have entered the English language in the last 10 years.

Suggested Activities

1. In any social setting there are many opportunities to watch nonverbal communication (i.e., gestures, facial expressions, body language). Use one of these opportunities to be an observer of interaction. Look carefully. What do you see? Can you find any recurrent gestures and/or facial expressions? What do they mean? Make a list of nonverbal communication elements and what they mean. Also, watch for any misunderstandings caused by nonverbal communication.

Does nonverbal communication constitute a language? Explain your answer with examples from your observations. What do your observations indicate about the elements that are necessary for communication to take place?

2. Ask two teachers and two adults who are not teachers to tell you what they think of when they hear the term *language disorder*. Ask them to describe the kinds of problems that a child with a language disorder would face. Ask what should be done to help such children.

What do the responses indicate about the term *language disorder?* How closely does their understanding of this term match the definitions that were presented in the chapter?

References

de Villiers, J. G., & de Villiers, P. A. (1978). *Language acquisition.* Cambridge, MA: Harvard University Press.

Gardner, R., & Gardner, B. (1969). Teaching sign language to a chimpanzee. *Science, 165,* 664–672.

Leonard, L. (1990). Language disorders in preschool children. In G. Shames & E. Wiig (Eds.), *Human communication disorders* (pp. 159–192). Columbus, OH: Merrill.

Lorenz, K. (1971). *Studies in animal behavior.* Cambridge, MA: Harvard University Press.

Owens, R. (1992). *Language development: An introduction.* New York: Macmillan.

Premack, D. (1972). Teaching language to an ape. *Scientific American 227,* 92–99.

Rumbaugh, D. (1977). *Acquisition of language skills by a chimpanzee.* New York: Academic Press.

Savage-Rumbaugh, E. S. (1990). Language acquisition in a nonhuman species: Implications for the innateness debate. *Developmental Psychobiology, 23* (7), 599–620.

Terrace, H. (1980). *Nim.* New York: Knopf.

Von Frisch, K. (1967). *The dance language and orientation of bees* (L. E. Chadwick, Trans.). Cambridge, MA: Belknap.

Chapter 2

The Elements of Language

Language has been described as consisting of several elements. In this chapter we will look in depth at the elements of language. We will see how linguists have described each element and the rules that govern its use. Knowing these elements forms the framework for understanding language disorders and for differentiating language disorders from language differences.

After reading this chapter, you should be able to:

1. Describe the basic elements of language.
2. Understand the terms *phoneme* and *morpheme* and know how they differ from each other.
3. Understand the rules that underlie syntax.
4. Understand some of the challenges in developing rules for semantics.
5. Understand the concept of *pragmatics* and its application in communication.

Human language is extremely complex. In order to simplify and better understand language, linguists have developed various systems for dividing language into its components (or elements). Most linguists identify five major elements: phonology, morphology, syntax, semantics, and pragmatics (e.g., Gleason, 1993). Alternatively, Bloom and Lahey (1978) describe language as consisting of three components: form, content, and use. This model recognizes the interrelatedness of language elements. Within the component they call "form," Bloom and Lahey include the elements of phonology, morphology, and syntax (see Figure 2.1). It is often difficult to separate morphology from phonology (for example, when children are learning that the plural from of *cats* makes an "s" sound while the plural of *dogs* has a "z" sound). Similarly, morphology and syntax are closely related in the emergence of language in young children. Nevertheless, in this chapter we will use the model that includes five language elements because it describes language in its most elemental form. As you read the chapter you should, however, keep in mind the interrelated nature of these elements.

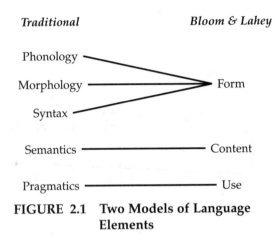

**FIGURE 2.1 Two Models of Language
Elements**

Phonology

As an exercise to illustrate the interrelatedness of language elements, imagine that your task is to program a computer to understand and use spoken language. This is a formidable task but one that has been pursued for some time and has begun to yield very promising results. What would you include in your program? What would the computer need to know in order to process language?

Since computers work best with the most elemental sort of information, the first step might be to input the sounds of the English language. This would not be a terribly difficult task. Linguists have identified approximately 45 distinctive sounds in English (Owens, 1992). These elemental units of language are called *phonemes*. A **phoneme** has been defined as "the smallest linguistic unit of sound that can signal a difference in meaning" (Owens, 1992, p. 18). Linguists can determine whether a sound is a phoneme in a particular language by asking native speakers of that language whether the sound, when added to a root word, makes a new word that they recognize. For example, let's say that we have already established that *bill* is a word in English. Now, if we substitute a *p* sound for the initial *b* sound, will speakers of the language recognize this as a new word? Yes, they recognize the new word as *pill*. Therefore, it appears that *p* is a phoneme in English. Now, let's say that we have determined that the word, *row* is a word in English. If we substitute a rolled *r* for the flat *r* in *row*, have we made a new word that speakers of English recognize as having a different meaning? No. Although the rolled *r* is a phoneme in Spanish, it is not in English.

Having programmed your computer with the 45 or so sounds of English, you are ready to go. The first word your computer produces is *tphj*. Oh no! Something seems to be missing. In fact, what is missing are the rules that govern phonology (there are rules that govern all of the other elements of language, as well). Remember, our definition of language said that it was a *rule-governed* system. In phonology there are rules that determine which sounds can (and cannot) occur together. There are rules that tell when and how vowels must be used and how sound combinations are pronounced. For our computer to process language, its program must include these rules. But this is possible, for the rules are finite and can be discovered.

Phonology, the first of the form elements, is the study of the sound system of language. Linguists who are interested in phonology attempt to identify the phonemes of a language and the rules that govern the combination and pronunciation of these phonemes. Knowledge of these rules enables linguists to understand how native speakers of a language know which sound combinations are possible in their language.

Morphology

So it looks as though we are ready to proceed with our task of developing a computer program to process language. With the rules governing sound our computer is now producing combinations that look a lot more like English. Some of them may not be words that we recognize (e.g., *blif* and *ulop*), but they are at least *possible* English words. But then we notice that we are getting some larger words such as *unpossible* and *deerses,* and we realize that something else is missing. Although these combinations of sounds conform to the rules of phonology, speakers of the language reject these combinations.

The problem is that there must be another set of rules—a set of rules that govern how words are made. In fact there is such a group of rules. They are called *morphological rules.* **Morphology** is the study of words and how they are formed. Morphological rules determine how sounds can be put together to make words; they govern the structure of words.

Consider the word *base.* Any speaker of English would acknowledge this as a word in English. What about *baseball?* Of course this is a word, too, but it is different. It consists of two words—*base* and *ball.* Moreover, each of these words has a meaning that is related to the compound word. That is, both *bases* and *balls* are used in the game of *baseball.* Well, what about *basement?* Can *basement* be separated into two words? In trying to do so we are left with *base* and *ment.* There is no problem with *base* (we have already agreed that it was a word), but just what is a *ment?* No, it appears that *basement* cannot be broken down any further. What do these examples suggest?

From evidence such as the above, linguists have concluded that there are elemental building blocks of language, called *morphemes.* **Morphemes** are the smallest units of meaning in a language (Gleason, 1993). To better understand morphemes let us go back to the previous example. The word *base* is a morpheme. It cannot be broken into smaller pieces while retaining its original meaning. So what about *baseball?* As discussed previously, this *can* be divided into two parts, which retain the meaning of the whole—*base* and *ball.* Therefore each of these words is a morpheme. Although *basement* might also be divided into two parts, doing so would leave a unit that has no meaning, *ment.* Therefore, *basement* is one morpheme.

Actually, linguists say that there are two kinds of morphemes. To illustrate, let us return again to the example. We have already said that *baseball* consists of two morphemes. Each of these is called a *free* morpheme. In other words, each morpheme can stand on its own as a word with meaning. Now let us add a plural *s* to create the word *baseballs*. How many morphemes do we have now? There must be three, since we have already established that *baseball* alone has two morphemes. But what is this new morpheme? What does *s* mean? In this context the *s*, since it is used as a plural, means "more than one." Therefore, there are three morphemes in the word *baseballs*—*base, ball*, and *s* (plural). However, the plural *s* is a special kind of morpheme. It cannot stand alone but has meaning only when it is attached to other morphemes. It is called a *bound* morpheme. Prefixes (such as *un* and *pre*) and suffixes (such as *ing* and *able*) are examples of bound morphemes.

If all of this seems a bit complicated, just consider the kind of problems that linguists have with words such as *cranberry*. For years linguists thought that this was one word, since there is no such thing as a *cran*. Then along came *cranapple* juice. This demonstrated that *cran* can be separated from *berry* and still retain its meaning. Therefore, maybe *cranberry* was really two morphemes all along. This is the sort of debate that linguists love to pursue (see Fromkin & Rodman, 1978, for more).

For our purposes, the point of this discussion is that there *are* rules that determine what a word is and how words can be formed. Thus, native speakers of English recognize that *unlikely* is fine but *inlikely* does not mean anything, that even though *boy* is pluralized as *boys*, more than one man is not *mans* but *men*.

Morphology, then, as the study of words and how they are formed, includes the identification of morphemes (the basic *meaningful* units of language) and the rules for constructing words. With our computer programmed to identify and use morphemes, we can eliminate many of the strange sound combinations we were getting previously. Unfortunately, now we are getting sentences such as the following: *car the man hit the; the sweet is very child.* Clearly, there is still something wrong with our computer program. We need another set of rules. This additional group of rules is called *syntax*.

Syntax

Look at the following first stanza from Lewis Carroll's "Jabberwocky":

Twas brillig, and _____ slithy
toves did _____ and gimble in
the _____. All mimsy were the borogoves
and the mome raths outgrabe.

Can you guess what goes in each blank? You may not always get the exact word *(the; gyre; wabe)*, but, even though this is a lot of nonsense, you probably guessed accurately about the *type* of word that must go in the blank. You undoubtedly knew that the first word was an article. You probably guessed that the second word was a verb, and so on. How did you do this? The answer is that you have *rules* of grammar (syntax) that help you to accomplish tasks like this. You may or may not be able to formally state the rules. You may not even be aware that you possess these rules (until you are forced to use them in some ridiculous exercise), but they are there. These are *syntactic* rules. **Syntax** is the study of the rules that govern how words are put together to make sentences. What do these rules look like?

How would you describe the structure of the following sentences:

1. The dog is running.
2. The girl is reading a book.

For the first sentence, you might say that there is an article (*the*) and a noun (*dog*), an auxiliary verb (*is*) and a main verb (*running*). These are elements of the syntactic rules that linguists call **phrase structure rules.** These rules describe the structure of sentences.

Linguists have devised a shorthand code to describe these rules. For the first sentence, the code would look like the following:

$$
\begin{aligned}
S &\rightarrow NP + VP \\
NP &\rightarrow Art + N \\
VP &\rightarrow Aux + V
\end{aligned}
$$

This notation says that the sentence consists of two elements—a noun phrase and a verb phrase. The noun phrase, in turn, consists of two elements—an article and a noun. The verb phrase also consists of two elements—an auxiliary verb and a main verb.

If this were all that we knew about the English language, we could say that these were the rules of English syntax. But then we might find a sentence like the second example. Since this sentence is not completely explained by our original set of phrase structure rules, we must modify the rules somewhat. Sentence two could be rewritten as:

$$
\begin{aligned}
S &\rightarrow NP + VP \\
NP &\rightarrow Art + N \\
VP &\rightarrow Aux + V + NP \\
NP &\rightarrow Art + N
\end{aligned}
$$

This sentence introduces a new element into our phrase structure rules—a noun phrase that *follows* a verb phrase. If we were to continue examining sentences and refining our rules, we would end up with the finite (and surprisingly small) set of rules for the English language. While small in number, these rules can be used to generate an infinite number of sentences, because of the **recursive** feature of phrase structure rules. This feature permits phrases to be joined together without limit.

For example, in conjoined sentences (sentences that include a conjunction such as *and* or *but*), two or more noun phrases may be joined, as in the following example: *The boy and the girl sat outside the school.* Other nouns (e.g., *teacher, man, friend*) could be added to our sentence without limit. Similarly, more than one verb phrase may be embedded in a single sentence as in: *The girl who is here is my niece.*

For many years it was thought that phrase structure rules were all that were needed to describe a language. But there are certain kinds of sentences that are not easily explained by phrase structure rules. These include imperative sentences *(Go to bed!)* and questions *(Why are you crying?).* Such sentences bothered linguists for many years but could not be adequately explained away. Finally, Noam Chomsky (1957, 1965) developed a theory to account for sentences such as these. Called *transformational grammar,* his theory suggests that there are two levels in all languages—a surface structure and a deep structure. The surface structure is what we actually hear, but the deep structure is the underlying linguistic structure of the utterance. In between the deep structure and the surface structure, according to Chomsky, there is a set of rules *(transformational rules)* that can convert a deep-structure sentence to something else.

For example, take our question sentence, *Why are you crying?* The underlying (deep) structure of this sentence would be *You are crying* (deep-structure sentences are always simple, declarative sentences). In order to get the surface question, a question-transformation rule has to be applied, inverting the subject *(you)* and auxiliary verb *(are)* and adding the appropriate *wh* word *(why).* This entire operation occurs subconsciously. In the case of the imperative, the deep-structure sentence is actually *You go to bed.* The imperative-transformation rule says that when the first noun is in the second person *(you)* it can be deleted, leaving the surface structure *(Go to bed).*

Transformational rules have served us well for many years; however, they have been found to have some limitations. Some problematic sentences can be generated by the theory and its rules. For example, the ambiguity apparent in the sentence *The duck is ready to eat* (Is it the duck that is preparing to eat or is someone about to consume the duck?) cannot be resolved by reference to phrase structure and transformational rules. Additionally, the theory does not adequately explain the universality and learnability of languages (Leonard & Loeb, 1988). The most recent revision of transformational grammar theory, known as **government and binding theory** (Chomsky, 1981, 1982), attempts to account for the universality of language by describing the rules that relate the language we hear to the underlying mental representations we hold in our minds. In addition, Chomsky has identified additional sets of rules that provide limits to the interpretation of sentences. While a complete discussion of this theory is beyond the scope of this book, research in linguistics is continuing to try to describe the universal rules of grammar.

So we can now program our computer with syntactic rules, including phrase-structure and transformational rules. These will help us to organize the words of English into coherent sentences that will easily be interpreted by native speakers of the language—sentences such as *Colorless green ideas sleep furiously*. Oh no! It looks like we have another problem.

The sentence *Colorless green ideas sleep furiously* was actually used by Chomsky (1957) to support his theory of the importance of structure in language. As he noted, there is nothing wrong with the syntax of this sentence. All of the words are in the right order. Still, the sentence does not *mean* anything (at least not in the literal sense). If we are to program our computer to understand and produce both grammatically correct *and* meaningful sentences, we will have to include another set of rules—semantic rules.

Semantics

Let's look at that *green ideas* sentence again—*Colorless green ideas sleep furiously*—to determine what, exactly, is wrong with this sentence. First of all, something cannot both *have* color (*green*) and be *colorless*. Additionally, ideas cannot have color and they cannot sleep. Even if they could sleep, it is not actually possible to sleep furiously. That this sentence makes no sense suggests that there must be rules that govern which words can meaningfully go together. These rules are called *semantic rules*. **Semantics** is the study of the meaning of words.

The search for these rules has not been easy. There are several theories of semantics, none of which seem to fully describe how words are linked to ideas. One of the most widely accepted and well-researched theories is the *semantic component theory* (Katz & Fodor, 1963). This theory claims that there are certain fundamental features of all words. For example, the word *husband* might consist of the features: + (is) male; + adult; + human; – (is not) married. There are also **selection restrictions.** These rules govern which words can appear together. For example, someone would not be described as a *married bachelor* or *my sister the bachelor* or *my 2-year-old the bachelor* because of the component features of the word *bachelor.* You cannot be both married and a bachelor. Neither can you be a female nor a child and also be a bachelor.

Of course, it *is* possible to talk about child bachelors and married bachelors in a nonliteral sense. Similarly, it is possible to interpret a phrase such as *colorless green ideas.* Surely many of us have had nights when we *slept furiously.* But we have to work to make sense of these expressions. They are not *literally* true; they have truth only in a metaphorical sense. It is this metaphorical feature of semantics that at times is what makes poetry interesting, and even beautiful.

Our fundamental-feature and selection-restriction rules could also be applied to the *colorless green ideas* sentence. Since one feature of green is that it is a color, it cannot be both a color and lack color. Since ideas are not animate, it is not possible for them to sleep. Fundamental-feature and selection-restriction rules help account for the contradiction that speakers find in a sentence such as *My sister is married to a bachelor,* and for the ambiguity that we found previously in the sentence *The duck is ready to eat.* However, it is not altogether clear that children use a semantic feature approach in *learning* the meanings of words. In Chapter 4 we will examine the debate over semantic acquisition.

Now, after including some semantic rules in our computer program, we should be done. Although it may be difficult to describe all of the semantic rules, those that we have do a very good job of delivering meaningful sentences. Every once in a while, we might get a sentence that is difficult to interpret, but that happens in natural language as well.

Now, imagine trying to hold a two-way conversation with your computer. You type in statements or questions, and it types back responses. Suppose you type in "Can you use a sentence with the word *dog?* It types back "Yes." But that is not what you intended. You had wanted the computer to respond with a sentence using the word *dog.* Is there a problem? You bet there is. And you discover another problem. When you type a sentence such as "How are you today?" the computer might respond with almost anything—"The cat is on the mat," or "The car is at the shop." The response does not make any sense. What is wrong?

Pragmatics

So far our computer programming task has been relatively simple. We tried something. When it did not work, we changed the program and added another set of rules that got us closer to our goal of simulating human language. The rules could be discovered and were relatively few. Rules for semantics turned out to be a bit more difficult, but still it was possible to include these rules. But now we are faced with a major problem. Our computer seems insensitive to some of the subtle rules that govern conversation. It is misinterpreting the intent of some sentences and not responding to the content of other sentences. In short, we are having difficulty getting our computer to *use* language in conversation, suggesting that there must be yet another element of language. In fact, there is. This element is called **pragmatics**—the use of language for communication, or, as Gleason (1993) put it, "the use of language to express one's intentions and to get things done in the world" (p. 24).

Pragmatics includes the study of the rules that govern the use of language for social interaction. There are rules that govern the reasons for communicating, as well as rules that determine the choice of codes used in communication (Bloom & Lahey, 1978). Let's look more closely at one of these rules.

Recently I was observing a student teacher in her placement in a classroom with 6- and 7-year-old children with language and communication disabilities. The student teacher was seated at a table at the front of the room, and the children were at their desks. Wanting the children to join her at the table, the student teacher asked, "Can you come to the table?" The children looked at the student teacher, then at each other, but they did not move. Naturally, this wanton disobedience angered the student teacher, so she raised her voice and quite sharply said, "Can you come to the table!" Once again, the only response was some puzzled looks and some foot shuffling. Finally, in exasperation the student teacher said, "Please come to the table now." The children immediately got up and went to the table. What happened in this episode? Why were these children so reluctant to come forward?

The answer is that they were probably having difficulty interpreting the communicative intent of the student teacher. Like our computer, they may have interpreted the correct answer to the question, "Can you come to the table?" as "Yes." But, in fact, this was not meant to be a question at all though it had the form of a question. This is an example of an **indirect speech act**—an utterance for which the syntactic form does not match the communicative intention. In the context in which this sentence was uttered, the intent was clearly that of a command. Unfortunately, the intent may not have been so clear to the children, because indirect speech acts tend to be more difficult to interpret than **direct speech acts.** Direct speech acts are those in which the communicative intention *is* reflected in the syntactic form, such as, *Can I have some cake?* (question) and *Stop that car!* (imperative). Every utterance, however, is a speech act, and linguists such as Searle (1965) and Dore (1974) have identified speech acts and the rules that determine whether a conversation is intelligible.

Pragmatics also includes the study of the rules of conversation, in addition to including the communicative functions (or speech acts). You may recall what happened when we tried to engage the computer in conversation. It did not respond appropriately to what we had typed. Our computer violated one of the principles (rules) of conversation identified by Grice (1975)—specifically, the **relation** principle. This principle says that a response must be relevant to the topic. Other principles involve the **quantity** of information provided by the speaker, the **quality** (or truthfulness) of that information, and the **manner** (directness) of the information. When these principles are violated, we know that something is wrong with the conversation. Similarly, there are rules of conversation that govern how one speaks to persons of different levels of social status and rules that determine how conversations are repaired.

It would be difficult, if not impossible, to program our computer with such pragmatic rules because these require not only a solid understanding of language but an understanding of people and their social environment, as well. How do we tell the computer to talk one way to someone wearing a black coat and white collar and another way to someone wearing jeans and a T-shirt? The wonder is that we are able to make these subtle distinctions ourselves and that children are able to develop these skills fairly quickly.

Summary

This chapter examined the elements of language in detail—considering how form (phonology, morphology, and syntax), content (semantics), and use (pragmatics) relate to language and noting the rules characterizing each in determining the structure and use of language. The rules, considered individually, seem manageable enough, but discussion of the interrelatedness of the elements in language reveals the complexity of the language system.

Review Questions

1. Which of the following are *possible* words in English?

glix   nrzwt
fmdab   flim
smedder   blumpt
slirt   slwtr

Make up five more possible words for English.

2. Add the appropriate ending to each of the following nonsense words:

lod (plural):   _____   gack (past):   _____
lotch (plural):   _____   nop (past):   _____
flim (progressive):   _____   nug (plural):   _____

3. Mike's teacher said to Mike, "Can you raise your hand?" Mike said "Yes," and he was given a detention. What was wrong with Mike's response?

4. List the semantic features of the following pairs of words. Compare your answers with those of a partner.

dog/wolf   fruit/vegetable   table/desk

5. What is the message in the following statements? Is it a direct or an indirect speech act?

Statement	Message	Direct/Indirect
Can you pass the salt? (Uttered by someone seated at dinner table)		
Can you raise your hand? (Uttered by doctor examining a patient following an injury)		
Can you raise your hand? (Uttered by teacher in classroom who is upset with a student who is acting out)		

Suggested Activities

1. Select two children between the ages of 8 and 12. One of the children should be younger than the other, or one child should have a language disorder.
Read the following complex sentences to each child, and ask the accompanying question. Then try teaching the individual children any of the items they missed. Report on:

a. The number of errors each child made and on which sentences they were made.
b. What the errors indicate about the syntactic development of these children.
c. What happened when you tried to teach the child the missed items.

Complex Sentence Activity

(1) Before the cat was fed, the girl gave him some water.
Q: When did the girl give some water?
A: Before the cat was fed.
(2) The boy who kissed the girl ran down the street.
Q: Who ran down the street?
A: The boy.
(3) The lion that the tiger bit jumped over the giraffe.
Q: What jumped over the giraffe?
A: The lion.
(4) The horse jumped over the fence after the man hit him.
Q: When did the horse jump?
A: After the man hit him.
(5) The boy saw the man who was wearing a green hat.
Q: Who was wearing a green hat?
A: The man.
(6) The car that was hit by the truck was driven by the man.
Q: What did the man drive?
A: The car.
(7) The lady asked the man who was watching which hat to wear.
Q: Who wore the hat?
A: The lady.
(8) The cat that was chased by the dog was caught by the boy.
Q: What did the boy catch?
A: The cat.
(9) The baby crawled to the couch after her mother called her.
Q: When did the baby crawl?
A: After her mother called her.
(10) The girl asked the child who was sick to leave the room.
Q: Who left the room?
A: The child.

References

Bloom, L., & Lahey, M. (1978). *Language development and language disorders*. New York: Wiley.

Chomsky, N. (1957). *Syntactic structures*. The Hague: Mouton.

Chomsky, N. (1965). *Aspects of the theory of syntax*. Cambridge, MA: MIT Press.

Chomsky, N. (1981). *Lectures on government and binding*. Dordrecht, Netherlands: Foris.

Chomsky, N. (1982). *Some concepts and consequences of the theory of government and binding*. Cambridge, MA: MIT Press.

Dore, J. (1974). A pragmatic description of early language development. *Journal of Psycholinguistic Research, 3*, 343–350.

Fromkin, V., & Rodman, R. (1978). *An introduction to language*. New York: Holt, Rinehart, & Winston.

Gleason, J. B. (1993). Language development: An overview and a preview. In J. B. Gleason (Ed.), *The development of language*. New York: Macmillan.

Grice, H. (1975). Logic and conversation. In P. Cole & J. Morgan (Eds.), *Syntax and*

Semantics, Volume 3: Speech Acts. New York: Academic Press.

Katz, J., & Fodor, J. (1963). The structure of a semantic theory. *Language, 39,* 170–210.

Leonard, L., & Loeb, D. (1988). Government-binding theory and some of its applications: A tutorial. *Journal of Speech and Hearing Research, 31,* 515–524.

Owens, R. E. (1992). *Language development: An introduction.* New York: Macmillan.

Searle, J. (1965). What is a speech act? In M. Black (Ed.), *Philosophy in America.* New York: Allen & Unwin; Cornell University Press.

$$C \quad h \quad a \quad p \quad t \quad e \quad r \quad \textit{3}$$

Language Acquisition
Bases and Models

The why *and* how *of language acquisition are discussed in this chapter. The first section presents the physical and cognitive bases for language acquisition and development, describing the major structures of the speech and language system and the theories about the relationship between cognition (thought) and language.*

The second half of the chapter presents four theories of language acquisition, detailing how each theory explains the phenomenon of language acquisition and discussing both the contributions and limitations of each theory.

After reading this chapter, you should be able to:

1. Understand the physical structures that produce speech.
2. Understand the role played by the central nervous system in human comprehension and production of language.
3. Explain the possible relationships between *cognition* and *language.*
4. Describe the four major theories of language acquisition and their limitations.

Physiological Bases of Language Development

You may recall that despite intensive efforts to raise chimpanzees in a manner similar to that of human infants, the chimps failed to develop more than a few garbled words (see Box 1.1). Why did these experiments fail? The answer lies primarily in the physiological structures that allow us to learn and develop language. We will look at two types of structures that contribute to language development and use: those of speech production and the regions of the brain that control language.

Speech Production Structures

The speech production system is quite complex, and a thorough discussion of the physiology of speech would go beyond the scope of this book. There are several texts, however, that give a detailed description of the physiology of the speech production system (e.g., Shames, Wiig, & Secord, 1990; Hulit & Howard, 1993). Here we will briefly look at the structures that contribute to the four processes of speech production—respiration, phonation, resonation, and articulation—and at how these processes and structures together produce speech sounds. Under the control of the brain, they function almost simultaneously in the speech production process (see Figure 3.1).

Respiration

How is sound produced? First, we need air, for it is a stream of shaped and guided air that forms sounds. As a normal part of the breathing cycle, air is taken into the lungs (i.e., inhaled) for about 2.5 seconds per breath and expelled (i.e., exhaled) for about an equal amount of time. However, during speech something very different happens. Muscles that control respiration, namely, the **diaphragm** (see Figure 3.2), work to control the air stream so that the exhaling stage can last 15 seconds or more. Just imagine what speech would be like if we were limited to 2 or 3 second bursts.

Phonation

In addition to their maintaining a longer stream of air, the respiratory muscles allow air to be forced under pressure through structures in the **larynx.** The **vocal folds** contained in the larynx act as a valve that prevents foreign matter from entering the lungs and also obstructs the flow of air from the lungs, thus, causing the vibrations necessary for speech. As the air stream is restricted and buffeted, it creates a buzzing sound.

Resonation

Moving upward from the larynx, the air resonates in the mouth, the nasal cavities, and/or the pharynx (see Figure 3.2). The tone of the resulting sound is affected by the size and shape of the resonating structures into which the air is expelled. In general, the larger the resonating cavity, the lower the tone. Try making a vowel sound. This is the sound created by resonated air.

Articulation

Articulation of sound takes place when the air stream is further impeded by structures such as the lips, tongue, and/or teeth. The production of consonants requires the action of articulation. In fact, each phoneme has a unique combination of articulators and resonators that work together to form the sound. For example, the *b* sound can be described as a voiced (vocal folds vibrate) phoneme that is resonated in the anterior (forward) portion of the mouth, with the lips closed. The *p* sound is produced in exactly the same way, except that it is unvoiced (Shames, Wiig, & Secord, 1990).

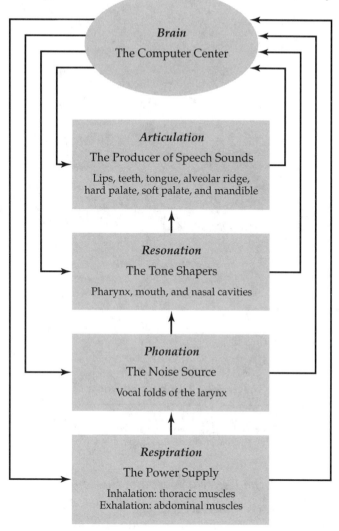

Motor Pathways   *Sensory Pathways*

FIGURE 3.1   The Processes of Speech

Source: From L. M. Hulit and M. R. Howard, *Born to Talk.* Copyright © 1993 by Allyn and Bacon. All rights reserved. Reprinted by permission of Allyn and Bacon.

In essence, when a sound is produced, air is expelled from the lungs through the larynx, where vibration through the vocal folds takes place. The sound is then resonated and articulated to create the speech sound that is actually heard. All of this happens quite automatically several times a second, hundreds of times each minute during speech. With so many structures involved and such precise timing required, it is a wonder that more children do not have speech production problems.

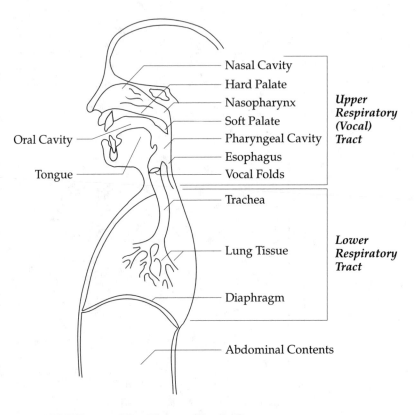

FIGURE 3.2   The Human Vocal Organs

Source: From G. H. Shames, E. H. Wiig, and W. A. Secord, *Human Communication Disorders: An Introduction* (4th ed.). Copyright © 1990 by Allyn and Bacon. Reprinted by permission.

Control of the Central Nervous System

Control of speech production is governed by the central nervous system. The human nervous system can be divided into two major divisions: the peripheral nervous system and the central nervous system.

The **peripheral nervous system** is made up of the cranial and spinal nerves that carry sensory information *to* the brain while relaying motor information *from* the brain to the muscles of the body. The twelve cranial nerves directly connect from the brain to the ears, nose, and mouth, while the spinal nerves are connected to the spinal cord via long pathways.

The **central nervous system** includes the brain and spinal cord. The brain is divided into three major regions—the hindbrain, the midbrain, and the forebrain (see Figure 3.3). The **hindbrain** consists of structures of the brain stem, such as the medulla oblongata, the pons, and the cerebellum, which control functions such as respiration, digestion, and large motor movement. This part of the brain is sometimes called the most primitive, because these structures were the first to develop

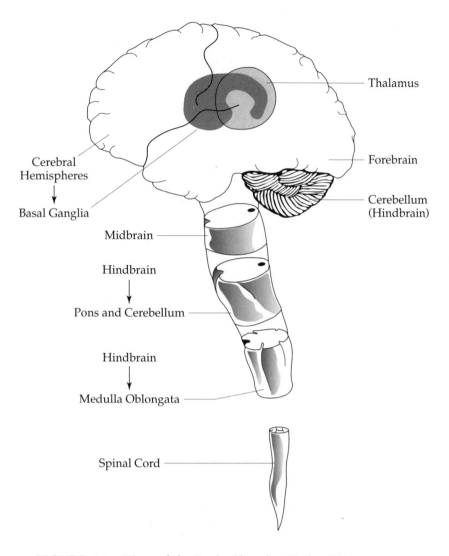

Thalamus

Forebrain

Cerebral
Hemispheres

Basal Ganglia

Cerebellum
(Hindbrain)

Midbrain

Hindbrain

Pons and Cerebellum

Hindbrain

Medulla Oblongata

Spinal Cord

FIGURE 3.3   View of the Brain Showing Major Regions

Source: From G. H. Shames, E. H. Wiig, and W. A. Secord, *Human Communication Disorders: An Introduction* (4th ed.). Copyright © 1990 by Allyn and Bacon. Reprinted by permission.

in animals and are the first to develop in the neonate. The **midbrain** consists of structures that assist in relaying information to and from the brain and the visual and auditory nerves.

The **forebrain** (cerebrum) is the largest part of the brain. The cerebrum is divided into two nearly equal hemispheres connected by a bundle of fibers called the *corpus collosum.* For purposes of study, each hemisphere of the cerebrum is

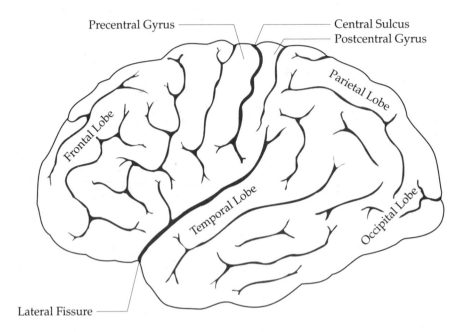

Precentral Gyrus
Central Sulcus
Postcentral Gyrus
Parietal Lobe
Frontal Lobe
Temporal Lobe
Occipital Lobe
Lateral Fissure

FIGURE 3.4   Left Cerebral Hemisphere

Source: From G. H. Shames, E. H. Wiig, and W. A. Secord, *Human Communication Disorders: An Introduction* (4th ed.). Copyright © 1990 by Allyn and Bacon. Reprinted by permission.

divided into four regions—frontal lobe, parietal lobe, temporal lobe, and occipital lobe (see Figure 3.4).

Each hemisphere of the cerebrum, and each region within the hemisphere, is believed to have a special function. In most people, language processing, both comprehension and production, takes place in the left hemisphere, though the right hemisphere *does* have a role to play in the processing of language. For example, research has shown that people who have suffered brain damage to the right hemisphere have difficulty understanding humor and nonliteral language (Obler, 1993).

Two areas in the left hemisphere are thought to be especially important in language production and comprehension: Broca's area and Wernicke's area. **Broca's area** is located near the middle of the left cerebral hemisphere, where the frontal, parietal, and temporal lobes meet. This is the area where organization of the complex motor sequences necessary for speech production goes on. **Wernicke's area** lies closer to the rear of the left cerebral hemisphere in the temporal lobe and is the area involved in the comprehension of language. When these regions of the brain are damaged, the effect on language use can be devastating (see Box 3.1).

Knowing what happens during a conversation is a help in understanding the role of the central nervous system in language processing. Sound enters the ears and is conducted to the brain along the auditory nerve. The sound is initially

BOX 3.1   Types of Aphasia

In his book *The Shattered Mind* (1974), Howard Gardner describes the devastating effects that brain damage can have on language. He gives some of the following examples:

David Ford (Broca's Aphasia)

Mr. Ford was a 39-year-old Coast Guardsman who had suffered a stroke. In response to a question about his work (radio operator), Mr. Ford said: "I'm a sig . . . no . . . man . . . uh,well, . . . again." When asked what had happened to his speech, Mr. Ford replied: "Head, fall, Jesus Christ, me no good, str, str . . . oh Jesus . . . stroke."

Mr. Ford's language was slow and produced with a great deal of effort. He seemed to know what he wanted to say, but was not able to get it out. This is characteristic of persons with Broca's aphasia.

Philip Gorgan (Wernicke's Aphasia)

A 72-year-old retired butcher, Mr. Gorgan's language difficulties were quite different from, though no less severe than, Mr. Ford's. In response to a question about why he was in the hospital, Mr. Gorgan replied: "Boy, I'm sweating, I'm awful nervous, you know, once in a while I get caught up, I can't mention the tarripoi, a month ago, quite a while, I've done a lot well, I impose a lot, while, on the other hand, you know what I mean, I have to run around, look it over, trebbin and all that sort of stuff."

Mr. Gorgan's rambling, incoherent response is characteristic of Wernicke's aphasia, where the ability to understand and produce *meaningful* language is impaired.

processed in the midbrain and relayed to the cerebrum. Here it is identified as speech and analyzed in Wernicke's area. If a response is required, a message is sent to Broca's area, where the motor plan for articulation is developed. This plan is sent to the motor area of the parietal lobe, where messages are then relayed to the appropriate muscles for a response (see Figure 3.5). Of course, this is a highly simplified version of what happens in the brain during conversation. It ignores both the important role played by memory areas and the emotional aspects of language processing. Even without including these factors, language processing is still a very complex activity. Considering the speed with which all of this is happening, it is truly an amazing feat.

Why is the ability to understand and use language not fully developed at birth? The most likely explanation is that the brain is not fully developed. Over time, the combination of physiological maturation and experience causes the brain to develop. However, there appears to be a time limit within which this brain development must take place. Lenneberg (1967) proposed that there is a "critical period" for brain development, as it relates to language functioning. After this period (which ends with the onset of puberty), acquisition of a first language is difficult, if not impossible.

These findings about brain development and language have important implications for those interested in helping children with language learning difficulties. Since brain development continues throughout childhood, it may be possible, through appropriate experiences, to have some effect on development in those children. The critical period theory, however, suggests there is limited time to influence language acquisition, supporting the need for early intervention.

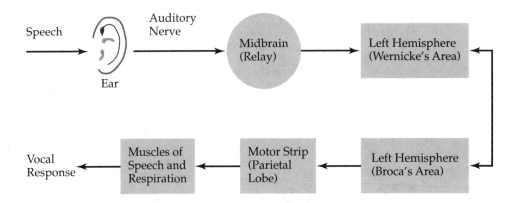

FIGURE 3.5   Comprehension and Production of Speech in the Brain

Cognitive Bases of Language Development

What do you see when you see snow? You may see a beautiful blanket of white, sparkling in the moonlight. On the other hand, you may see a gray, grungy mess that is causing monumental traffic jams. If you were an Inuit you might recognize several types of snow. In fact, the Inuits have many words to describe the different qualities of snow. Skiers make similar distinctions. They talk about *powder, granular, popcorn snow,* and the like. What determines what you see—the thing itself, or the words you have to describe it? This is one of the major problems in understanding the relationship between language and cognition.

Some researchers, such as Benjamin Whorf (1956), have argued that language affects our perception of the world. They claim that having a word to describe something makes it possible to perceive the thing itself. Consider colors, for example. When you were first learning about color you probably learned about the primary colors—*red, blue,* and *green.* As your experience broadened, you learned to identify *purple, maroon, peach.* If you have ever painted a house, you may have encountered names such as *azure, ice, melon,* and so on. Proponents of the view that *language determines thought* argue that your perception of these fine color distinctions occurred only after you had acquired a language label for these colors.

On the other hand, many theorists argue that *language is dependent upon cognition,* a view whose theoretical basis was provided by the Swiss psychologist Jean Piaget and his followers (Piaget, 1954; Sinclair-DeZwart, 1973). According to this view, cognitive development precedes language development. Piaget claimed that "language is not enough to explain thought, because the structures that characterize thought have their roots in action and in sensori-motor mechanisms that are deeper than linguistics" (1954, p. 98).

Piaget believed that language was only one of several symbolic functions a child develops through growth and interaction with the environment. Language developed, Piaget claimed, only after prerequisite cognitive accomplishments had occurred. These accomplishments include development of such principles as distancing and object permanence. **Distancing** involves the gradual movement away from actual physical experiences to symbolic or representational behavior. **Object permanence** is the idea that objects exist even when they are not being touched, tasted, or seen. These and other developments of the sensorimotor period (see Table 3.1) help move the child from being dependent on the physical world to relying more on the symbolic—a necessary prerequisite to language development, according to Piaget.

The theory that language development is dependent on cognitive development has not gone unchallenged. Chomsky (1980), for example, pointed out that language comprehension begins before language production and long before the cognitive developments that Piaget claimed must precede language. Even though such criticism may be valid, Piaget's theories about cognition and language reveal the importance of cognition in the language learning process.

A third model of language and cognition claims that *language and cognition are interdependent*. The great Russian psychologist Lev Vygotsky most clearly stated this view (1962). According to Vygotsky, language and cognition develop as separate and independent systems. Initially language development occurs because of interaction with others, but, eventually, language becomes internalized. It is at this point that language and thought begin to merge, allowing the child to engage in abstract thought and symbolic reasoning. Without language, according to Vygotsky, thinking could not progress beyond the earliest stages of development.

There may even be a fourth model of language and cognition, although this theory has not been as clearly articulated as the three preceding models. It is possible that *language and cognition are both dependent on physical maturation;* that is, language and cognition may develop independently of each other (as Vygotsky claimed), but both are dependent on physical development. As the central nervous system matures, so too do language and cognitive abilities. According to this model, disorders of language and cognition could be explained by physiological dysfunction.

In examining the relationship between language and cognition, we have found that some researchers claim that language determines cognition, while others claim that cognitive development must precede language development. It may be that language and cognition are interdependent or that they are both dependent on physical maturation. At this point there is no definitive answer regarding the relationship between language and thought. All of the theoretical models have contributed to our understanding of this relationship, but none have put the issue to rest.

So far, in examining the physiological and cognitive foundations for language acquisition, we have seen how cognitive and physical developments set the stage for language acquisition. We will now look at the process of language acquisition.

TABLE 3.1 Highlights of Sensorimotor Development

Substage (and Months)	Object Permanence	Causality	Means-Ends	Imitation	Play	Communication
1 (0 to 1)	Out of sight, out of mind.	No concept of causality.	No understanding of means-ends.	None.	None.	No communicative intent.
2 (1 to 4)	Uses senses to make and maintain contact with objects.	No concept of causality.	No understanding of means-ends.	Preimitation. Repeats own behavior that has been imitated by someone else.	Produces behaviors preliminary to play including grasping and looking at objects.	Cries, coos, and laughs.
3 (4 to 8)	Watches object move and anticipates its future postition. Reaches for partially hidden object.	Does not understand cause-effect. Behaves as though the cause of all actions.	Produces goal-oriented behaviors but only after activity has begun.	Imitates only behaviors has spontaneously produced at an earlier time.	Still very sensory but begins to interact with other people.	Babbles.
4 (8 to 12)	Looks for an object if sees it being hidden.	Externalizes causality. Knows other people and objects can cause activities.	Evidence of planning and the production of intentional behaviors.	Imitates behaviors has not spontaneously produced.	Uses developing concepts in his play activities.	Links gestures and vocalizations to convey fairly specific messages.
5 (12 to 18)	Follows sequential displacement to find hidden object.	Sees other people and objects as agents for causality in new situations.	Uses experimentation to solve problems.	Uninhibited imitation to facilitate own understanding.	Play reflects cognitive growth. Figures out how to make toys work.	Produces first meaningful words. Communication is intentional but still heavily nonverbal.
6 (18 to 24)	Fully developed concept of object permanence. Can now accommodate invisible displacements.	Causality enhanced by ability to represent objects and cause-effect relationships in his mind.	Can mentally represent a goal and his plan for achieving the goal.	Deferred imitation. Imitates a behavior has represented mentally and stored in his memory.	Progresses from autosymbolic to symbolic play.	Imitates and spontaneously produces multiple word utterances.

Source: From L. M. Hulit & M. R. Howard, *Born to Talk*. Copyright © 1993 by Allyn and Bacon. Reprinted by permission.

Models of Language Acquisition

How do children acquire their first language? A satisfactory answer to this question has eluded linguists and psycholinguists (persons who study the relation of thought to language) for many years. The reason that this is such a difficult question lies with the phenomenon of language acquisition itself. Lindfors (1987) described the problem as follows:

> *The Problem:*
> *How are we to account for the fact that:*
>
>   − *virtually every child*
>   − *without special training*
>   − *exposed to surface structures of language in many interaction contexts*
>   − *builds for himself (in a short period of time and at an early stage in his cognitive development)*
>   − *a deep-level, abstract, and highly complex system of linguistic structure and use. (Lindfors, 1987)*

In her statement of the problem, Lindfors challenges us to explain how it can be that **virtually every child** learns language. Not only do almost all children learn language, but they learn it at approximately the same rate. This is true, as Lindfors points out, whether children live on an isolated island or in an urban area, in a high-tech or stone-age civilization. All children, no matter what their language, go through a series of very similar stages of language acquisition.

Lindfors further points out that this language acquisition process goes on with **no direct training.** That is, most children do not have the benefit of special schooling for the development of language. We do not expect parents to take a systematic approach to teaching language to their child. For instance, we would not expect parents to begin teaching words that begin with the letter *a* and proceed through the alphabet to *z*. We would hardly expect parents to sit down with their year-old child and say something like, "Now, the singular past tense form of the verb *be* is *was*." If parents did such things, we would think them more than a bit odd. Yet, despite a lack of systematic training, most children do acquire a first language.

What children do hear from their parents is the **surface structure** of the language. They hear all of the stops and starts, the ungrammatical sentences, and the colloquial and slang expressions that are a part of the language of normal conversation. Somehow, through this torrent of words, they discover the rules of language (the deep-level, abstract, and highly complex system). They do all of this in a very short time (most of the important work is completed by age 5) and at a stage of cognitive development when, according to Piaget, they should not be able to form abstract rule systems at all.

This is the miracle of language acquisition—a miracle that linguists and *psycholinguists* have tried to explain. In developing their explanations (theories) of language acquisition, theorists have considered factors that influence language acquisition and development. These factors include:

- the linguistic environment
- inherited abilities
- the individual's experiences
- the individual's opportunities for interaction

Each of these factors has been emphasized in one of the major theories of language acquisition, and each contributes to the entire process of language acquisition. We will examine four theories or models of language acquisition. Each of these explains part of the phenomenon of language acquisition, but none alone gives a completely adequate explanation.

The Role of the Environment: The Behavioral Model

Most people's response to the question of how children learn language is that they learn it through imitation. When pressed to describe how this might occur, people will say that the child hears what the adult says and tries to imitate it. The imitations become more and more like adult language, and eventually children sound just like adults.

In a very simplified form, this common-sense explanation is very similar to the actual process described in behavioral theories of language acquisition. This particular theory was set forth most completely by B. F. Skinner in his book *Verbal Behavior* (1957). As described by Skinner, the behavioral theory of language acquisition places a great deal of emphasis on the role of the environment in language acquisition. The child is seen as a relatively passive recipient of external influences—from parents, siblings, and others.

Language, according to behavioral theory, is learned like any other behavior. Children begin with no language. Gradually they begin to imitate (or model) sounds of those individuals to whom they are most frequently exposed. These individuals respond to the sound outputs (operants) by doing one of three things: reinforcing the verbal behavior (*Good!*), punishing the behavior (*Shut up!*), or ignoring the behavior. If reinforcement occurs, there is a good chance that the behavior in the child will occur again. If either of the other two responses happens, the likelihood of the verbal behavior recurring is reduced. Over time, as the child's verbal behavior is repeated, the parents (or others) become less responsive and force the child to produce a verbal output that is closer to the adult model (successive approximation). As Skinner put it, "Any response which vaguely resembles the standard behavior of the community is reinforced. When these begin to appear frequently, a closer approximation is insisted upon" (pp. 29–30). Eventually the child produces the adult word. Through the process of chaining, the child learns to string together several verbal behaviors to make a sentence. The actual process might go something like this:

Mother says: See Daddy. There goes Daddy.

Child responds: Da.

Mother: Yes, there's Daddy.

(Later Mother says)

Mother: Wave bye-bye to Daddy.

Child: Da Da.

Mother: Yes, that's right. There he goes.

(Still later)

Mother: Say goodbye to Daddy.

Child: Bye-bye Da Da.

Mother: Good girl.

Notice how, in this example, the initial simple response, "da" becomes more fully formed ("bye-bye da da") as Mother prompts a response. According to the behavioral theory, the mother is helping to build a response chain in her child by reinforcing more complex language behaviors.

There is a good deal of support for the behavioral theory of language acquisition. This support comes both from structured research and from the less formal, but no less important, observations of parents and others. There *does* appear to be a process of imitation and reinforcement at work in the child's acquisition of language. Over time the child's verbal output does change in a way similar to that described by the theory. Moreover, people *believe* that imitation is a critical component of language learning.

However, there are serious limitations to the behavioral explanation of language acquisition. First, the theory makes the wrong prediction about what children will learn—particularly the *order* of word acquisition. If imitation were the primary process involved in word acquisition, then one would expect that the child's first words would be those heard most frequently. In English the words *a* and *the* are the most frequently heard words. But these words rarely, if ever, are found in the language of young children. A second problem for this theory of language acquisition is its difficulty in explaining the phenomenon of **novel productions.** Young children have been found to use constructions that they have *never* heard previously. Children may say things like *I wented* when they want to use the past tense of *go* and *womans* when they want to pluralize the word *woman*. Behavioral theory alone does not account for novel productions such as these. A third problem with the behavioral theory of language acquisition is that systematic observations of parents indicate that parents actually tend to *ignore* grammatical errors and are more concerned about the truth value of what their children say. For example, if a child says "I eated ice cream at grandma's," the parents are more likely to respond "No you didn't, you ate Jello" than to say "No, we don't say *eated*. Say *ate*" (Brown and Hanlon, 1970). Finally, behavioral theory cannot account for the observation that comprehension usually precedes production of language in children—that is, children can understand words and sentences before they can produce them. If language learning occurs by a process of reinforcement for language production, then how can it be that children can understand language before they can produce it?

Although behavioral theory is limited in its ability to explain all language acquisition, there is still some value to the theory. First, the theory highlights the essential role that parents and significant others play in the child's language learning. Second, the theory's description of the process of language learning, though flawed, has inspired others to develop alternative theories. Finally, the behavioral approach has been a successful tool in the development of intervention approaches to enhance the language skills of many persons with significant language disorders. For these reasons, it is important to know about the behavioral theory of language acquisition and to use the observations of behaviorists as one source of information for the language intervention process.

The Role of Inheritance: The Psycholinguistic (Nativist) Model

Chomsky (1968) and others developed the **psycholinguistic** (or nativist) theory of language acquisition partly in response to the behavioral theory of language acquisition. In developing this theory, Chomsky noted several interesting phenomena. First, it seemed highly unlikely to him that 4-year-old children could have learned all the language they know simply by being exposed to it and remembering what they heard. The memory load required for such a feat would seem to be well beyond that available to a child. Second, Chomsky and others (such as Lenneberg, 1967) noted the *universality* of language. That is, they pointed out that language is learned by people of all cultures, in all environments, and in very similar stages. Moreover, language appears to be *unique* to humans—Washoe and her cousins notwithstanding (see Box 1.1). Third, it seemed clear to Chomsky that children were doing more than memorizing chunks of language—they were learning language *rules*. This point is evident in the cute but revealing mistakes that children make as they are learning language.

Putting these pieces of information together, Chomsky concluded that language must be innate (hence the *nativist* label). Language, according to Chomsky, is inborn in the human species—"hard-wired" at birth. Babies are born ready to learn language. Not only are they ready to learn, they possess a mechanism that Chomsky called the **language acquisition device (LAD),** which consists of basic grammatical categories and rules that are common to all languages. These basic rules might look something like the operating principles described by Slobin (1979) (see Table 3.2). In order for the LAD to operate, the child must merely be *exposed* to language. The quality of the adult language does not really matter nor do adults have to actively teach or reinforce language use. Upon a child's exposure to language input, according to the theory, the child's LAD will take over to help the child discover the underlying rules of language. Once the rules are mastered (and a certain amount of vocabulary is acquired), the child will be able to understand and produce language.

This theory addresses well some of the unexplained phenomena associated with language acquisition. The nativist theory accounts for the fact that virtually all children learn language and do so without special training. The LAD model explains how children learn language rules merely by being exposed to lan-

TABLE 3.2   Slobin's Operating Principles of Language

Principle A: Pay attention to the end of words.
Principle B: There are linguistic elements which encode relationships between words.
Principle C: Avoid exceptions.
Principle D: Underlying semantic relationships should be marked overtly and clearly.
Principle E: The use of grammatical markers should make semantic sense.

Source: Adapted from D. Slobin (1979).

guage—that babies are programmed from birth to search out and discover the generalizations (rules) of language. The theory also accounts for the speed with which language is acquired, since it represents that children are able to process language rules right from birth.

There are, however, some significant limitations to this psycholinguistic theory. One of the most troublesome is the diminished role given to language input. We will see later that recent investigations of parent-child interactions have found that parents alter their language for their children in systematic ways—simplifying and clarifying. If mere exposure to language were all that was needed for language acquisition, why would parents continue to go to the trouble of altering their language for children? A second problem stems from the theoretical underpinnings of the model itself. Chomsky was interested in explaining the acquisition of *syntax* in children. He was much less interested in explaining the acquisition of the other elements of language. While the theory adequately explains the acquisition of syntax, it does not account for the child's acquisition of semantic, morphophonological, or pragmatic rules. Finally, the theory poses a dilemma to those who are interested in helping children improve their language performance, as it seems to suggest that there is little hope for children experiencing significant difficulty with language. If language is innate, perhaps these children simply lack the ability to learn language. However, we know from experience supported by research that it is possible to enhance language skills. Therefore, there must be more to language learning than this biological component.

Chomsky's development of a model of language acquisition essentially marks the start of the field of *psycholinguistics*—the study of the psychology of language. His nativist (or psycholinguistic) model sparked a flood of research on language learning that continues to this day. Some of the subsequent research has supported Chomsky's claims, but some has supported competing theories of language acquisition. Although the nativist model is a no more complete explanation of language acquisition than the behavioral theory, it too has made an important contribution by addressing some of the most challenging questions about language learning and by advancing our knowledge about language and language acquisition.

The Role of the Environment: Semantic-Cognitive Model

"Mommy, sock." These two words helped lead Lois Bloom (1970) to contribute to a new interpretation of child language acquisition. Bloom had observed a child using this expression on two occasions. One time, the child used this expression to note that the sock belonged to her mother (possessive). The second time, she appeared to be making a request (e.g., "Put my sock on, Mommy"). Although we do not know precisely what the child meant to say, it is clear from this context that the same words were being used to express two different meanings. Observations such as these led Bloom to conclude that semantics precedes syntax in child language acquisition. In other words, children develop syntax because they already have something to talk about rather than because they have the grammar to express themselves. In this case the child used one syntactic form ("Mommy, sock") to express two semantic functions (possessive and requesting).

The semantic-cognitive model of language acquisition was developed from evidence such as the above, as well as from linguistic and cognitive theory. At about the same time Bloom was conducting her observations of children, Fillmore (1968) was publishing his ideas about the role of semantics in language structure. Fillmore noted that the selection of a word to be used in a sentence is determined more by the *meaning* of the sentence than by the syntactic structure of the sentence. Thus, in a sentence such as *The _____ hit the ball*, rules of syntax tell us that the word that goes in the blank must be a noun, but semantics tells us that only certain nouns will do. The words *boy* or *girl* would be fine but *clock* or *desk* would not do. Fillmore's theory—**case grammar**—forced linguists to rethink their assumptions about the relationship between syntax and semantics.

While Fillmore's and Bloom's work focused on the role of semantics in language acquisition, the Swiss cognitive psychologist Jean Piaget was interested in the relationship between cognition (thought) and language. Piaget did not propose a theory of language development as such, but his work was seen as implying that language development is secondary to cognitive development. According to Piaget (1954), language is but one of many symbol systems. Also, according to Piaget and his associates (chiefly Sinclair-deZwart), cognitive developments such as object permanence *must* precede language development.

The combined influences of Fillmore's case grammar, Piaget's cognitive theories, and observations by researchers such as Bloom led to the development of the **semantic-cognitive theory** of language acquisition. This theory gives preeminence to the semantic aspect of language. The theory proposes that young children pay particular attention to the *meanings* of things. When they use language, they do so to talk *about* something they have already experienced. In other words, the experience comes first, then the language follows. According to this theory, syntax develops as the result of the need to talk about more and more things or experiences. In addition, certain cognitive accomplishments must take place before language can be acquired at all.

Like the other language-acquisition theories we have reviewed, the semantic-cognitive theory has some strong support. It seems logical that children will talk when they have something to talk *about*. As they acquire more experiences, they need more sophisticated language to express their ideas. In addition, there is evidence that certain cognitive development steps usually do precede the emergence of language. This theory helps to explain how it is that children tend to talk about the same kinds of things no matter what their socioeconomic background and environment.

This theory also has its shortcomings. Like the nativist theory, the semantic-cognitive model gives little attention to the role of input language. These theoretical models would have us believe that adult input matters little, if at all. A second problem is that the relationship between cognition and language is not as simple as Piaget claimed. Some children attain the cognitive prerequisites for language but do not develop language skills. Other children are more advanced in language than would be predicted by their cognitive skills. Therefore, it may not be essential for cognitive development to precede language.

Like the other language-acquisition models, the semantic-cognitive model has made important contributions to our understanding of language acquisition. It has forced theorists to look beyond syntax and consider other aspects of language development. It has also had an impact on intervention practices, as we will see later. However, like the other models, while it has contributed pieces to the puzzle, it does not solve the entire enigma of language acquisition.

The Role of Communication: Pragmatic-Interactionist Model

The pragmatic-interactionist model of language acquisition is based on a very simple observation—people talk in order to communicate. Therefore, the model places greatest emphasis on the communicative function of language. According to this theory, language development takes place as children learn to choose the linguistic form that will best express their communicative intent.

This model is grounded in two areas of research. On the one hand, linguists such as Searle (1965), and later Dore (1974) and Halliday (1975), began to identify and classify the rules of pragmatics. At the same time, psychologists and psycholinguists such as Bruner (1975) and Bates (1976) were observing and describing communication between parents and their children. These two areas of research—theoretical and applied—came together in the pragmatic-interactionist model of language acquisition.

An additional stimulus to the development of this model was the identification of a phenomenon called "motherese" (Newport, 1976; Newport, Gleitman, & Gleitman, 1977) or, more accurately, *child-directed speech (CDS)* (Bohannon, 1993). A number of researchers have observed that parents (and other adults) tend to alter their language in the presence of young children. These alterations include using shorter and less complex sentences, slowing the rate of their speech, using a more limited range of semantic functions, and engaging in shorter conversations.

It is hypothesized that parents make these changes because they somehow intuitively know that children need this in order to learn language. In any case, children are more responsive when language is adjusted to their level. According to Bruner (1977), adjustments in adult language such as those described previously provide the framework, or "scaffolding," for language development. By engaging in communication with their parents (and other significant adults), children learn that language can be used for communication and they indirectly pick up structural aspects of language. Communication—especially repetitive, routine communication—makes it possible for children to hear and model the adult language forms.

With the pragmatic-interactionist theory of language acquisition we have, in a sense, come back to where we started in our examination of language acquisition. Like the behavioral model, this model puts a great deal of emphasis on events that take place in the environment around the child. Children learn language by being exposed to language. Unlike the behavioral model, however, the pragmatic-interactionist model does *not* claim that overt reinforcement is necessary in order for language to be acquired. Instead, it is similar to the nativist model in acknowledging the role of physiological maturation in determining the level of communicative interaction that can be handled by the child. The pragmatic-interactionist model can be seen as an attempt to account for both the role of the environment (nurture) and the role of biological processes (nature) in language development.

The pragmatic-interactionist model of language acquisition has much going for it. Any parent can attest to the fact that young children can communicate their needs long before they have the language to express themselves. This supports the claims of the pragmatic-interactionist model that communication precedes language. Moreover, there is evidence that children who have limited opportunities for interaction with adults have more difficulty acquiring language.

One of the limitations of the pragmatic-interactionist model, though, is in how it accounts for the acquisition of specific syntactic structures. In other words, how is it that almost all children follow the same sequence of language development at about the same time? If children rely primarily on the adults in their environment for language input, then it would be logical to expect that both the quality and quantity of input (and thus the child's output) would vary widely. Yet, this is not the case. Clearly there must be other factors at work. There is also limited research on just how much interaction is needed to stimulate language development. Is there a minimum amount? Is there an optimal amount? Until these questions are answered, we cannot be sure about the role of communicative interaction in early language development.

The pragmatic-interactionist model of language learning is relatively new, yet it has had a significant influence on language intervention techniques. Today many clinicians are emphasizing the importance of engaging children in communication—especially in repetitive, routine interactions. Rather than breaking language down into small parts and teaching each part, some are using indirect methods of language stimulation, stressing the wholeness of language and the essential role of communication in the language learning process.

Conclusion

Perhaps it is not possible to completely account for the phenomena of language development described at the beginning of this chapter. Although such a conclu-

TABLE 3.3   Major Models of Language Acquisition

Model	Principles	Limitations
Behavioral	Language learned through imitation and reinforcement	Makes wrong predictions about word acquisition
	Language learned like other behaviors	Cannot explain novel utterances
		Parents reinforce meaning, not structure
		Comprehension precedes production
Psycholinguistic (Nativist)	Inborn ability for language	What is role of input?
	Language acquisition device (LAD)	What about parts of language other than syntax?
Semantic-Cognitive	Meaning precedes stucture (Fillmore)	What is role of input?
	Same utterance can have multiple meanings (Bloom)	Relationship of cognition and language very complex
	Cognition precedes language (Piaget)	
Pragmatic-Interactionist	Need to communicate precedes language structures	How to account for specific structures
	Parents alter language for their child	

sion may seem discouraging, it may be that what is important is the search for answers itself. As a result of this search our ideas about language have been clarified and the debate about language learning has been sharpened. Additionally, the search for answers has led to the development of language intervention methods.

Summary

Language acquisition is a complex, wondrous, and still somewhat mysterious phenomenon. The physiological and cognitive foundations for language acquisition presented in the first part of this chapter laid the groundwork for the second part of the chapter, discussion of four theories of language acquisition: behavioral, psycholinguistic (nativist), semantic-cognitive, and pragmatic-interactionist (see Table 3.3). The support, both theoretical and observed, for each of these models was presented, as were shortcomings of the models. Each of these models has contributed something to our knowledge of language acquisition, yet none of them can completely account for the remarkable achievement that we call *language*.

Review Questions

1. A child says, "I goded to the store." What does an utterance such as this suggest about the role of imitation in child language? What does it indicate about rule learning?

2. Chomsky proposed that children have an innate linguistic mechanism that he called a *language acquisition device*. What is the LAD? What does the LAD do?

3. What is the significance of Bloom's discovery that her child said "Mommy, sock?"

4. What are two limitations of the behavioral theory of language acquisition?

5. Match the language acquisition model to the name of the researcher associated with that model by filling in the number of your answer next to the model:

_____ Psycholinguistic	1. Skinner
_____ Pragmatic-Interactionist	2. Bloom
_____ Semantic-Cognitive	3. Chomsky
_____ Behavioral	4. Bruner

Suggested Activities

1. Observe a parent and child (2½–4 years old) in a natural setting in the home. You might ask the parent to provide some favorite toys for the child. Tape record and observe the interaction between the parent and child. As you observe, try to note what the parent and child are doing and any nonverbal interaction (gestures, facial expressions) that may be going on.

Later, transcribe the tape. Try to write down *exactly* what each participant said. Analyze the tape for the following:

   a. Is there evidence of rule acquisition by the child? (Look for errors in words and/or sentence structure.)
   b. What does the parent do to alter spoken language to the child?
   c. What do the parent and child talk about?

2. In order to test whether receptive language does, in fact, precede expressive language, find a child (12–18 months) who is just beginning to use expressive language. Ask the child's parent to pick five toys or objects that the child likes to play with or uses frequently. Place the child on the floor with the objects between yourself and the child. Say:

(Child's Name), touch the *(Object 1)*
(Child's Name), pick up the *(Object 2)*
(Child's Name), get the *(Object 3)*

Continue like this through the five objects. Now, ask the child to name each object.

   a. What happened? Did the child respond correctly when asked to touch the objects? Was the child able to say the name of each object?

b. What do the results indicate about the child's language abilities?

c. What do the results suggest about thought and language?

References

Bates, E. (1976). *Language and context: The acquisition of pragmatics.* New York: Academic Press.

Bloom, L. (1970). *Language development: Form and function of emerging grammars.* Cambridge, MA: MIT Press.

Bohannon, J. (1993). Theoretical approaches to language acquisition. In J. B. Gleason (Ed.), *The development of language.* New York: Macmillan.

Brown, R., & Hanlon, C. (1970). Derivational complexity and order of acquisition. In J. Hayes (Ed.), *Cognition and the development of language.* New York: Wiley.

Bruner, J. (1975). The ontogenesis of speech acts. *Journal of Child Language, 2,* 1–19.

Bruner, J. (1977). Early social interaction and language acquisition. In R. Schaffer (Ed.), *Studies in mother-infant interaction.* New York: Academic Press.

Chomsky, N. (1968). *Language and mind.* New York: Harcourt, Brace, & World.

Chomsky, N. (1980). On cognitive structures and their development: A reply to Piaget. In M. Piattelli-Palmarini (Ed.), *Language and learning: The debate between Jean Piaget and Noam Chomsky* (pp. 35–52). Cambridge, MA: Harvard University Press.

Chomsky, N., & Halle, M. (1968). *The sound pattern of English.* New York: Academic Press.

Dore, J. (1974). A pragmatic description of early language development. *Journal of Psycholinguistic Research, 3,* 343–350.

Fillmore, C. (1968). The case for case. In E. Bach & R. Harmas (Eds.), *Universals in linguistic theory* (pp. 1–88). New York: Holt, Rinehart, & Winston.

Gardner, H. (1974). *The shattered mind.* New York: Random House.

Halliday, M. (1975). *Learning how to mean: Explorations in the development of language.* New York: Arnold.

Hulit, L., & Howard, M. (1993). *Born to talk.* Columbus, OH: Merrill.

Lenneberg, E. (1967). *Biological foundations of language.* New York: Wiley.

Lindfors, J. (1987). *Children's language and learning.* Englewood Cliffs, NJ: Prentice-Hall.

Mercer, C. (1991). *Students with learning disabilities.* Columbus, OH: Merrill.

Newport, E. (1976). Motherese: The speech of mothers to young children. In J. Castellan, D. Pisoni, & G. Potts (Eds.), *Cognitive theory* (Vol. 2). Hillsdale, NJ: Erlbaum.

Newport, E., Gleitman, A., & Gleitman, L. (1977). Mother I'd rather do it myself: Some effects and non-effects of maternal speech style. In C. Snow & C. Ferguson (Eds.), *Talking to children: Language input and acquisition* (pp. 109–149). New York: Cambridge University Press.

Obler, L. (1993). Language beyond childhood. In J. B. Gleason (Ed.), *The development of language* (pp. 421–449). New York: Macmillan.

Piaget. J. (1954). *The construction of reality in the child.* New York: Basic Books.

Searle, J. (1965). What is a speech act? In M. Black (Ed.), *Philosophy in America* (pp. 221–239). New York: Allen & Unwin; Cornell University Press.

Shames, G., Wiig, E., & Secord, W. (1990). *Human communication disorders: An Introduction.* 4th ed. Boston: Allyn & Bacon.

Sinclair-DeZwart, H. (1973). Language acquisition and cognitive development. In T. Moore (Ed.), *Cognitive development and the acquisition of language.* New York: Academic Press.

Skinner, B. F. (1957). *Verbal behavior.* New York: Appleton-Century-Crofts.

Slobin, D. (1979). *Psycholinguistics* (2nd. ed.). Glenview, IL: Scott, Foresman.

Vygotsky, L. (1962). *Thought and language.* Cambridge, MA: MIT Press.

Whorf, B. (1956). *Language, thought, and reality.* New York: Wiley.

$$C\ h\ a\ p\ t\ e\ r\quad 4$$

The Development of Language

Language development, from birth through the school years, is described in this chapter. Beginning with a description of the early communicative attempts of newborns, the chapter then examines the emergence of language and developments in the preschool years, describing the stages of syntactic and semantic development. The chapter ends with a description of language development in the school-age years.

After reading this chapter, you should be able to:

1. Describe the development of communicative skills in the newborn.
2. Describe the stages of language development in the preschool years.
3. Understand the various perspectives on the emergence of semantic abilities.
4. Describe the major language developments accomplished during the school years.
5. Understand the concept of metalinguistics and how it relates to school tasks.

Having examined the physiological and cognitive bases for language development, we are ready to turn our attention to describing the course of language development itself. For those interested in understanding and teaching children with language disorders, knowledge of patterns of language development is important. Imagine what it would be like if you had no idea about the progression of language development. Where would you begin teaching? What would you teach? What would you teach next? What examples would you use? How would you develop reasonable goals for instruction? Gaining knowledge of language development is the best way to answer these questions.

Prelinguistic Development

When does language use begin? When a child's first words emerge? When the child begins to use more than one word? Perhaps it begins much earlier. Newborns have been found to have some surprising language abilities. For example, they are able to distinguish their mothers' voices from those of other women (De Casper & Fifer, 1980) and discriminate speech sounds (Eimas, Siqueland, Jusczyk, & Vigorito, 1971). Findings such as these have led some researchers to wonder whether speech recognition may go on in the womb (De Casper & Spence, 1985).

In order to determine when language use begins, it is necessary to say what we mean by *language.* If we think of language only as expressive then, clearly, this language does not emerge in most babies until approximately the end of the first year of life. However, if we broaden our definition of language to include comprehension, then there is evidence that the infant may be processing language soon after (or even before) birth.

Although babies may appear to be passive recipients of language, in fact, they may actually be actively engaged in language processing. For example, a considerable amount of research has found that infants are active participants in communicative exchanges. They initiate an interaction by turning toward their parent and end the exchange by turning away. They smile and coo and burp in ways that parents interpret as communicative (Murray & Trevarthen, 1986). At first, these actions by the infant are probably not intentional, but parents react as if they were. This early stage of communication has been called the **perlocutionary stage** (Bates, Camaioni, & Volterra, 1975). Consider the following interaction:

Baby cries. Mother enters the room and says: "Are you hungry? Do you want something to eat now?"

Baby quiets and turns toward mother. Mother says: "Yes, you are hungry, aren't you?"

Baby stretches, touching rattle lying in crib. "Do you want to play?"

Mother picks up rattle and shakes it. Baby gurgles. "Yes, that's what you wanted, isn't it?"

Note how much the mother is reading into this conversation. She is interpreting her child's behaviors as communicative attempts. At 10 to 15 months old, the child will be at the **illocutionary stage** of communication. At this stage, children begin to use intentional communication. They use objects to get the attention of adults (*protodeclarative*) or use an adult to get a desired object (*protoimperative*). When children begin to use words to express communicative intentions, they have reached the **locutionary stage**, according to Bates et al. (1975). By the time babies are 9 months old (prior to the emergence of spoken language), they can express a wide range of communicative intentions, including requests, demands, and rejection.

Infants are active participants in early communicative interaction, and adults perform in ways that seem meant to enhance their child's participation in communicative interaction. Careful research during the past 20 years has found that adults do not talk to their children in the same way that they talk to other adults. In fact, with children they do things like reduce the complexity of their language, use a greater range of pitch in their voice, and use more limited vocabulary

TABLE 4.1   Characteristics of Child-Directed Speech (Motherese)

Higher overall pitch; greater range of pitch
Exaggerated intonation and stress
Slower speech
More restricted vocabulary
More reference to *here* and *now*
Fewer broken or run-on sentences
Fewer complex sentences
More questions and imperatives
Shorter conversations

(Newport, Gleitman, & Gleitman, 1977; Sacks, 1993) (see Table 4.1). This alteration of parents' language with their children has been called *motherese* or *parentese*. As their child grows older, parents make adjustments to their own language to fit the changing needs and abilities of their child (Newport et al., 1977).

It seems that children and adults are engaged in communicative interaction right from the beginning. Babies are active participants in communication, performing in ways that get the adults' attention and prompt a response. Adults are engaging their children in communication by altering their own language to fit the linguistic and cognitive abilities of their child. At this early stage of communication, the child is not yet verbal. Now we will look at what happens when the child begins to talk.

Emergence of Expressive Language

Most parents can remember the excitement of hearing their baby's first words. But this remarkable achievement did not happen overnight. Indeed, babies do not wake up one morning speaking in full sentences (at least most do not). In fact, the progression from the shrieking first heard in the hospital nursery to the controlled utterance of *da-da* or *ma-ma* is slow, systematic, and predictable for most children. Stark (1979) developed a framework for describing prelinguistic development consisting of five stages. We will use Stark's model to guide us through these early stages of language development. But first, a caution. Language development is quite individual. Although generalizations can be made about development, these generalizations are not true of *every* child. There is wide variation in language development among children. Therefore, one should be very cautious about concluding that a child is language disordered because the child does not conform to the stages described below. It may also be a mistake to get overly excited about a child who develops ahead of these stages. There should be concern, however, when a child deviates significantly from the normal developmental sequence.

Stage I (0–8 Weeks)

At this stage newborns are making reflexive cries and vegetative sounds. That is, they are opening their mouths and emitting whatever comes out. What comes out is generally a loud, piercing cry that does wonders for getting a parent's attention. It is difficult, even painful, to ignore this cry. The crying is typically in short, rapid bursts, although there are individual differences. Some babies are relatively quiet; others seem to cry all the time. Some have a loud, piercing cry; others whimper. In addition, babies produce sounds—such as burps, coughs, and sneezes—that parents may respond to as if they were attempts to initiate communication.

Stage II (8–20 Weeks)

This period is one in which the infant gains increasing control over its sound-producing apparatus. Crying becomes differentiated, so that parents begin to identify different kinds of cries (hunger, discomfort, demands). The bursts of crying begin to smooth out in more sustained (but usually less frequent) occurrences. By the end of this period, most babies are making cooing sounds. These are vowel-like utterances that are often interpreted by parents as sounds of pleasure. Many babies also begin to laugh at this stage.

Stage III (16–30 Weeks)

Vocal play characterizes this stage. This is a period in which there is continued control over the vocal mechanism. Consonant sounds begin to enter the baby's vocalizations. These may be added to the cooing sounds heard previously. By the end of this stage, the baby is beginning to produce the sounds we call *babble.*

Stage IV (25–50 Weeks)

This is the true babbling stage. The baby is producing combinations of consonants and vowels such as *ba* and *na*. By the end of this period, these consonant-vowel (CV) combinations are being repeated in long strings (*ba ba ba ba*), often with changes in pitch and intonation.

Stage V (9–18 Months)

Now the child's babbling becomes increasingly complex. The range of consonant sounds increases. *Jargon* emerges in most children. This is a type of vocalization that sounds very much like language, because the sounds and intonation are quite languagelike. In fact, when listening from another room, one might almost think that the baby is actually talking, since these strings of sounds take on the sound characteristics of sentences.

Stage V marks a transition to true language production. This is the age when parents detect first words being uttered. Sometimes these are heard within the flow of jargon speech. Sometimes the words are articulated clearly, not to be heard again for days or weeks. Some children may use *protowords,* CV combinations that are used consistently to mean something. For example, one of my children used the combination *na* to indicate that she *wanted* something. What makes this a protoword and not just babble is that the sounds are used *consistently,* in *appropriate contexts* to signal their meaning.

Our review of early vocalizations has taken us from the reflexive crying of the newborn to the emergence of true first words. We have noted the universality of this progression, while keeping in mind the individual variations that are found

TABLE 4.2   Prelinguistic Development

Stage	Form	Content	Use
I (0–8 wks)	Reflexive crying Vegetative sounds Sound discrimination	Biological and physical needs	Eye contact Body movement
II (8–20 wks)	Cooing and laughing Vowel-like sounds Cry more controlled	Differentiated crying: Hunger, distress	Games Routines
III (16–30 wks)	Increased control over speech Prolonged vocalizations Babble	Beginning of semantic functions	Intent to communicate
IV (25–50 wks)	Repeated syllable clusters Jargon speech Some words	Expansion of semantic functions	Illocutionary stage
V (9–18 mos)	Protowords Transition to language	Overextensions Underextensions	Locutionary stage

Source: Adapted from R. Stark. (1979). Prespeech segmental feature development. In P. Fletcher & M. Garman (Eds.), *Language Acquisition* (pp. 15–32). New York: Cambridge.

in developing children. Table 4.2 summarizes the development of vocalizations (form), as well as communication (use) and content.

Language Development in the Preschool Years

In his pioneering book on language development, Roger Brown described a longitudinal study of the language development of three children—Adam, Eve, and Sarah. Working with a group of remarkably talented assistants, Brown and his colleagues observed, recorded, and analyzed each step in the language growth of these children. Their observations were reported in the book *A First Language* (Brown, 1973). This is still the most comprehensive description of language development available. One of Brown's key observations was that the *length* of a child's utterance is a better indicator of language development (especially syntactic development) than is the child's age. Brown developed a measure of syntactic development called **mean length of utterance (MLU)**. MLU is relatively simple to calculate and has become a widely used measure of language development. MLU is calculated by counting the total number of morphemes in a sample of language and dividing by the number of utterances in the sample. For example, if there were 100 morphemes used in a sample of 50 utterances, the MLU would be 2.0 (100/50). Brown and his colleagues used MLU to describe the stages of language they observed in their subjects (see Table 4.3). Brown's stages are used in the following description of language development in the preschool years.

TABLE 4.3   Brown's Stages of Morphological Development

Linguistic Stage	MLU	Approximate Chronological Age (months)	Characteristics
I	1.0–2.0	12–26	Use of semantic rules
II	2.0–2.5	27–40	Morphological development
III	2.5–3.0	31–34	Development of variety of sentence types: negative, imperative, interrogative
IV	3.0–3.75	35–40	Emergence of complex constructions: coordination, complementation, relativization
V	3.75–4.5	41–46	
VI	4.5+	47+	

Source: From D. K. Berstein and E. T. Tiegerman, *Language and Communication Disorders in Children.* Copyright © 1993 by Allyn and Bacon. Reprinted by permission.

Stage I (MLU = 1.0–2.0; Age = 12–26 Months)

This stage marks the emergence of true words, examples of which are listed in Table 4.4. Notice which kinds of words are there (and which are not). Note that nouns predominate; Nelson (1973) found that 65 percent of first words were nouns. The next most frequent words are action words (*hi, bye-bye*), then modifiers (*hot, cold*). Nelson also found that there were clear individual differences among children. Some children tended to use language to describe and categorize, while others used language primarily for interpersonal interaction. What else can we note about these first words? They are usually one or, at most, two syllables, and certain sounds tend to predominate (*b, p, m*). In addition, children often make systematic phonological errors at this stage. These include:

Reduction of consonant clusters (*green* becomes *geen*)
Deletion of unstressed syllables (*banana* becomes *nana*)
Devoicing of the final consonant (*bed* becomes *bet*)

By the end of Stage I, children are beginning to use multiword utterances. Like first words, these utterances have a typical pattern which has often been described as *telegraphic*. That is, they are characterized by the deletion of prepositions, conjunctions, articles, and pronouns (see Table 4.5). In their utterances, children typically talk about a limited set of items—objects, agents, and actions.

Stage II (MLU = 2.0–2.5; Age = 27–30 Months)

According to Roger Brown, the major accomplishment of Stage II is the emergence of **grammatical morphemes** (prefixes, suffixes, prepositions). Although

TABLE 4.4   Representative Early Words

juice	mama	all gone
cookie	dada	more
baby	doggie	no
bye-bye	kitty	up
ball	that	eat
hi	dirty	go
car	hot	do
water	shoe	milk
eye	hat	cap
nose		

Source: From R. E. Owens, Jr., *Language Development: An Introduction* (4th ed.). Copyright © 1996 by Allyn and Bacon. Reprinted by permission.

these begin to appear in Stage II, the development of the use of grammatical morphemes continues through Stage V. Brown found that there was a highly predictable sequence of acquisition of grammatical morphemes (see Table 4.6). Pronoun use also begins to develop in Stage II. The earliest pronouns used are *I* and *my*. Later (Stage III), *he, she,* and *you* emerge in usage. By Stage V (approximately 4 years old), most children are using even the most sophisticated pronouns.

TABLE 4.5   Examples of Two-Word Utterances

Andrew	Eve
more car	bye-bye baby
more cereal	Daddy bear
more high	Daddy book
more read	Daddy honey
outside more	there Daddy
no more	there potty
no pee	more pudding
no wet	Mommy stair
all wet	Mommy dimple
all gone	Mommy do
bye-bye Calico	Mommy bear
bye-bye back	eat it
bye-bye car	read it
bye-bye Papa	see boy
Mama come	more cookie
see pretty	

Source: From J. B. Gleason, *The Development of Language* (4th ed.). Copyright © 1993 by Allyn and Bacon. Reprinted by permission.

Note: Examples in Column 1 are from Braine, 1976. Examples in Column 2 are from Brown & Fraser, 1963.

**TABLE 4.6   Average Order of Acquisition of
Fourteen Grammatical Morphemes
by Three Children Studied by Brown**

1.	present progressive
2/3.	prepositions (in/on)
4.	plural
5.	irregular past tense
6.	possessive
7.	copula, uncontractible
8.	articles
9.	regular past tense
10.	third person present tense, regular
11.	third person present tense, irregular
12.	auxiliary, uncontractible
13.	copula, contractible
14.	auxiliary, contractible

Source: From J. B. Gleason, *The Development of Language* (4th ed.).
Copyright © 1993 by Allyn and Bacon. Reprinted by permission.

Stage III (MLU = 2.5–3.0; Age = 31–34 Months)

The major developments of Stage III are the emergence of sentence types such as negation, imperative, and question and the elaboration of the basic sentence elements (noun phrase and verb phrase). Each of the sentence types has a developmental progression.

We will examine negation as an example of the steps in sentence development. Any parent can tell you that long before 31 months of age, children can express negation. They do so by pushing the bottle away, by scrunching up their faces, and by using the word *no*. However, at Stage III we begin to see the emergence of more adultlike ways of saying *no*. At first, the child simply adds the word *no* to the beginning of a sentence (*No the kitty eating*). Next, the child learns to place the negative marker inside the sentence, just before the verb (*The kitty no eating*). Still later, auxiliary verbs are used (*The kitty is not eating*). The appearance of negation, like that of other sentence types, begins at Stage III and continues to develop through the preschool years.

As a variety of sentence types are beginning to emerge, the young child is adding elements to basic noun and verb phrases. Up to this point, noun phrases have generally consisted of a noun and, perhaps, a determiner (article). Now the child begins to add adjectives, initiators (*all, both, only*), and postmodifiers (prepositional phrases and clauses) to the basic noun phrase. Similarly, verb use expands from simple verbs to inclusion of auxiliary verbs, the progressive (*ing*), and modals (*can, will, may*).

Stage IV (MLU = 3.0–3.75; Age = 35–40 Months)

Stage IV marks the emergence of complex sentence types. Complex sentences are formed when two or more *clauses* (a group of words with a subject and predicate) are joined together. The first type of complex structure to emerge is that of **coordination.** Children begin by linking ideas with the word *and* (*I am going to the store and my dad is going to work*). Later the child learns to use coordination of multiple ideas as a way to *shorten* sentences (***My mom and I** are going to the bank*). Still later, children begin to use other conjunctions (*but, because, since*). At Stage IV children also typically begin to use embedded sentences. These are sentences in which a subordinate clause (*who is my friend*) is embedded in an independent clause (*The boy is here*) to form a complex sentence (*The boy who is my friend is here*).

Stage V (MLU = 3.75–4.5; Age = 41–46 Months)

There are no major new structures that emerge in Stage V. Instead, this stage is marked by elaboration and refinement of structures that emerged in earlier stages. The child continues adding grammatical morphemes; more frequently uses adjectives, adverbs, and embedded sentences; and more consistently uses inversion in questions (*Are you going to the store?*). In short, the child is learning to become a more effective (and more social) communicator.

This description of the syntactic development of children between 1 and 4 years of age is complete for the purpose intended here, though there has been no attempt to describe every feature that develops during this period. The references at the end of this chapter are sources for more detailed descriptions of syntactic development. Instead, the goal has been to describe major accomplishments that illustrate the general course of development and provide background for an understanding of what happens when children fail to develop in the expected ways.

By the time most children enter kindergarten, they are able to understand and use quite complex and sophisticated language. They have mastered the use of pronouns and grammatical morphemes and can use all adult sentence forms, including compound and complex sentences. But they have not learned everything there is to know about language. There is still much to be learned after children enter formal schooling. Before examining syntactic development during the school years, however, we need to look at the development of another aspect of language in the preschool years—semantics.

Learning to Mean: The Development of Semantics

By the time they are 8 years old, most children have a receptive vocabulary of about 8,000 words (Gleason, 1993). How did they acquire so many words and how did they learn what each means?

Although no one can say exactly how children learn about word meaning, there are several prominent theories. One of these theories is the **semantic-feature hypothesis.** Eve Clark (1973) suggested that children develop meaning by adding features to their understanding of a particular concept. As they learn more, their concept becomes more like that of adults. As evidence for this theory, consider the child who calls all things with four legs either *doggy* or *kitty*. Later, the child learns that doggies not only have four legs, but they bark—while cats meow. At first, the child will **overextend** the word to include a broad class of items. Gradually, the child refines a concept until it matches the adult meaning. Occasionally, children **underextend** meanings. Then they restrict a word to only one object (usually something they treasure, such as a cup or pacifier). In this case, they will only use the word when that particular object is present.

The semantic-feature theory of the acquisition of meaning makes a lot of sense. Parents can often observe their children overextending words. However, the semantic-feature theory may not be sufficient to explain what is going on with the acquisition of meaning. In her observation of children, Katherine Nelson (1974) noted how they seemed to pay more attention to the *action* related to objects rather than to the perceptual features of the object. She pointed out that children's first words tended to be items that moved or could be manipulated by the child. Her **functional-core** hypothesis claims that children learn about meaning by interacting with things, much as Piaget claimed that cognitive growth is spurred on by experience.

Bowerman (1978) proposed still another theory of semantic development—one that incorporates features of both of the preceding theories. Bowerman's theory has come to be called the **prototype** hypothesis. She claimed that children learn word meanings by developing a cognitive model based on both perceptual and functional characteristics. For example, a child would learn the meaning of the word *dog* by encountering a dog and extracting features that would enable him or her to build a cognitive concept of *dog*. Encountering different types and sizes of dogs would then oblige the child to refine the original model through comparison of the new examples to the original model. Research by Rosch and Mervis (1975) found that adults appear to have cognitive prototypes that are quite consistent across individuals. They found, for example, that a group of adults asked to choose pictures of a "typical" dog will usually choose something that looks like a collie.

Although a complete understanding of semantic development remains elusive, the three models described above give us some insights into the process children use to develop the semantic aspect of language. Each of the models views children as *active* participants in the language-learning process, constantly adding new concepts and refining old ones. As their understanding of the world changes, they develop new words or adjust the meanings of existing words to match their new knowledge. This process is gradual, at first, but builds in intensity as the child enters school.

You may wonder how researchers, observing the same phenomenon of semantic development, could have reached such different conclusions about the way children learn meaning. Several factors may explain the differing models that have been proposed. First, there are individual differences in children. Some children pay more attention to physical features of objects while others are more action oriented. Second, at different stages of development children may prefer one strategy over another. A third factor that may affect how children acquire meaning is the object itself. Some objects (e.g., pets and toys) are more likely to be discovered through action while others (e.g., walls and clouds) are more likely to be viewed at some distance. So, in a sense, each of the models of semantic development may be right at a particular time, for specific children, for particular objects or items.

Language Development in the School Years

By the time most children enter school they have acquired an enormous number of language skills. They can talk in complete sentences and use many different types of sentences, including complex sentences. They can talk about past and future, as well as present, events, and they have a large and varied vocabulary. They are competent communicators, able to take their part in a conversation. One might ask, then, whether there is anything left to learn. The answer is yes—plenty.

The beginning of formal schooling marks a period in which there are new demands on language ability. Now the child is expected not just to talk but to *understand* language itself. In school, children are asked to take language that for several years they have used without much thought and to now become aware of the sounds and structures that underlie that language. Further, they must then apply their language skills to reading and writing. Every day they are presented with new words to learn and relate to prior knowledge. At the same time, because of the social structure of school, they face new demands on their skills as communicators. Success in classroom discussions, playground negotiations, and lunchroom conversations all require maximum skills in communication. It should come as no surprise that children with minimal language skills begin to fall behind soon after beginning school.

Syntax

During the school years children complete their development of many of the syntactic structures that emerged earlier. For example, elaboration of noun and verb phrases continues in this period, as children use more modifiers and learn to use them in new ways (e.g., as sentence starters, *Suddenly the sun came out*). Embedded sentences and compound sentences are used more frequently.

While much syntactic development during the school years can be characterized as elaboration of previous structures, Menyuk (1977) pointed out that several new language forms emerge during (and even after) the school years. For example, children begin to understand and use gerunds—verbs that are turned into nouns by the addition of an *ing* ending (*Swimming is lots of fun*). School-age children begin to understand and use new types of embedded sentences, such as center-embedded sentences (*The cat that chased the rat ran into the barn*). After age 5, children begin to use and understand passive sentences (*The ball was hit by the girl*). These and other developments in language structure generally emerge after the child has entered school.

Semantics

Rapid expansion of vocabulary is one of the major developments of the school years. New vocabulary comes from exposure to a wide array of literature, as well as to new concepts from the sciences and social studies. In addition to learning more words, school-age children deepen their understanding of words already in their vocabulary and are better able to define words (Litowitz, 1977). They can compare and contrast words, synthesize meanings, and begin to understand that some words have more than one meaning (e.g. table).

During the school years, a new development in the semantic domain is the ability to understand and use **nonliteral** (or figurative) language. To use nonliteral language (metaphors, idioms, jokes, proverbs), one must have a firm grasp on the literal meanings of words, for only then can the beauty and humor of figurative language be properly used and appreciated. During the school years, children are asked to write poems and stories that go beyond the literal use of language to incorporate more and more figurative language. Social interaction also requires children to understand words used in nonliteral ways (*He is cool* does not mean that he is cold) and to understand increasingly sophisticated forms of humor.

Research has found that the ability to understand and use nonliteral language begins to develop around age 5 and continues through the school years. For example, the comprehension of idioms (*He put his foot in his mouth*) has been found to develop slowly throughout childhood and even into the adult years (Nippold, 1985). Similarly, children often have a difficult time understanding proverbs (e.g., *One swallow does not a summer make*) and at first struggle to find literal explanations for them. They might say something like "It gets hot in the summer, so it is hard to swallow." Gradually, they are able to move away from the literal meaning of the words to the correct nonliteral interpretation (Billow, 1975).

The use of humor by children is a fascinating area of study (see Bernstein, 1986). If you have ever heard a 5-year-old try to tell you a joke, you know the difficulty children have learning to use humor. There is actually a developmental sequence to the understanding and use of humor. For example, Fowles and Glanz (1977) found that children begin to use riddles between ages 6 and 9 years but often do not understand what they mean. Children may say things like:

Question: Why did the chicken cross the road?

Answer: Because it was there.

This is followed by a howl of laughter from the child and a puzzled look by the adult. The child is able to understand the *form* of a riddle but does not yet understand the point of the joke. Between 9 and 12 years of age, children begin to use and understand humor that is based on the sound and meaning of words. For example, they are able to understand the humor in the old joke:

Question: What is black and white and red (read) all over?

Answer: A newspaper.

Although the ability to tell jokes and understand humor may seem a trivial matter, in fact it is an important component of social acceptance and an essential social skill. Children who lack the language skills to appreciate humor may be at risk for social rejection.

Pragmatics

Some of the most dramatic language developments in the school years are in the area of pragmatics. Although most kindergarten-age children can express their wants and needs, they are not yet truly sophisticated communicators. They do not have command of some of the subtleties of communication. For example, a preschool child may launch into a conversation about Sally, forgetting to tell you that Sally is the name of her teddy bear. In any case, the child's entire conversation may be irrelevant to the topic being discussed.

During the school years, children continue to develop **conversational competence.** They learn, for example, to make their contributions *relevant* to the conversation and to listen to others so they can *maintain* the topic of the conversation. They also learn how to *establish* the topic of conversation and to *initiate* and *close* conversations, as well as what to do when they do not understand something in the conversation. These strategies—called **repair sequences**—include asking for clarification, asking to have something repeated, and asking for more information (Konefal & Folks, 1984). Children also learn to become more sensitive to the conversational context. Research evidence shows that by 8 years of age, children speak differently to their peers than they do to younger children or to adults (Berko Gleason, 1973).

As you read the paragraph above you may have wondered who these children are who possess such good conversational skills. You may have thought about children you know who butt into conversations, who seem insensitive to the give-and-take of conversation, who talk to teachers just as they talk to each other. But this is the point. We *expect* school-age children to be more competent and more sensitive conversational partners. When they let us down, we are justifiably disappointed. However, keep in mind that, as with other aspects of language, *competence* may exceed *performance*. In other words, although students may possess the language *ability*, they may fail to utilize their skill—for a variety of reasons.

In addition to their developing communicative competence, school-age children are developing other pragmatic skills. For example, their ability to understand and use **indirect requests** is increasing. This is a critical skill for school success. When a teacher says, "It's getting noisy in here," she is really saying, "Be quiet." The child who is not able to *understand* indirect requests may misunderstand the message and be punished for misbehavior. Indirect requests take place when the communicative *intent* differs from the linguistic *form*. In the example above, the linguistic form is that of a declarative sentence (*It's getting noisy in here*). But the communicative intent is a command (*Be quiet*). During the school years, children become more adept at using indirect requests, recognizing that they are more likely to get what they want by saying, "Gee, I'm hungry," than by saying, "Give me another cookie."

Metalinguistic Ability

When we ask children to sound out words, to analyze sentences into their constituent parts, to complete a map of story elements, or to identify rules of language we are asking them to use **metalinguistic** abilities. Metalinguistic ability allows the child to go beyond language use and to *think about* language.

By the time they enter school, children have a substantial amount of language ability, but they are generally not aware of what they know. Have you ever tried asking a first grader to differentiate grammatical from nongrammatical sentences? Many first graders can tell you which ones are the "bad" sentences, but when asked to explain their reasoning, they encounter difficulty. They may look at you with a blank stare or say something like, "It just doesn't sound right." They *know* the rules of grammar, but they cannot *say* them. By second or third grade, however, most children can state a rule to support their answer. They can tell you that nouns must come before verbs or that word endings must agree in number. This observation has been confirmed by research such as that by Sutter and Johnson (1990).

The example discussed above focused on *syntactic* awareness. Another aspect of metalinguistic awareness that is critical for success in school is *phonological* awareness. By the time they enter school, most children can recognize all the phonemes of English. Once in school, they are required to become *aware* of these sounds and use them in reading. That is, they must bring to conscious awareness their underlying knowledge of the sound system of their language. This is what is meant by phonological awareness. Children are asked to divide words into sounds, to become aware of rhyme, and to count the number of sounds in a word. In order to perform tasks such as these, children must have awareness of the phonological characteristics of their language. Research has found that children who are more skilled in phonological awareness are usually better readers (Blackman & James, 1985), while children with reading disorders are often deficient in phonological skills (Kamhi & Catts, 1986). These findings suggest that phonological abilities are important skills for reading.

Conclusion

Language development in the school years evolves in two ways: elaboration of existing structures and acquisition of new structures. During the school years children build upon their earlier language development—refining previous structures and broadening their use of these structures—while at the same time, they continue to develop new structures. They can understand and use ever more complex sentences, passive sentences, nonliteral language, and subtle conversational rules (see Table 4.7). During the school years children also develop metalinguistic ability—the ability to think about language and apply language to other purposes (e.g., reading and writing). It would be incorrect to think of language development as ending at age 5 or 6. In fact, language continues to change and develop throughout life.

TABLE 4.7   **Language in the School Years**

Syntax	Semantics	Pragmatics
Continued expansion of NP and VP	Expansion of vocabulary	Development of conversational competence
Use of new types of embedded sentences	Elaboration of definitions	Comprehension and use of indirect requests
Understanding and use of passive voice	Understanding multiple-meaning words	
Use of gerunds	Use of nonliteral language	

Summary

In this chapter we have seen how language development begins at birth (or even before birth) and continues through the school-age years, reviewing evidence that babies are active participants in early communicative interaction and that parents simplify the language they use with their children. We have examined the course of spoken language development—from the early vocalizations through the emergence of first words and sentences to the further refinements and elaborations that take place in later childhood—also considering three theories that attempt to account for semantic development. Finally, we have examined the continuing development of language in the school years, with an emphasis on the development of the semantic, pragmatic, and metalinguistic skills that are essential for success in school and in society.

The information in this chapter and the preceding three chapters describes the course of language development from birth through the school years and provides the background for understanding language and communication disorders. These chapters examined the components of language and defined speech and communication and reviewed the physiological and cognitive bases for language development and the four theories that have attempted to explain language acquisition. With this background in language theory and development, we are ready to examine the language difficulties of school-age children.

Review Questions

1. At which stage of communicative development (perlocutionary, illocutionary, locutionary) is each of the following children:

    _____ **a.** Baby bangs on crib with rattle to get mother's attention
    _____ **b.** Baby gurgles. Mother says, "Oh, are you hungry?"
    _____ **c.** Child says: "More cookie."

2. Describe what adults do to alter their language for young children.

3. What happens during the transition period as young children are beginning to use recognizable words?

4. What is MLU? How is it related to syntactic development?

5. Match the MLU stage to the appropriate syntactic development:

_____ Emergence of grammatical morphemes ıı

_____ Emergence of negation and questions   ııı

_____ Use of telegraphic language   ı

_____ Emergence of complex sentences   ıⅴ

6. According to the semantic-feature theory, how does a child learn to differentiate a cow from a dog?

7. List three syntactic structures that are usually developed in the school years.

8. Why is metalinguistic ability important for success in school?

Suggested Activities

1. Examine children's understanding of nonliteral (figurative) language. For this activity you should use two children—one about 5 years old, the other about 8 years old. Ask each child to tell you what the following sentences mean:

A stitch in time saves nine.
The cat's fur was as smooth as silk.
She put her foot in her mouth.
People who live in glass houses shouldn't throw stones.

What do you observe?
Do the children interpret the sentences literally?
Do they understand the nonliteral meaning of each statement?

2. To examine children's growth in communicative abilities, set up a *referential communication* activity. Put a barrier (a large box will do) in the middle of a table so that a person seated on one side of the table cannot see the other side. Have two piles of blocks (various sizes and shapes work best). Ask children of different ages (6–7 and 9–10) to help each other assemble the blocks into a pattern. Have the pattern set up on one side of the barrier. Ask one child to give directions to the other, using only language (no gestures or peeking allowed). After one or two attempts switch the children so that the one giving the directions is now the listener.

What happened?
Was the speaker able to direct the listener to assemble the blocks accurately?
Were directions specific?
Did the listener ask for help?
Did you notice any age-related differences?

References

Bates, E., Camaioni, L., & Volterra, V. (1975). The acquisition of performatives prior to speech. *Merrill-Palmer Quarterly, 21,* 205–224.

Berko Gleason, J. (1973). Code switching in children's language. In T. Moore (Ed.), *Cognitive development and the acquisition of language* (pp. 159–167). New York: Academic Press.

Bernstein, D. (1986). The development of humor: Implications for assessment and intervention. *Folia Phoniatrica, 39*, 130–144.

Billow, R. (1975). A cognitive developmental study of metaphor comprehension. *Developmental Psychology, 11*, 415–423.

Blackman, B., & James, S. (1985). Metalinguistic abilities and reading achievement in first grade children. In J. Niles & R. Lalid (Eds.), *Issues in literacy: A research perspective.* Thirty-fourth Yearbook of the National Reading Conference. Clemson, NC: National Reading Conference, Inc.

Bowerman, M. (1978). The acquisition of word meaning: An investigation in some current conflicts. In N. Waterson & C. Snow (Eds.), *The development of communication.* New York: Wiley.

Brown, R. (1973). *A first language: The early stages.* Cambridge, MA: Harvard University Press.

Clark, E. (1973). What's in a word: On the child's acquisition of semantics in his first language. In T. Moore (Ed.), *Cognitive development and the acquisition of language* (pp. 65–110). New York: Academic Press.

De Casper, A., & Fifer, W. (1980). Of human bonding: Newborns prefer their mothers' voices. *Science, 208*, 1174–1176.

De Casper, A., & Spence, M. (1986). Prenatal maternal speech influences newborns' perception of speech sounds. *Infant Behavior and Development, 9*, 133–150.

Eimas, P., Siqueland, E., Jusczyk, P., & Vigorito, J. (1971). Speech perception in infants. *Science, 171*, 303–306.

Fowles, B., & Glanz, M. (1977). Competence and a talent in verbal riddle comprehension. *Journal of Child Language, 4*, 433–452.

Gleason, J. B. (1993). Studying language development: An overview and preview. In J. B. Gleason (Ed.), *The development of language* (pp. 1–37). New York: Macmillan.

Kamhi, A., & Catts, H. (1986). Toward an understanding of developmental language and reading disorders. *Journal of Speech and Hearing Disorders, 51*, 337–348.

Konefal, J., & Folks, J. (1984). Linguistic analysis of children's conversational repairs. *Journal of Psycholinguistic Research, 13*, 1–11.

Litowitz, B. (1977). Learning to make definitions. *Journal of Child Language, 4*, 289–304.

Menyuk, P. (1977). *Language and maturation.* Cambridge, MA: MIT Press.

Murray, L., & Trevarthen, C. (1985). Emotional regulations of interactions between 2 month olds and their mothers. In T. Field & N. Fox (Eds.), *Social perception in infants.* Norwood, NJ: Ablex.

Murray, L., & Trevarthen, C. (1986). The infant's role in mother-infant communication. *Journal of Child Language, 13*, 15–31.

Nelson, K. (1973). Some evidence for the cognitive primacy of categorization and its functional basis. *Merrill-Palmer Quarterly, 19*, 21–39.

Nelson, K. (1974). Concept, word, and sentence: Interrelations in acquisition and development. *Psychological Review, 81*, 267–285.

Newport, E., Gleitman, A., & Gleitman, L. (1977). Mother I'd rather do it myself: Some effects and non-effects of maternal speech style. In C. Snow & C. Ferguson (Eds.), *Talking to children: Language, input, and acquisition* (pp. 109–149). New York: Cambridge University Press.

Nippold, M. (1985). Comprehension of figurative language. *Topics in Language Disorders, 3*, 1–20.

Rosch, E., & Mervis, C. (1975). Family resemblances: Studies in the internal structure of categories. *Cognitive Psychology, 7*, 573–605.

Sachs, J. (1993). The emergence of intentional communication. In J. Berko Gleason (Ed.), *The development of language.* New York: Macmillan.

Stark, R. (1979). Prespeech segmental feature development. In P. Fletcher & M. Garman (Eds.), *Language acquisition* (pp. 15–32). New York: Cambridge University Press.

Sutter, J., & Johnson, C. (1990). School-age children's metalinguistic awareness of grammaticality in verb form. *Journal of Speech and Hearing Research, 33*, 84–95.

Part **II**

Language and Communication Problems

Language and communication problems are found in all kinds of children—those with and without disabilities, rich and poor, English speaking and non-English speaking. Frequently, though not always, difficulties with learning language and in communicating with others are associated with specific disabilities. In the next five chapters we will examine the impact of specific disabilities on language development.

Each chapter discusses the nature of the disability itself, the language and communication characteristics of children with this disability, and the implications for classroom instruction.

As you read this unit, you may want to keep in mind two major points. First, there is considerable debate within the field of special education about the usefulness of disability labels. Some have argued that current labels are largely meaningless (e.g., Reynolds, Wang, & Walberg, 1987). On the other hand, labels are a convenient way of grouping children who have similar characteristics. Research, educational programs, and textbooks are often organized on the basis of disability. This unit is organized by disability labels, because these labels are widely used by schools to identify children with disabilities and to deliver services to children. The second point is that we should be careful not to assume that because a particular problem is associated with a disability label, all of the children with that label have the problem. Each child is an individual, with an individual pattern of abilities and limitations. It should also be understood that when generalizations about a particular population of children are made, this generalization does not apply to every child with that disability label.

The purpose of this unit is to describe the language and communication characteristics of children with a variety of disabilities. Increasingly, these children are being educated in regular, as well as special education, settings. There are many other children who may not be labeled but who may, however, share some of the language and communication problems experienced by children with identified disabilities.

Chapter 5

Language and Students with Learning Disabilities

Students with learning disabilities comprise a large, if somewhat poorly defined, segment of the population of children with special needs. This chapter describes both the specific language characteristics of children with learning disabilities and the effects of these language difficulties on the academic and social performance of the children with them. Some suggestions are provided for teaching children with learning disabilities.

After reading this chapter you should be able to:

1. Understand the difficulties in defining *learning disabilities.*
2. Describe several major language difficulties experienced by many students with learning disabilities.
3. Discuss the effects of specific language difficulties on reading, writing, thinking, and interpersonal interaction.
4. Choose appropriate instructional approaches for students with language-learning disabilities.

_____ **Case Study: Janice W.** _____

Janice W. is an 8-year-old African American girl who is a student in a regular second-grade class. Janice's teacher is concerned about her lack of progress in reading and her poor socialization, feeling that Janice understands more than she is able to show. At this time Janice is reading at an early first-grade level, and her reading is slow and hesitant. Her teacher also reports that Janice is pleasant and cooperative but is very shy and reluctant to participate in groups. Janice's first-grade teacher noticed similar problems with reading and socialization but hoped that Janice would outgrow these problems.

Janice comes from a single-parent family; her mother has struggled to provide for her three children, Janice and her two brothers, since her husband left her three years ago. Mrs. W. has held a succession of low-paying jobs and has been unemployed several times. The W. family lives in public housing in a high-crime neighborhood. Mrs. W. has reported that

Janice's early development was normal, although she remembers that Janice had frequent colds and earaches and was always a quiet child.

Janice was observed in the classroom during a group reading lesson and during group work on a writing assignment that followed the reading lesson. When called on to read, Janice read very quietly. She hesitated frequently and misread a number of words. She needed a great deal of assistance to complete a paragraph. However, when asked a question about the passage, she responded correctly. During the group activity Janice kept to herself; she joined in only when prompted to do so by her teacher.

Janice was tested for possible classification for special educational services. Her full-scale IQ score on the WISC-III was in the 92 to 95 range. Her performance subscore was in the 108 to 110 range, while her verbal subscore was in the 84 to 86 range. The Test of Language Development—2 (Primary) was administered and yielded a spoken language quotient (SLQ) of 84. This score placed Janice in the below-average range. Her test profile indicated that her lowest scores were in word articulation and word discrimination—elements of phonology. Janice scored highest in grammatic understanding and picture vocabulary.

What are we to make of a case like Janice's? Here is a child who seems to be bright and is not a behavior problem, yet is struggling to succeed in school. What is wrong? It is because of cases like Janice's that the term *learning disability* was developed. Janice must have a disability that diminishes her ability to learn, some would argue. As a result, she is not achieving to her potential. Yet, calling her "learning disabled" certainly does not solve Janice's problems. We want to know more about her. What exactly is wrong? What can be done?

In this report there are several hints that Janice has some sort of language-based learning disability. For example, her difficulty reading words, her reluctance to talk, and results from the language testing could indicate a language-based disability. Yet, Janice talks normally and can communicate when she is encouraged to do so. Her language disorder, if indeed there is one, is really quite subtle. In order to better understand Janice and other children like her, we will examine the term *learning disabilities* and the relationship between language disorders and learning disabilities.

The Dilemma of Learning Disabilities

What is a learning disability? How do we know that such a thing even exists? In 1960 there were no classes for children labeled *learning disabled,* since the term had not even been coined yet. By 1991, however, 2,144,377 children (or almost 4% of the entire school population) were identified as having learning disabilities. Where did these children—and their disabilities—come from?

History of Learning Disabilities

In order to answer these questions it is necessary to know something about the history of learning disabilities. Lerner (1993) has described the history of learning disabilities as occurring in four phases: foundation phase (about 1800–1930), transition phase (about 1930–1960), integration phase (about 1960–1980), and contemporary phase (since 1980). The **foundation** phase was characterized by basic medical research on the functioning of the adult brain. This early medical research demonstrated that brain damage could cause a specific and limited disability. For example, Paul Broca, a French physician, demonstrated that damage to a specific region of the brain (later known as Broca's area) could cause loss of the ability to speak, though other functions remained intact. During the **transition** phase the results of these early studies of the brain were applied to children and methods of instruction were developed. It is during this period that the term *brain damaged* was coined by Werner and Strauss (1940) to describe children who had learning disorders but who were not mentally retarded. During what Lerner has called the **integration** phase, the various research developments in the domains of spoken language, written language, and perceptual-motor functioning became integrated into the newly coined term *learning disabilities*. This term represents the commonalities between children with a variety of learning difficulties, without drawing any firm conclusions about the origin of these problems.

In the present **contemporary phase,** there are a number of issues facing the field of learning disabilities. However, two questions predominate. One question involves the issue of placement. Where should children with learning disabilities be taught—in regular education classrooms, in resource centers, in self-contained classes? This is a highly emotional issue and one not likely to soon go away (see Fuchs & Fuchs, 1994). The other major issue is, in a sense, related to the first. It is the issue of definition. Ever since Samuel Kirk coined the term *learning disabilities*, there has been a debate about what it means. This discussion continues even today. The truth is that our definitions of learning disabilities lack specificity and are difficult to apply. As a result, it can be difficult to determine who actually has a learning disability and which children may benefit from special education.

Definition of Learning Disabilities

The federal definition of learning disabilities, incorporated in the *Individuals with Disabilities Education Act* (IDEA), states:

> The term "children with specific learning disabilities" means those children who have a disorder in one or more of the basic psychological processes involved in understanding or in using language, spoken or written, which disorder may manifest itself in imperfect ability to listen, think, speak, read, write, spell, or to do mathematical calculations. Such disorders include such conditions as perceptual handicaps, brain injury, minimal brain dysfunction, dyslexia, and developmental aphasia. Such term does not include children who have learning problems which are primarily the result of visual, hearing, or motor handicaps, of mental retardation, of emotional disturbance, or of environmental, cultural, or economic disadvantage.

For our purposes, it is important to note that the federal definition of learning disabilities cites the understanding and use of *language* as the prime characteristic of learning disabilities. The definition was designed to be broad and inclusive, although its last section was meant to exclude other causes of learning problems from the category of learning disabilities. The definition, however, has been difficult to apply in practice. Other definitions for learning disabilities have been developed, but significant problems with definition still remain.

If we are to understand the language and communication problems of students with learning disabilities, we must first establish who we are talking about. This is no easy task. This briefly reviewed history of the development of the field of learning disabilities—and of the origins of the term—is designed to give an understanding of the difficulties in defining the subject and illustrate why the term *learning disabilities* should be used with caution.

Language Characteristics

Over the past 20 years or so there has been increasing interest in and emphasis on the relationship between language difficulties and learning (especially reading) disabilities. We know from our brief historical survey of this field that research on language disorders was one of the paths of study that led to the term learning disabilities. However, the role of language in learning disabilities was for may years largely ignored, as the focus shifted to perceptual and motor problems. By the late 1970s there was a steadily increasing research base that was suggesting that language is an important factor in understanding reading and learning disabilities. The studies published in 1977 in a special issue of the *Harvard Educational Review,* entitled "Reading, Language, and Learning," and Frank Vellutino's 1979 book, entitled *Dyslexia: Theory and Research,* made the case for the importance of language in reading and in understanding reading disorders. Vellutino's book, in particular, systematically examined and destroyed the arguments for a visual-perceptual basis for reading disorders. Since the 1970s, a large volume of research has confirmed the link between language problems and reading disabilities (e.g., Aram & Nation, 1980; Menyuk, Chesnick, Liebergott, Korngold, D'Agostino, & Belanger, 1991; Vellutino & Scanlon, 1987).

Having established the central role of language in reading and reading disabilities, researchers have been trying to identify the specific language difficulties that underlie both reading and other learning disabilities. It seems that the more they have looked for these language difficulties, the more they have found. For example, Gibbs and Cooper (1989) found that more than 96 percent of a large sample of students with learning disabilities had some type of communication deficit. More than 90 percent of their sample had a language impairment, while 23 percent had articulation disorders. Yet, only 6 percent of this group of students with learning disabilities were receiving services from a speech-language specialist.

While findings such as those in the Gibbs and Cooper study support the conclusion that most students with learning disabilities have language difficulties, these problems are often subtle and may go unrecognized. Donahue (1986) has suggested that within the population that is sometimes called *reading disordered* there may be three subgroups of children with language disabilities:

1. **Students with relatively severe language problems** who are usually identified at an early age as having a language disability—often before entering school.
2. **Students with less severe language problems** who are usually not identified as having a language difficulty until they are in school. Often their problems emerge as they attempt to perform school tasks such as listening, reading, and writing.
3. **Students whose language problems are identified later** who come to school with apparently intact spoken language but experience difficulty in reading, due to factors other than language (e.g., attention and/or motivation).

The relationship between language difficulties and learning disabilities is complex. There is increasing evidence that most students with reading difficulties have problems in language development. This does not mean, however, that these language disabilities necessarily cause reading disabilities. We will examine evidence about causation in the next section. It is likely, however, that language difficulties play an important role in other learning disabilities. Language is essential for thinking, socialization, and classroom interaction. Since most students with learning disabilities have problems in one or more of these areas, it is not surprising to find that difficulties in understanding and using language might at least contribute to the learning problems experienced by children with learning disabilities. In the next section, we examine the research on specific language disorders experienced by children with learning disabilities.

Phonology

There is a great deal of research evidence that suggests that many, if not most, children with reading disabilities have significant difficulty processing phonological information (see Table 5.1). In particular, children with learning difficulties have been found to be deficient in something called *phonological awareness*. Phonological awareness, according to Blachman (1994), can be defined as "an awareness of, and the ability to manipulate, the phonological segments represented in an alphabetic orthography" (p. 253). In other words, the written form of English is composed of alphabetic bits called letters. Each letter has a sound attached to it. Unfortunately for speakers and readers of English, a single letter may represent several different sounds. For example, the letter *c* may sound like *k* as in *cake* but sound like *s* in the word *celery*. Similarly, a single sound (such as *s*) may be represented by more than one letter (sometimes by *s*, at other times by *c*). In order to figure out which sounds go with each letter, children must first learn to identify the sounds (phonological awareness) within speech, then learn to match these sounds to letters (phonics).

Phonological awareness is not the same as auditory perception, although the two are sometimes confused with each other. A study conducted by Brady, Shankweiler, and Mann (1983) demonstrated this fact. In their study, good and poor readers were asked to identify both speech (real words) and nonspeech (environmental sounds) stimuli. The poor readers made many more errors than

TABLE 5.1   Research Findings on the Phonological Skills of Children
with Learning Disabilities

Bradley & Bryand (1978)	Reading disabled children were insensitive to rhyme.
Fox & Routh (1980)	Children with reading problems had difficulty dividing words into phonemes.
Brady, Shankweiler, & Mann (1983)	Poor readers had problems with speech sounds but not with environmental sounds.
Catts (1989)	Children with severe reading problems repeated phrases more slowly than others and made more speech errors.

the good readers in identifying the speech sounds, especially when there was background noise. However, there were no differences between the groups on their perception of the environmental sounds. The authors concluded that poor readers do not have a general problem with auditory input but do have a specific difficulty processing language sounds.

Phonological awareness appears to be an ability that develops over time. By 5 years of age most children can divide words into syllables but they are just beginning to be able to divide words into sound units (phonemes). Research has found that by the end of first grade, about 70 percent of children can perform this latter task (Liberman, Shankweiler, Fischer, & Carter, 1974). Numerous studies have found that those children who are better at phonological awareness tend to be better readers (e.g., Bradley & Bryant, 1983; Liberman & Shankweiler, 1985; Vellutino & Scanlon, 1987).

A growing number of research studies have found that children with reading disabilities have difficulty acquiring phonological awareness. A typical study was one conducted by Fox and Routh (1980) with first-grade children who had average, mildly depressed, and severely depressed reading abilities. They asked these children to "say just a little bit" of spoken syllables. The children with severe reading problems were generally unable to divide the syllables into phonemes, while the other children were able to perform this task. Other studies have found that children with reading disabilities are insensitive to rhyme (Bradley & Bryant, 1978) and to the length of words (Katz, 1986) (see Box 5.1 for examples of how phonological awareness ability can be assessed). After examining the research, Catts (1989) concluded that "children with limited awareness of these aspects of language (rhyme, alliteration, and syllable structure) often experience difficulties in learning to read, whereas those with a high degree of sound awareness often excel at reading" (p.115).

This research on phonical awareness is very interesting because it suggests that we may have found a cause (although not the only one) for reading disabilities. However, the evidence presented so far, while compelling, is mostly circumstantial. That is, it indicates that there is a relationship between phonological awareness and reading disabilities, but it does not confirm which is the cause and which is the outcome. What would be more convincing would be to demonstrate

BOX 5.1   Assessing Phonological Awareness

How can phonological awareness be assessed? Kamhi and Catts (1986) used four techniques to evaluate the phonological awareness of children from 6 to 9 years of age, with and without reading and language impairments. The four methods were:

1. Division of bisyllabic words into CVC (consonant/vowel/consonant) monosyllables

The children were given some examples of how to divide the words into parts, using a puppet that modeled the correct response. Then the children were told to divide the following words into parts:

airplane	doctor
football	monkey
hotdog	pencil
pancake	window

2. Division of monosyllabic words into sounds (phonemes)

The same preparation was used as that described above. Then the children were told to divide the following words into their sounds:

plane	doc
foot	key
hot	pen
cake	dow

3. Elision task

The children were told "I'm going to say a word to you. You say the word just like I do. Then I'm going to tell you a part to leave off, either at the beginning or the end of the word. You say the word, leaving off the part I tell you to." The children were given several examples; then were given the following words:

(t)old	sun(k)
(b)lend	bus(t)
(t)all	pin(k)
(n)ice	ten(t)
(s)top	far(m)
(n)ear	car(d)
(b)ring	for(k)
(s)pin	star(t)

4. Segmentation (tapping) task

The children were told "Now we're going to play a tapping game. I'm going to say something to you—some play words—and then tap them after I say them. You need to listen carefully, so you can learn how to play the game."

Example: The tester says "oo" and taps one time.

Then, the tester says "boo" and taps two times.

Then "boot" and taps three times.

The experimental items were:

ap	leb
em	kest
niz	feh
blim	sput
zan	piv
ib	kel
polt	kii
wog	mik

Source: Test Items from A. Kamhi & H. Catts, "Toward an Understanding of Developmental Language and Reading Disorders." *Journal of Speech and Hearing Disorders, 51*(1986), 336–347. © American Speech-Language-Hearing Association. Reprinted by permission of the American Speech-Language-Hearing Association and the authors.

that teaching children to enhance their phonological skills improves their reading. This is just what Bradley and Bryant (1983) found when they looked at the effects of sound-categorization training on the reading development of beginning readers. Children who were poor at sound categorization were taught to recognize and group words by their sounds. Children who were taught this skill did better on reading and spelling tests than other children who were taught to group by word meaning or who received no training. Blachman (1987) taught students with learning disabilities how to enhance their phonological awareness. As a result, their reading scores increased significantly. Results such as these would seem to support the conclusion that phonological awareness difficulties are a cause of reading disabilities. However, the research support is still limited, and we must be cautious in drawing any firm conclusions.

Not only is phonological awareness (or encoding) a problem for children with reading disabilities, but, for many, phonological production is a problem, as well. You may recall that in their study, Gibbs and Cooper found that about 23 percent of their sample of students with learning disabilities had articulation problems. This compares to the 4 to 6 percent frequency of articulation problems they say are generally found in the student population without disabilities. Catts (1989) found that children with severe reading disabilities repeated phrases more slowly than good readers and made more errors in their speech. Studies such as these suggest that students with reading disabilities have an increased risk for speech-production problems. However, many children with speech-production problems do not have serious reading difficulties. Likewise, many children with reading disabilities have no significant speech-production problems. Therefore, we should be careful not to jump to conclusions that speech-production difficulties cause reading disabilities.

Now, let's go back and have another look at Janice, the child described in the case study at the beginning of this chapter. Janice's difficulty with reading words, coupled with her relatively good comprehension and intact communicative abilities, suggest that Janice may be having difficulty with phonological awareness. This hypothesis has been supported by results from standardized testing. These results indicated that Janice has problems with language—especially with word discrimination and articulation. Both the test results and the classroom observations point to phonological processing as a likely contributor to Janice's reading problems.

Morphology

Given the problems many children with learning disabilities have with the sound system of the language, it should not be surprising to find that they also have difficulty with word parts. In fact, most studies of the morphological abilities of children with learning disabilities have found this as an area of difficulty. For example, Vogel (1977) found that on two tests of morphological knowledge 7- and 8-year-old poor readers did significantly worse than children of the same age who were good readers. The poor readers did especially poorly with the more complex rules. According to Wiig (1990), children with learning disabilities have difficulty with parts of words that are hard to hear (such as word endings and unstressed syllables). As a result, these children are slow to acquire the rules for using grammatical markers. Wiig and Semel (1984) identified numerous morphological problems commonly found in children with learning disabilities (see Table 5.2).

TABLE 5.2   Morphological Problems of Students with Learning Disabilities

1. The formation of noun plurals, especially the irregular forms *(s, z, ez, ren)*
2. The formation of noun possessives, both singular and plural *('s, s')*
3. The formation of third-person singular of the present tense verbs *(t, d, ed)*
4. The formation of the past tense of both regular and irregular verbs *(t, d, ed)*
5. The formation of the comparative and superlative forms of adjectives *(er, est)*
6. The cross-categorical use of inflectional endings *(s, 's, s')*
7. Noun derivation *(er)*
8. Adverb derivation *(ly)*
9. The comprehension and use of prefixes *(pre, post, pro, anti)*

Source: Adapted from E. Wiig and E. Semel. (1984). *Language assessment and intervention for the learning disabled.* Columbus, OH: Merrill.

Although it may seem as though problems with morphology may be rather unimportant, these problems often show up in students' writing and may also affect their reading comprehension.

Syntax

Many students with learning disabilities have difficulty understanding and using the syntactic component of language. As was the case with morphology, the higher-level components often are the most problematic. In a number of studies it was found that the more complex sentences became, the more difficulty students with learning disabilities experienced in understanding such sentences (Vogel, 1974; Wallach & Goldsmith, 1975; Wiig, Lapointe, & Semel, 1977). Typically, students with learning disabilities have problems understanding sentences that contain relative clauses, that use the passive voice, and that use negation. Young children with learning disabilities appear to be developing through the same stages of syntactic development as other children, but do so more slowly (Roth & Spekman, 1989). However, even older children with learning disabilities have difficulty with some of the higher-order syntactic structures.

Studies that have examined spoken language production have also found a number of difficulties in syntactic development among children with learning disabilities. Simms and Crump (1983) examined the language used by students with and without learning disabilities as they discussed two films they had just viewed. The researchers analyzed language samples for the length and complexity of language used by the students and found that although their sample of students with learning disabilities actually used longer sentences than other students, their sentences were significantly less syntactically complex than those of the other students. This is really not surprising, since the use of complex structures, such as compound and embedded sentences, usually reduces sentence length. Other studies have usually found that students with learning disabilities

TABLE 5.3   Research Findings on the Morphological and Syntactic Skills of Children with Learning Disabilities

Morphology

Vogel (1977)	Poor readers perform worse on tests of morphological knowledge.
Wiig & Semel (1984)	Poor readers have numerous specific morphological problems.

Syntax

Vogel (1974)	Those with learning disabilities (LD) use shorter sentences and make more grammatical errors.
Simms & Crump (1983)	Children with LD use less complex sentences.
Roth & Spekman (1989)	Children with LD have delays in syntactic development.

use shorter sentences and make more grammatical errors than children without disabilities (Vogel, 1974; Wiig & Semel, 1975; Wiig, LaPointe, & Semel, 1977).

In general, research on the syntactic abilities of students with learning disabilities has found that these students experience difficulties both in understanding and using complex syntactic structures. These difficulties could also contribute to problems in understanding and producing written language (see Table 5.3).

Semantics

Since many, if not most, students with learning disabilities have difficulties with aspects of cognition such as planning, organizing, and evaluating information, it should not be surprising to find that they also have difficulty with semantic concepts. After all, semantics involves the development of relationships between ideas and language. In fact, semantics is a significant problem for many students with learning disabilities. In particular, research has discovered two main problem areas: word finding and the use of figurative language (see Table 5.4).

Many studies have found that the expressive vocabulary skills of children with learning disabilities lag behind those other children (e.g., Rudel, Denckla, & Broman, 1981; Wiig & Semel, 1975). Although the exact cause of word-retrieval problems is not clear—some claim the problem is the result of a general language disorder, others, of a memory disorder—there is evidence that problems with word retrieval contribute to reading disabilities (Mann, 1991).

In addition to their word-finding problems, students with learning disabilities have been reported to have difficulty understanding words with multiple meanings (Wiig & Semel, 1984). For example, during a math class if these students are told to make a table using numbers from their book, they may wonder how they are supposed to build something with four legs out of numbers. Both word-

TABLE 5.4   Research Findings on the Semantic Skills of Children with Learning Disabilities

Word Finding

Wiig & Semel (1975)	Have slow word-retrieval speed
Wiig & Semel (1984)	Misunderstand multiple-meaning words

Figurative Language

Nippold & Fey (1983)	Are poor at interpreting metaphor
Seidenberg & Bernstein (1986)	Have reduced comprehension of similes
Fowles & Glanz (1977)	Have less appreciation of humor in riddles
Wiig & Semel (1984)	Have difficulty interpreting proverbs

finding problems and difficulties with multiple-meaning words are examples of semantic difficulties.

Children with learning disabilities have also been found to have difficulty with nonliteral (or figurative) language. For example, they have problems understanding and using metaphor (Nippold & Fey, 1983) and simile (Seidenberg & Bernstein, 1986). Difficulties with nonliteral language can show up in reading and writing. Similarly, students with learning disabilities have been found to have difficulty understanding and using humor. In one study (Fowles & Glanz, 1977), students with reading disabilities, age 6 to 9 showed less appreciation for humor than did their peers without reading disabilities. They were also less able to retell riddles in their own words or explain why they were funny. Wiig and Semel (1984) described some of the problems that students with learning disabilities experience in understanding proverbs. They tend to be very literal in their interpretations. For example, if asked to explain the following proverb, *A bird in the hand is worth two in the bush,* they may tell you that it means that someone is holding a bird in their hand.

Problems understanding and using nonliteral language may reflect the rigidness with which many students with learning disabilities seem to approach language. That is, it seems as though they become attached to the most concrete meaning of words—even when this clearly makes no sense in the context. Nonliteral language is often an important part of the curriculum; metaphor and simile are important language devices that are used in many stories. Students are asked to use such devices in their own writing (and are graded accordingly). Proverbs are often used in the elementary reading curriculum, and humor is an essential skill in school (as any teacher will tell you). Students who have difficulty understanding and using humor are at risk for misunderstanding both teachers and their peers and of being misunderstood by others. It may help if teachers are aware of the sort of semantic problems that students with learning disabilities may encounter. In addition, by providing examples of the use of nonliteral language and pointing out when such language is used, teachers may be able to help students improve their skills in this area.

Pragmatics

Research has consistently found the area of pragmatics to be a major problem for children with learning disabilities (Boucher, 1986; Lapadat, 1991). Not only do students with learning disabilities have difficulties with language, they often lack the ability (or the knowledge) to analyze social situations, to plan their responses, and to evaluate the consequences of their actions (Bryan, 1991; Vaughn, 1991). Both language and social-cognition skills contribute to pragmatics.

Research on the pragmatic skills of children with learning disabilities has focused mostly on their conversational skills. A number of specific problems have been identified. For example, when asked to participate in a TV talk show format, students with learning disabilities tended to be less effective interviewers than did their peers without disabilities. They asked fewer open-ended questions—that is, questions that would give the "guest" the opportunity to discuss the topics in detail (Bryan, Donahue, Pearl, & Sturm, 1981). Look at the example below of two students who were asked to pretend to be part of such an interaction:

Host: Welcome to the show. Today we have Doogie Howser with us.

Guest: Hello.

H: Well, we're going to ask him a few questions. Doogie, what time did you start being a doctor?

G: When I was four.

H: What? When is the first time that you delivered a baby?

G: Twelve.

H: What time is it now?

G: 9:37.

H: Did you ever have a girlfriend?

G: Yes.

Now, contrast this example to the next one:

Host: Good morning America! Today we have Doogie Howser on our show.

Guest: Hello.

H: How did you do in medical school?

G: I did good. That's how I became a doctor so early. I delivered a baby when I was 13.

H: Is being a doctor scary?

G: Yeah, because you don't know what kind of patient you're going to get or if it's going to be overreactive or something like that.

These conversations were taken from two fourth-grade students. In the first sample, the host is a student who has been classified as having learning disabilities. The guest is a peer without a learning disability. In the second sample the students switched roles. You can see that the host in the second sample asked questions that elicited longer, more elaborate answers. We do not usually ask students to host talk shows in school, but we do ask them to participate in communication with peers. These examples suggest that students with learning disabilities are less competent conversational partners.

Several studies have found students with learning disabilities to be less sensitive to the conversational needs of their partners. For example, studies of referential communication have usually found that children with learning disabilities provide incomplete and inaccurate descriptions (Spekman, 1981). In referential communication tasks, children are required to verbally guide a partner in completing a task (such as assembling blocks) when the partner is unable to see the array in front of the speaker. Although this is a somewhat artificial task, it has been found to be a good way to evaluate conversational abilities. Students with learning disabilities typically have a difficult time with this task. Other studies have found that children with learning disabilities have difficulty adjusting their language to the level of their conversational partner (Bryan & Pflaum, 1978) or to speakers of different levels of authority (Donahue, 1981). The latter difficulty can present a problem, for example, when a student needs to speak differently to the principal than to a buddy on the playground.

In summary, it appears safe to conclude that children with learning disabilities frequently have significant difficulties with pragmatics—especially with conversational skills. They have difficulty clearly expressing themselves to others, they frequently fail to adjust their language to the needs and/or level of their listener, and they are not sure what to do when they do not understand something being said to them. These difficulties have consequences for classroom interaction, social relationships, and the ability to understand and use written language.

Metalinguistic Skills

Metalinguistic skill, according to van Kleeck (1994), "refers to the ability to reflect consciously on the nature and properties of language" (p. 53). When children play word games, use rhyme, or recognize nongrammatical sentences, they are using metalinguistic skills. As van Kleeck points out, metalinguistic skills are not essential for the development of spoken language. We don't ask young children to tell us what parts of speech they just used (at least not before they enter school). However, many researchers believe that metalinguistic skills are essential for learning how to read and write.

We have already discussed one type of metalinguistic skill—phonological awareness. As children progress from the initial stages of reading to become more proficient readers, other types of metalinguistic skills become important. For example, they develop awareness of the grammatical rules that underlie language and the pragmatic rules that govern conversation.

Children with learning disabilities have been found to have difficulty developing metalinguistic skills. This is most evident in the area of phonological awareness. But researchers have also found that children with learning disabilities have difficulty recognizing grammatical and morphological errors and making the appropriate corrections (Kamhi & Koenig, 1985). In a study of predictors of reading difficulty, Menyuk et al. (1991) found that measures of metalinguistic abilities (including word retrieval, phonological, and semantic) were the best predictors of later reading problems, but that different metalinguistic skills predicted the performance of different children. Although the relationship between higher-order metalinguistic skills and reading is not entirely clear, some research (e.g., Menyuk & Flood, 1981) has suggested that these skills are an important contributor to success in reading and writing.

Effects of Language Impairments

It is essential that teachers and other professionals intervene as soon as possible to help students who are experiencing language learning disabilities. Research has found that children with language disabilities are clearly at risk for academic failure. In fact, the incidence of reading disabilities in children with early language difficulties has been estimated to be between 4 and 75 percent (Bashir & Scavuzzo, 1992). There is some evidence that children with language learning disabilities are also at risk for emotional problems (Baker & Cantwell, 1982).

For those who think that if we just wait long enough, children with language disabilities will get better, the news is not good. Although some studies have found that children with early language problems improve over time, most researchers have concluded that their learning continues to be significantly impaired when compared to their peers (Rissman, Curtiss, & Tallal, 1990). In one study (Aram, Ekelman, & Nation, 1984) a group of children with early identified language disorders was examined ten years later. Most adolescents (70 percent) continued to have difficulties with academic tasks and social acceptance. Although some children with early language problems do, indeed, grow out of them (30 percent of the children in the study cited above), it appears that most continue to experience significant problems. Therefore, it is important for teachers to recognize language disorders and use effective intervention approaches.

Intervention

So, just what *are* some effective intervention approaches for enhancing the language skills of students with learning disabilities? In this section our focus will be on two instructional methods. Although these intervention methods were designed to address specific problems experienced by students with learning disabilities, they can be applied to other children experiencing similar problems. Chapters 11 and 12 provide more discussion of intervention procedures.

Training in Phonological Awareness

Earlier in this chapter we discussed the large research base that has implicated phonological awareness as a cause of the reading difficulties faced by most students with learning disabilities. Several research studies have found that it is possible to teach phonological skills and have a positive effect on reading. For example, Bradley and Bryant (1983; 1985) conducted large-scale training studies in England, using kindergarten and first-grade children who scored low on a sound-categorization test. In their first study, they simply taught their subjects to group pictures on the basis of shared sounds. For example, the children were taught to group *hen* with *pen* and *men* because these words rhymed. They also taught a group of their children to associate sounds with letters. They found that children trained in this way outperformed untrained children on reading and spelling and that these positive outcomes persisted for several years. Ball and Blachman (1988) found similar results when they taught phonological skills to a group of kindergarten children in the United States.

Blachman (1991) has described an instructional approach that many teachers may find useful in teaching phonological skills. Her approach uses a three-step lesson plan:

1. **Say-It-and-Move-It Activity.** This is a phonological segmentation task in which children were taught to represent sounds by using manipulatives (such as disks, tiles, or buttons). The children were taught to represent, with a disk, each sound they heard. The child was given a card that was divided in half. The top half was a disk storage area. On the bottom half of the card there was an arrow pointing from left to right. If the teacher said "Show me the *a*," the children were to move a disk from the top half of the card to the left-hand end of the arrow and say the sound. After demonstrating mastery of this skill, the teacher progressed to two phoneme words (*up, it, am*) and three phoneme words (*sun, fat, zip*).

2. **Segmentation-Related Activity.** One of several segmentation activities is used in the second step of this lesson. For example, children might learn to group words based on rhyme, or they were taught to segment words using *Elkonin* cards. In this activity, the children were taught to identify the number of sounds in words using picture cards developed by the Russian psychologist Daniel Elkonin. The cards have a picture of a common word at the top (e.g., *sun*) and a series of boxes below the picture that represent the number of *phonemes* (not letters) in the word. Children were taught to move a disk along the boxes that correspond to each sound as they said the word (see Figure 5.1).

3. **Letter Names/Letter Sounds.** Children were taught to use key words and phrases to help them remember the sounds made by each letter. For example, they might see a card for the letter *t* that showed *t*wo *t*eenagers *t*alking on a *t*elephone. Another activity described by Blachman was a post office game in which children selected a picture that illustrated a word with a target letter (e.g., *pot* for *p*) and placed it in the correct letter pouch. Later, as children learned the letter-sound relationships, letters were placed on the manipulatives used in the Say-It-and-Move-It activity.

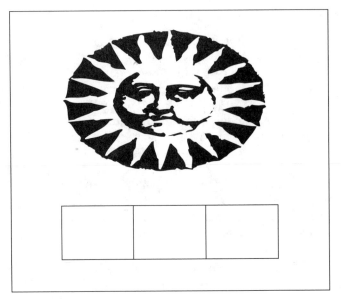

"Sun"

FIGURE 5.1   An Example of an Elkonin Card

When Blachman taught teachers to use these techniques, their kindergarten students outperformed others on several measures of phonological awareness and letter names.

If you decide to use phonological training techniques, the following suggestions may help:

- **Begin with sounds that are easy to hear:** Blachman suggests that "continuous" sounds (like *s, z,* and *l*) are good because they can be held for a long time. Avoid blends *(pr)* and dipthongs *(ow)*.
- **Start with a limited number of sounds:** Introduce new sounds slowly.
- **Teach to mastery:** That is, don't move on until the child has demonstrated mastery in identifying the sound.
- **Individualize instruction:** Although much instruction can be done in groups, some individuals will require additional practice.
- **Integrate with reading and writing:** As soon as possible, try to incorporate phonological tasks into the children's reading and writing activities.

Key Word Method

Phonological training has generally been used with young children who are beginning readers. What about older children with language learning problems?

What can we do for them? One type of approach that has been frequently found to be useful in helping older students learn a variety of skills is **strategy training.** With strategy training, students are taught *how* to learn, not just what to learn. In other words, they are taught a strategy to use as they are learning.

Many students with learning disabilities have difficulty learning new vocabulary words. Mastroprieri (1988) described a strategy for vocabulary learning that she and her colleagues have applied successfully in a number of academic areas (Scruggs & Mastroprieri, 1992). The key word strategy includes the following steps:

1. Recoding: The new vocabulary word is recoded into a key word that sounds similar to the target word, is familiar to the student, and can be easily pictured. For example, *forte* (meaning "loud") could be recoded as *fort*.

2. Relating: The student relates the key word to the target word, using an illustration. A sentence that relates the word to the drawing is created. In our example, a picture of a fort during a battle might show guns firing. The sentence might read *The guns at the fort are loud.*

3. Retrieving: The definition of the new vocabulary is recalled by thinking of the key word, creating the drawing (either actual or imagined), thinking of the related sentence, and stating the definition—*forte* means "loud."

Although this technique may seem slow and cumbersome, it works; it has been applied successfully in a number of studies. In addition, teachers who have used the key word method with many different student populations, including secondary-age, inner-city students with learning problems have found that their students were able to recall many more definitions than they were previously able to.

The key word method is just one example of a learning strategy that may be used to help older students with language-learning difficulties. The research on this and other instructional techniques suggests that it is possible to help these students overcome at least some of their learning difficulties.

Summary

In this chapter we have examined the language difficulties of children with learning disabilities, also discussing some of the difficulties in defining this population. In describing the specific problems associated with learning disabilities, we examined research that suggests that language difficulties are an important cause of learning disabilities and that they do not usually get better on their own. Finally, two instructional approaches—phonological training and the key word strategy—were presented. Having read this chapter, you should be better able to identify language disorders in the classroom and understand some of the consequences of language disabilities.

Review Questions

1. How did the transition phase of research in learning disabilities differ from the research conducted during the foundation phase?

2. What evidence suggests that language disabilities are an important contributor to learning disabilities? Consider evidence from definitions, research, and observations.

3. Give two examples of techniques that could be used to evaluate phonological awareness in children.

4. Many children with language-learning disabilities have difficulty understanding and using figurative language. How could difficulty with figurative language affect academic performance?

5. List and briefly describe three specific conversation-skill problems that have been identified in students with learning disabilities.

6. Some have suggested that the language-learning problems of children with learning disabilities would improve even if nothing were done. Is this true?

_____ **Case Study**_____

Student: Henry S.   Grade: 4
Sex: Male   C.A.: 9:6

Reason for Referral

Henry is a 9-year-old boy who presently attends a regular fourth grade class. Henry's parents have expressed concern about the placement of their child. They believe that he is potentially gifted, although the school has not recognized their son's potential. Henry's teachers, on the other hand, have expressed concern over Henry's slow progress in school and his difficulties in interpersonal relationships. Therefore, it is necessary to evaluate Henry so that an appropriate placement can be made.

Background Information

Henry is an only child who at age 6 months was adopted by his present parents. Both parents teach at a local college. There is little information available on Henry's birth mother—other than the fact that she was quite young when Henry was born. Henry fell from a horse at age 4 and was hospitalized for a few days, but his doctor's prognosis was for a complete recovery.

Henry's attainment of developmental milestones, as reported by his mother, was generally within the expected range. He crawled at 6 months, spoke his first word at 12 months, and put two words together at about 2 years. His parents describe their child as very active and energetic—he loves to play all types of games but is clumsy and a poor athlete. He particularly enjoys Karate. Henry has had some difficulty with eye coordination, but this was reported to have been corrected through exercises.

Education Background

A review of Henry's school records and an interview with his present teacher provided the following school-related information: Henry did not attend any preschool because his parents preferred that he be educated at home. He attended a Montessori kindergarten program and later entered the public schools in the first grade at age 6. He had many adjustment problems when he began to attend school, refusing to sit in his chair and follow normal classroom rules. Henry's academic skill development soon fell behind that of his classmates, especially in reading, and the school officials considered his retention. Upon the request of his parents, Henry was not retained but was promoted to the second grade.

Since first grade Henry's behavior has improved, although he continues to have behavior problems on occasion. His academic record is irregular. He is currently reading at a 2.5 grade level, according to his teacher, and is a slow reader. Though able to match letters to sounds in isolation, Henry has difficulty combining the sounds into words. His sight vocabulary is limited, but his comprehension is better than his word attack skills. Henry can recall most of the ideas he reads and is very good at inferring meaning from the text. He is achieving at a third grade level in math and has had problems with place value and regrouping and has particular difficulty with word problems. Henry enjoys science and social studies and does well in these subjects, despite difficulties reading the books.

Henry was observed while playing with his classmates at recess. It was observed that Henry attempted to join in activities but that his attempts were frequently rejected. In the testing situation Henry was attentive and cooperative. He talked openly with the examiner and easily established rapport. He demonstrated a large vocabulary and an adequate grasp of spoken language, with excellent articulation. His language was, however, somewhat formal and he did not seem to relax at any point. His approach to the various tasks presented was impulsive. He responded quickly with little thought given to the problem. He wrote equally well with both hands and said he had no hand preference.

Test Results

The WISC-III-R (a test of intelligence) was administered to assess Henry's general level of intellectual functioning. Henry earned a verbal score of 110–115 and a performance score of 86–90. His full-scale score was 99–102. Subtest scores were:

General Information	15	Picture Completion	10
Comprehension	16	Picture Arrangement	7
Arithmetic	10	Block Design	5
Similarities	15	Object Assembly	6
Vocabulary	11	Coding	6
Digit Span	11		

These scores indicate that Henry had measured intelligence in the normal range with strengths in the verbal as compared to the performance domain.

The Wechsler Individualized Achievement Test (WIAT) was administered to obtain standardized measures of academic achievement. The subtest scores are as follows:

Subtest	Standard Score	Percentile Rank
Basic Reading	80	9
Math Reasoning	115	84
Spelling	85	16
Reading Comprehension	110	78
Numerical Operations	105	63
Listening Comprehension	92	25
Oral Expression	105	63
Written Expression	95	37

These achievement test scores indicate that Henry's strengths are in mathematical reasoning and in reading comprehension. He scored poorly in basic reading skill, spelling, and listening.

Case Questions

1. What are Henry's major problems? Use evidence from the case to support your answer.

2. What language difficulties is Henry experiencing? How are they affecting Henry's school performance?

3. What are Henry's strengths? How could these be utilized in the development of an instructional program for Henry?

4. If you were a member of a teacher assistance team that was asked to assist Henry's teacher in developing appropriate instruction for Henry, what suggestions would you make? Be specific and give examples.

5. How would you respond to Henry's parents, who insist that he is gifted?

Suggested Activities

1. Several techniques for the assessment of phonological skills were described in this chapter. Develop two additional techniques for assessing phonological skills. One of these could focus on detection of rhyme. The other might deal with discriminating auditory perception from phonological awareness. Try out these techniques with at least two children between 6 and 8 years of age.

2. Select two children between 9 and 12 years old. One of the children should be classified as having disabilities, or is at-risk. Have this child pretend to be a talk show host. Be sure the child knows what that is and can give you an example. Tell the child to take five minutes to interview a guest. The other (without disabilities) child will play the guest. This child should be instructed to answer the questions as completely as possible.

Tape record the interaction. Then have the children switch roles. Transcribe the interviews later, and report on the following:

- What problems (if any) did the children have asking or responding to questions?
- Compare the conversational methods used by the two students, including opening of the interview, types of questions asked, completeness of answers, topic maintenance, conversational repairs, termination of the interview.
- What do the results say about the conversational skills of the students?

References

Aram, D., Ekelman, B., & Nation, J. (1984). Preschoolers with language disorders: 10 years later. *Journal of Speech and Hearing Research, 27,* 232–244.

Aram, D., & Nation, J. (1980). Preschool language disorders and subsequent language and academic difficulties. *Journal of Communication Disorders, 13,* 159–170.

Baker, L., & Cantwell, D. (1982). Psychiatric disorder in children with different types of communication disorders. *Journal of Communication Disorders, 15,* 113–126.

Ball, E., & Blachman, B. (1988). Phoneme segmentation training: Effect on reading readiness. *Annals of Dyslexia, 38,* 208–225.

Bashir, A., & Scavuzzo, A. (1992). Children with language disorders: Natural history and academic success. *Journal of Learning Disabilities, 25,* 53–65.

Blachman, B. (1987). An alternative classroom reading program for learning disabled and other low-achieving children. In R. Bowler (Ed.), *Intimacy with language: A forgotten basic in teacher education* (pp. 49–55). Baltimore, MD: The Orton Dyslexia Society.

Blachman, B. (1991). Early intervention for children's reading problems: Clinical applications of the research in phonological awareness. *Topics in Language Disorders, 12,* 51–65.

Blachman, B. (1994). Early literacy acquisition: The role of phonological awareness. In G. Wallach and K. Butler (Eds.), *Language learning disabilities in school-age children and adolescents* (pp. 253–274). New York: Merrill.

Boucher, C. (1986). Pragmatics: The meaning of verbal language in learning disabled and nondisabled boys. *Learning Disability Quarterly, 9,* 285–295.

Bradley, L., & Bryant, P. (1978). Difficulties in auditory organization as possible cause of reading backwardness. *Nature, 271,* 746–747.

Bradley, L., & Bryant, P. (1983). Categorizing sounds and learning to read: A causal connection. *Nature, 301,* 419–421.

Brady, S., Shankweiler, D., & Mann, V. (1983). Speech perception and memory coding in relation to reading ability. *Journal of Experimental Psychology, 35,* 345–367.

Bryan, T. (1991). Social problems and learning disabilities. In B. Wong (Ed.), *Learning about learning disabilities* (pp. 195–231). San Diego: Academic Press.

Bryan, T., Donahue, M., Pearl, R., & Sturm, C. (1981). Learning disabled children's conversational skills: The "TV Talk-Show." *Learning Disability Quarterly, 4,* 250–259.

Bryan, T., & Pflaum, S. (1978). Linguistic, cognitive, and social analysis of learning disabled children's social interactions. *Learning Disability Quarterly, 1,* 70–79.

Catts, H. (1989). Phonological processing deficits and reading disabilities. In A. Kamhi and H. Catts (Eds.), *Reading disabilities: A developmental language perspective* (pp. 101–132). Boston: College-Hill.

Donahue, M. (1981). Requesting strategies of learning disabled children. *Applied Psycholinguistics, 2,* 213–234.

Donahue, M. (1986). Linguistic and communicative development in learning disabled children. In S. Ceci (Ed.), *Handbook of cognitive, social, and neuropsychological aspects of learning disabilities* (pp. 263–289). Hillsdale, NJ: Erlbaum.

Fowles, B., & Glanz, M. (1977). Competence and talent in verbal riddle comprehension. *Journal of Child Language, 4,* 433–452.

Fox, B., & Routh, D. (1980). Phonemic analysis and severe reading disability. *Journal of Psycholinguistic Research, 9,* 115–119.

Fuchs, D., & Fuchs, L. (1994). Inclusive schools movement and the radicalization of special education reform. *Exceptional Children, 60,* 294–309.

Gibbs, D., & Cooper, E. (1989). Prevalence of communication disorders in students with learning disabilities. *Journal of Learning Disabilities, 22,* 60–63.

Kamhi, A., & Catts, H. (1986). Toward an understanding of developmental language and reading disorders. *Journal of Speech and Hearing Disorders, 51,* 337–347.

Kamhi, A., & Koenig, L. (1985). Metalinguistic awareness in normal and language-disordered children. *Language, Speech, and Hearing Services in Schools, 16,* 199–210.

Katz, R. (1986). Phonological deficiencies in children with reading disability: Evidence from an object-naming task. *Cognition, 22,* 225–257

Lapadat, J. (1991). Pragmatic language skills of students with language and/or learning disabilities: A quantitative synthesis. *Journal of Learning Disabilities, 24,* 147–158.

Lerner, J. (1993). *Learning disabilities: Theories, diagnosis, and teaching strategies.* Boston: Houghton Mifflin.

Liberman, I., & Shankweiler, D. (1985). Phonology and the problems of learning to read and write. *Remedial and Special Education, 6,* 8–17.

Liberman, I., Shankweiler, D., Fischer, F., & Carter, B. (1974). Reading and the awareness of linguistic segments. *Journal of Experimental Child Psychology, 18,* 201–212.

Mann, V. (1991). Language problems: A key to early reading problems. In B. Wong (Ed.), *Learning about learning disabilities* (pp. 130–163). San Diego: Academic Press.

Mastropieri, M. (1988). Using the keyword method. *Teaching Exceptional Children, 20,* 4–8.

Menyuk, P., Chesnick, M., Liebergott, J., Korngold, B., D'Agostino, R., & Belanger, A. (1991). Predicting reading problems in at-risk children. *Journal of Speech and Hearing Research, 34,* 893–903.

Menyuk, P., & Flood, J. (1981). Linguistic competence, reading, and writing problems and remediation. *Bulletin of the Orton Society, 31,* 13–28.

Nippold, M., & Fey, S. (1983). Metaphor understanding in preadolescents having a history of language acquisition difficulty. *Language, Speech, and Hearing Services in Schools, 14,* 171–180.

Reynolds, M., Wang, M., & Walberg, H. (1987). The necessary restructuring of special and regular education. *Exceptional Children, 53,* 391–396.

Rissman, M., Curtiss, S., & Tallal, P. (1990). School placement outcomes of young language impaired children. *Journal of Speech Language Pathology and Audiology, 14,* 49–58.

Rudel, R., Denckla, M., & Broman, M. (1981). The effect of varying stimulus context on word finding ability: Dyslexia further differentiated from other learning disabilities. *Brain and Language, 13,* 130–144.

Scruggs, T., & Mastropieri, M. (1992). Effective mainstreaming for mildly handicapped students. *The Elementary School Journal, 92,* 389–409.

Seidenberg, P., & Bernstein, D. (1986). The comprehension of similes and metaphors by learning-disabled and nonlearning-disabled children. *Language, Speech, and Hearing Services in Schools, 17,* 219–229.

Simms, R., & Crump, W. (1983). Syntactic development in the language of learning disabled and normal students at the intermediate and secondary level. *Learning Disability Quarterly, 6,* 155–165.

Spekman, N. (1981). A study of the dyadic verbal communication abilities of learning disabled

and normally achieving 4th and 5th grade boys. *Learning Disability Quarterly, 4,* 139–151.

Van Kleeck, A. (1994). Metalinguistic development. In G. Wallach and K. Butler (Eds.), *Language learning disabilities in school-age children and adolescents* (pp. 53–98). New York: Merrill.

Vaughn, S. (1991). Social skills enhancement in students with learning disabilities. In B. Wong (Ed.), *Learning about learning disabilities* (pp. 408–440). San Diego: Academic Press.

Vellutino, F. (1979). *Dyslexia: Theory and research.* Cambridge, MA: MIT Press.

Vellutino, F., & Scanlon, D. (1987). Phonological coding, phonological awareness, and reading ability: Evidence from a longitudinal and experimental study. *Merrill-Palmer Quarterly, 33,* 321–363.

Vogel, S. (1974). Syntactic abilities in normal and dyslexic children. *Journal of Learning Disabilities, 7,* 35–43.

Vogel, S. (1977). Morphological ability in normal and dyslexic children. *Journal of Learning Disabilities, 10,* 35–43.

Wallach, G., & Goldsmith, S. (1975, November). Sentence processing in normal and learning disabled children: A look at auditory-verbal and visual-verbal channels. Presented at the American Speech-Language-Hearing Association Convention, Washington, DC.

Werner, H., & Strauss, A. (1940). Casual factors in low performance. *American Journal of Mental Deficiency, 45,* 213–218.

Wiig, E. (1990). Language disabilities in school-age children. In G. Shames and E. Wiig (Eds.), *Human communication disorders* (pp. 193–221). Columbus, OH: Merrill.

Wiig, E., Lapointe, C., & Semel, E. (1977). Relationship among language processing and production abilities of learning disabled adolescents. *Journal of Learning Disabilities, 10,* 292–299.

Wiig, E., & Semel, E. (1975). Productive language abilities in learning disabled adolescents. *Journal of Learning Disabilities, 8,* 578–586.

Wiig, E., & Semel, E. (1984). *Language assessment and intervention for the learning disabled* (2nd ed). Columbus, OH: Merrill.

Chapter **6**

Language and Students with Mental Retardation

This chapter examines the language and communication problems associated with mental retardation. Ideas about mental retardation are changing, and teachers, as well as other education professionals, should be aware of these changes. Children with mental retardation are a diverse group, ranging from those with relatively minor developmental delays to those with severe impairments.

An examination of the range of language and communication problems experienced by students with mental retardation and the possible causes of these impairments leads, finally, to some approaches to helping students with mental retardation improve their language and communication skills.

By the end of this chapter you should be able to:

1. Explain how *mental retardation* is defined and how the definition has changed.
2. Describe the specific language and communication deficiencies of children with mental retardation.
3. List factors that might account for these problems with language and communication.
4. Explain what teachers (and other professionals) can do to enhance the language and communication skills of students with mental retardation.

―――――――――――――― **Case Studies** ――――――――――――――

Karen

Karen, a 10-year-old girl with a measured IQ of 65, presently attends a regular third-grade class in a public school. There is an aide in the classroom who assists Karen and two other children with mild disabilities. Karen has difficulty understanding directions, reading, and completing work independently. She reads at a late first-grade level, and her math achievement is at the second-grade level. Her teacher reports that Karen has made progress while in this classroom. She noted that Karen is reluctant to contribute during cooperative learning groups but will participate with prompting.

Karen's mother has reported that Karen had no apparent physical problems during her early development, although her development was a little slower than that of other children. Karen was late in crawling and could neither stand nor walk at 18 months. When Karen was about 2 years old, her parents became concerned about her lack of speech; however, the family physician told them not to worry—that Karen would catch up. Karen had persistent otitis media (middle-ear infections) as a young child and continues to experience occasional earaches.

Prior to this year, Karen was in a self-contained, special education classroom. She appeared to make considerable progress in that class. She began to read and opened up to other children in the class. Before being placed in the special education class, Karen had spent two years in a regular first-grade program. Her teachers there described Karen as quiet and a hard worker, but also as "slow and immature." She had particular difficulty with beginning reading skills and with working independently. She appeared to have few friends.

Karen's parents asked that she be returned to the regular education classroom after her year in special education. Although the district was reluctant to return her to regular education (since she appeared to be progressing in the special education classroom), they agreed to do so. At this point, Karen appears to be making slow, but steady, progress. It is likely that she will remain in regular education in the future.

Danny

Danny is a 14-year-old boy with Down syndrome (Trisomy 21). He presently attends a special education class for children with moderate mental retardation.

Danny has a history of significant cognitive and language delays. He did not speak until he was approximately 3 years old. Even then, his speech was difficult to understand. Significant problems with articulation persist.

Danny has a measured IQ in the 40 to 45 range. However, his language age of 4 years (as measured by the Peabody Picture Vocabulary Test) is below his mental age of 5.6. A language sample analysis completed by the speech/language pathologist indicated that Danny had an MLU of approximately 3.5. He used mostly simple, declarative sentences and he appeared to have a limited vocabulary, although his poor articulation made this difficult to determine.

Danny is a very talkative, very outgoing young man. He loves to hug his teachers and to dance. His school program is focused on functional skills and community-based training. The class makes frequent trips to local malls and restaurants, where students get the opportunity to practice their math and travel skills. Danny's speech and language instruction is focused on improving his articulation and on helping him to make appropriate requests. Danny's parents hope that he will be able to live in a group home or an apartment setting and, perhaps, work in a service-type job.

The stories of Karen and Danny illustrate the diversity of the population of children known as mentally retarded. Despite the widespread popular belief that individuals with mental retardation are more alike than different, children with mental retardation actually exhibit a diverse pattern of abilities and disabilities.

Today, most live at home, but some reside in state or private institutions. Many are educated in regular education classrooms, but many more continue to receive their education in separate classrooms or in special schools. While all children with mental retardation have deficits in cognition, each child has an individual pattern of strengths and weaknesses. In addition to deficits in cognition, most children with mental retardation have problems with language and communication (Long & Long, 1994).

As we examine the research on the speech and language difficulties of children with mental retardation, it is important to keep in mind the diverse nature of this population. This will help in understanding some of the inconsistencies of the research on mental retardation. It is important to also consider against whom children with mental retardation are being compared. Some studies compare children with mental retardation to nondisabled children of the same chronological age, other studies match children with mental retardation to children having the same mental age (MA) but who are chronologically younger, and still other studies use some measure of language age as the means of comparison. Each of these methods has drawbacks and each can give quite different results.

The Changing View of Mental Retardation

Our understanding of mental retardation and our expectations for persons with mental retardation are undergoing rapid change. Examples of this change in attitudes and beliefs abound. In the last 10 to 15 years, there has been a movement away from institutions as the primary sites for treatment and residence for persons with mental retardation toward smaller, community-based, and even family-centered, residences. At the same time, there has been growing pressure on schools to educate children with mental retardation in regular education classrooms. These trends challenge widely held beliefs about the ability of persons with mental retardation to live and function in society. For those of us in education, they challenge us to develop instructional techniques that will benefit students with mental retardation without having a negative impact on the education of nondisabled students.

Definition

Many of the changes in attitudes about mental retardation are reflected in the new definition of mental retardation suggested in 1992 by the American Association on Mental Retardation (AAMR). Prior to 1992, the prevailing definition of mental retardation in the United States was the 1983 AAMR definition. This definition defined *mental retardation* as follows:

> *Mental retardation refers to significantly subaverage intellectual functioning resulting in or associated with concurrent impairments in adaptive behavior and manifested during the developmental period. (Grossman, 1983)*

An earlier version of this definition was adopted by Congress as the definition of mental retardation in Public Law 94-142. The definition includes the four
levels of mental retardation that have become familiar to those who work in special education. These levels are:

Mild Retardation   IQ 50–55 to approximately 70
Moderate Retardation   IQ 35–40 to 50–55
Severe Retardation   IQ 20–25 to 35–40
Profound Retardation   IQ below 20 or 25

The 1992 definition of mental retardation adopted by the AAMR still uses
"significantly subaverage intellectual functioning" (i.e., IQ score) as a defining
feature of mental retardation. However, the definition puts considerably more
stress on functional abilities to determine whether an individual is mentally
retarded. The complete definition states that:

Mental retardation refers to substantial limitations in present functioning. It is
characterized by significantly subaverage intellectual functioning, existing con-
currently with related limitations in two or more of the following applicable
adaptive skill areas: communication, self-care, home living, social skills, commu-
nity use, self-direction, health and safety, functional academics, leisure and work.
Mental retardation manifests before age 18. (AAMR, 1992)

What is really different about the 1992 definition is the way in which it is
intended to be used. Once a diagnosis of mental retardation is made, the work has
just begun. The next step is to identify the individual's strengths and weaknesses
in four domains of functioning: intellectual and adaptive skills, psychological and
emotional, physical and health, and environment (living and work environment).
Finally, a matrix can be developed that includes the individual's strengths and
weaknesses on one axis and the level of support he or she requires (intermittent,
limited, extensive, pervasive) on the other axis (see Table 6.1). This matrix replaces
the levels of retardation that have been used previously to classify persons with
mental retardation.

The 1992 AAMR definition of mental retardation is an attempt to recognize
the individuality of each person with mental retardation, as well as acknowledge
that each individual with mental retardation has a unique pattern of strengths
and weaknesses. In so doing, the 1992 definition eliminates the concept of levels
of mental retardation, replacing it with a more complex evaluation that recognizes
that individuals will need different levels of support across various domains of
functioning.

Deinstitutionalization

A second development that has had profound implications for the care and treatment of persons with mental retardation has been *deinstitutionalization*. From the
mid-1800s to the 1970s, large residential facilities were the primary sites for hous-

TABLE 6.1   Domains of Functioning and Levels of Support

	Intermittent Support	Limited Support	Extensive Support	Pervasive Support
Dimension I Intelligence & Adaptive Skills				
Dimension II Psych/Emotional				
Dimension III Physical/Health/ Etiology				
Dimension IV Environmental Considerations				

Intermittent Support = support on an as-needed basis
Limited Support = consistent, time-limited support
Extensive Support = regular involvement, not time-limited
Pervasive Support = constant, high-intensity support, across environments

Source: Adapted from AAMR. (1992). *Mental retardation: Definition, classification, and systems of support* (9th ed.). Washington, DC: Author.

ing and treatment for most persons with moderate to severe mental retardation and even for many with mild mental retardation. Originally established as small residential communities where individuals could be "cured," many institutions became merely holding places where residents were kept away from the rest of society (Mac Millan, 1982).

By the early 1970s there was a growing debate about the role of institutions in the treatment of people with mental retardation. Two developments gave additional impetus to the deinstitutionalization movement. Wolfensberger (1972) and others promoted the principle of *normalization* in dealing with people with mental retardation. The idea behind normalization is that people with mental retardation should be treated like nondisabled persons as much as possible. That is, they should live, dress, and work like other people. The other development was court cases such as *Wyatt v. Stickney* (1971/1972/1974). In its settlement of this case in 1972, the court ruled that institutionalized residents had a right to appropriate care, including the right to live in less-structured settings.

Use of residential institutions for persons with mental retardation has declined by almost 50 percent (Scheerenberger, 1992) since the population high point in 1974. More and more, persons with mental retardation are residing in small, community-based living arrangements. While this dramatic change in residential services has not been accomplished without some pain and much debate, it appears that in the future most persons with mental retardation will be living in the community.

Inclusion

Paralleling the movement to return people with mental retardation to the community has been the debate on the best place to educate children with mental retardation. Since the passage of Public Law 94-142 in 1975, children with mental retardation have been entitled to a "free, appropriate public education in the least restrictive environment." For most children with mental retardation, this has meant education in a separate special education class or in a private school for children with disabilities. A few students have been mainstreamed into regular education classes for varying parts of the school day.

While concerns about the efficacy of special education and the wisdom of separateness for children with mental retardation have been expressed for some time (e.g., Dunn, 1968), it was not until the mid-1980s that the movement for their greater inclusion in regular education gained momentum. Now known as the *regular education initiative*, this proposal recommends that special and regular education be merged into one educational system that serves *all* children, regardless of their abilities.

One way in which the regular education initiative philosophy has been translated into action has been through *inclusion*—the placement of students with disabilities in regular education classrooms. Inclusion has set off a firestorm of debate. Proponents claim that special education has been ineffective and that placement in regular education settings can be more effective than special education is for children with disabilities (e.g., Skrtic, 1991). Opponents have argued that there is no evidence that regular education teachers are ready—or able—to teach children with disabilities and that much of the research on the effectiveness of special education is flawed (e.g., Kauffman, 1987).

While the debate on inclusion goes on, an increasing number of children with disabilities—including children with mental retardation—are being educated in regular education classrooms. The focus for education professionals should be to develop instructional methods that will enable children with mental retardation to be successful in the regular education classroom, without their handicapping nondisabled children. Additionally, there is a need to collect data on the learning outcomes of all children.

One very important way to enable children with mental retardation to be successful in regular education (or special education) settings is by helping them to enhance their understanding and use of language, the primary medium of instruction in the classroom. In the remainder of this chapter we will examine the specific language difficulties associated with mental retardation, the possible causes of these problems, and what teachers and other professionals can do to enhance the language and communication skills of students with mental retardation.

Language and Communication Characteristics

Impairments in the understanding and production of spoken language are frequently found among children with mental retardation. In fact, language and speech disorders have been found to be the most frequent secondary disability among children with mental retardation (Epstein, Polloway, Patton, & Foley, 1989). Deficits in language and communication have been found to "constitute major impediments to the social, emotional, and vocational adjustment of retarded citizens" (Swetlik & Brown, 1977, p. 39). Let's look at some of the specific language and communication characteristics of children with mental retardation.

Phonology and Morphology

Difficulties with speech production (articulation) are more common among children with mental retardation than among children without (Long & Long, 1994). However, according to Shriberg and Widder (1990), estimates of the incidence of these speech-production deficits have been reported as low as 5 percent and as high as 94 percent. Most studies have found that although there is an increased incidence of speech production problems among children with mental retardation, these children appear to follow the same course of development as children without retardation and make similar phonological errors (Shriberg & Widder, 1990). The most common phonological errors are reduction of consonant clusters (saying *bake* for *break*) and final consonant deletion (saying *cah* for *cat*) (Klink, Gerstman, Raphael, Schlanger, & Newsome, 1986; Sommers, Patterson, & Wildgen, 1988).

It appears that children with more severe mental retardation have a greater incidence of speech-production problems (Mac Millan, 1982; Thomas & Patton, 1994). However, some studies that have directly investigated the relationship between IQ and articulation have failed to find that children with lower IQ scores have more articulation difficulties. It may be that because children with more severe disabilities often have many related physical problems (such as cleft palate, protruding tongue, and the like), it is these problems, rather than IQ score, that relate to the higher incidence of speech-production problems.

Factors other than physical characteristics have also been suggested to cause speech-production problems. For example, Shriberg and Widder (1990) suggested that children with mental retardation appear to have difficulty with phonological encoding (similar to the problems experienced by many children with learning disabilities). Pruess, Vadasy, and Fewell (1987) noted that there is a higher incidence of otitis media (middle-ear infections) in children with Down syndrome. Otitis media has been found to cause fluctuating hearing loss, which can cause impairments in articulation. Therefore, hearing problems are another possible cause of the articulation problems frequently found among children with mental retardation.

The research on speech production in children with mental retardation suggests that education professionals should be prepared to help these children enhance their speech skills. Many children with mental retardation have articulation difficulties that interfere with their ability to be successful in school and in social interactions. However, as Shriberg and Widder (1990) point out, speech training for children with mental retardation is being deemphasized in schools.

There are concerns about the slow rate of progress of such instruction and about the amount of time that speech training takes away from the teaching of what may be more functional skills. They suggest that microcomputer training programs might be useful in delivering speech training to children with mental retardation. In addition, it may be possible for teachers to incorporate some articulation training into regular classroom routines.

Studies of the development of morphological skills in children with mental retardation have generally found that these skills develop in a manner similar to that of children without retardation but at a significantly slower rate (Newfield & Schlanger, 1968). In other words, although children with mental retardation appear to be delayed in their ability to form words, they follow the same sequence of development as nondisabled children.

Syntax

Research on syntactic skills development in children with mental retardation has also generally found that while there are delays in development of these skills, the pattern of development is the same as that found in nondisabled children. In a classic study, Lackner (1968) examined the syntax production of five children with mental retardation, ages 6 and 16. He found that their sentence length increased with mental age and was similar to that of nondisabled children of similar mental age. Lackner also found that the order of development of syntactic rules was similar. One difference that Lackner found in his sample of individuals with mental retardation was that they less frequently used the more advanced syntactic structures. Kamhi and Johnston (1982) found similar results in their study of the language development of children with mild mental retardation. When compared to that of nondisabled children of similar mental age, the syntactic development of the children with mental retardation appeared to be quite similar. Interestingly, the researchers also compared the children with mental retardation to children with specific language impairments but who had IQ scores in the normal range. They concluded that the language produced by the children with language impairments was less complex and contained more errors than that produced by the children with mental retardation.

Both the Kamhi and Johnston (1982) study and other studies (e.g., Naremore & Dever, 1975) found that children with mental retardation had more difficulty with more advanced language constructs. For example, Kamhi and Johnston (1982) found that the nondisabled children produced more sentences with questions and with conjunctions. These findings suggest that there may be limits to the syntactic development of children with mental retardation—that is, although their early development may be similar to that of nondisabled children (although with delays), there may be a plateau of development. After this plateau, further syntactic development may be difficult.

We cannot be sure there are limits to the syntactic development of children with mental retardation. One reason is that there may be methodological problems with the research, as Kamhi and Johnston (1982) themselves pointed out.

Another reason is that there is a great deal of variability within the population called mentally retarded. There are undoubtedly some individuals with mental retardation who are able to acquire more advanced syntactic skills. Thus, research results can be used as a guide for intervention but should never be used to justify the denial of services to any individual.

The research on syntactic skills of children with mental retardation suggests that education professionals may generally expect slow development of these abilities along a normal developmental course, with the possibility of students' having particular difficulty in the acquisition of more advanced syntactic skills. Teachers may need to simplify their own language, as well as written text, to point out some of the more advanced syntactic structures (such as the passive voice) when they occur, and to encourage the use of more complex syntactic skills in older children with mental retardation.

Semantics

There has been relatively little research on the semantic abilities of children with mental retardation. The research that has been done indicates that children with mental retardation tend to be more concrete in their understanding of words, having more difficulty, for example, interpreting idiomatic expressions (e.g., *he broke her heart*) (Ezell & Goldstein, 1991). This tendency to be more concrete may be the result of delays in development of semantic abilities (Rosenberg, 1982).

Some studies have found that an area of strength for children with mental retardation is that of vocabulary skills. In a study of the comprehension of syntax and vocabulary conducted by Chapman, Schwartz, and Kay Raining-Bird (1991), the authors found that their subjects with mental retardation performed significantly better on the vocabulary-comprehension task than on tests of syntactic skills, in fact, outscoring a mental-age-matched control group on their vocabulary comprehension. Other studies have found that examination of language produced in natural settings shows children with Down syndrome have a more diverse vocabulary than do nondisabled children matched for mental age (Miller, 1988). To understand these results, one should keep in mind that in these studies the children with mental retardation were older than the control group and, therefore, may have had more of an opportunity to learn vocabulary skills. Even so, their vocabulary skills are not equivalent to those of nondisabled children of the same chronological age.

Another aspect of semantics involves the organization of language information. If children are given groups of pictures and asked to remember them, they tend to organize the pictures in their minds and recall them in groups. These groups may be based on physical characteristics or function of the items or on the conceptual category to which the items belong (e.g., toys, animals). Children with mental retardation have been found to lag behind in their development of organizing strategies (Stephens, 1972) and to use more concrete concepts (Mac Millan, 1982), suggesting that children with mental retardation have some difficulty developing and using semantic concepts.

Pragmatics

Since there is a good deal of research on the pragmatic abilities of individuals with mental retardation, we will examine the research in three areas: speech-act usage, referential communication, and conversational skills.

Speech Acts

The concept of speech acts was described in Chapter 1. These acts occur whenever one has the intention to communicate. Requests, commands, and declarations (*I promise*) are examples of speech acts. Children with mental retardation have been described as having delayed understanding of speech acts (Abbeduto, 1991). In one study (Abbeduto, Davies, & Furman, 1988), children with and without mental retardation were asked to interpret sentences requiring either a yes-no response or an action. For example, *Can you close the window* could be either asking whether one is *able* to close the window or requesting that someone *actually close* the window. In their study, Abbeduto et al. found that in their ability to understand what the speaker actually wanted, adolescents with mental retardation were similar to younger, nondisabled children matched for mental age.

Speech-act usage also has been found to be delayed, although it is similar to that of nondisabled children of equivalent mental age (Owens & McDonald, 1982). In other words, this study found that the speech-act usage of individuals with mental retardation was similar to that of younger, nondisabled persons. It appears that by adulthood, individuals with mental retardation can produce all of the basic speech-act categories (Abbeduto & Rosenberg, 1980).

Referential Communication

In referential-communication tasks, children are evaluated on their ability to explain a task to another person. This procedure reveals their ability to take into account the information needed by someone else to complete this task. One way to test referential communication is with a *barrier* task. For this procedure, children are seated across from each other with a barrier between them that prevents their seeing each other. One child is the speaker; the other, the listener. Each has an array of blocks or other items. The speaker's blocks—the model—are arranged in a design. The speaker's task is to tell the listener how to arrange the blocks to match the model, using only verbal directions. Using just such a procedure to study the referential-communication abilities of adolescents with mental retardation, Longhurst (1974) found that when the individuals with mental retardation were in the speaker's role, they were remarkably unsuccessful in directing the listeners to complete the task. However, when they were the listener, the subjects were able to successfully perform the task when directions were given by nondisabled adults.

A second way to evaluate referential communication is by asking individuals to describe an activity (such as a game) to someone else. In one such study (Loveland, Tunali, McEvoy, & Kelly, 1989), adolescents and adults with Down syndrome were asked to explain a game to an experimenter. These individuals with mental retardation performed quite well, giving the necessary information to the listener without a great deal of prompting. However, as Abbeduto (1991) points out, since we do not know how nondisabled persons would have handled this task, it is difficult to judge how good these results really are.

It appears from the research on referential communication that persons with mental retardation have some difficulty getting their messages across to others; they may have difficulty putting themselves in someone else's place. On the other hand, they do better when they are in the listener role and, perhaps, in more natural tasks, like explaining a game.

Conversational Competence

How effective are persons with mental retardation as conversational partners? People with mental retardation have often been described as passive communicators who wait for others to take the lead in conversations (Bedrosian & Prutting, 1978). However, people who have worked or lived with individuals with mental retardation have often found them to be very outgoing—often to the point of being intrusive. How can we reconcile the research findings with experience?

Perhaps the answer lies in the selection criteria of the population to be studied. Kuder and Bryen reported the results of a study in which they observed residents in a private institution interacting with staff in a classroom and in a residential setting (1991). They found that, in general, the residents initiated interaction with staff. For their study, they selected subjects who were capable of verbal communication. Previous studies (e.g., Prior, Minnes, Coyne, Golding, Hendy, & McGillivray, 1979) had included *all* of the residents in an institution, including some who may have been unable to engage in verbal interaction. Not surprisingly, by selecting only subjects *who could talk*, Kuder and Bryen found much more frequent initiation of conversation than had been previously reported.

There is more to conversational competence than simply being involved in interaction; there are qualitative aspects as well, such as turn taking, topic management, and conversational repair. The conversational competence of persons with mental retardation has been studied in each of these areas. In normal conversations, participants take turns talking. Occasionally they talk at the same time, but imagine what it would be like if we all talked at the same time all of the time. Persons with mental retardation have been found to have few problems with turn taking. Studies of the conversational turn taking in young children with mental retardation (Tannock, 1988), as well as adults (Abbeduto & Rosenberg, 1980), have found that they take turns in conversations and make few errors, much as nondisabled people do.

Although people with mental retardation appear capable of taking their turn in a conversation, what is even more important is what they *do* with that turn. Typically, people with mental retardation do not make significant contributions to maintaining the conversation (Abbeduto, 1991). They may make comments, such as *ok* or *um-um*, but do not *extend* the topic by adding new information.

Research on the conversational skills of people with mental retardation has also found that they have difficulty *repairing* conversations that break down. If you are talking with someone else and do not understand what is being said, you will do something to clarify the conversation. You will say *what?* or *excuse me* as a signal to the speaker that you do not understand. People with mental retardation have been found to be *capable* of using such conversational repairs, but fail to use them when they are needed (Robinson & Whittaker, 1986; Abbeduto, Davies, Solesby, & Furman, 1991). Children with mental retardation have also been found to be slow in responding to clarification requests made by others (Scherer & Owings, 1984).

In considering all of the research on the communicative abilities of persons with mental retardation, Abbeduto (1991) concluded that "deficits in verbal communication are a defining feature of mental retardation and should figure prominently in assessments of adaptive behavior." (p. 108). Although problems with verbal communication do seem to be quite common among people with mental retardation, there is considerable variability within the population.

Obviously, the ability to engage in effective communication with others is a critical skill for classroom success. Teachers and other education professionals should be alert to the problems that students with mental retardation may have in expressing themselves and understanding others. Placing students in heterogeneous groups can be a good way to encourage communicative interaction, if the groups are well managed and the group activities carefully chosen.

Conclusion

Review of the research on the language and communication abilities of people with mental retardation has revealed several things. First, in most cases, the language skills of this population can be described as delayed rather than different. That is, children with mental retardation seem to develop through the same stages as nondisabled children, only much more slowly. There are some exceptions to this generalization—especially when it comes to the acquisition of more advanced syntactic skills—and some pragmatic skills. But, for the most part, language delays are characteristic of children with mental retardation (see Table 6.2 for a summary). Second, there is a good deal of variation in the language and communication skills of persons with mental retardation. These variations may be due to cognitive delays, physical characteristics, or to the underlying cause of the individual's developmental disability. Still, language and communication difficulties are characteristic of most persons with mental retardation. Why is this so? In the next section, we will examine some factors that may help answer this question.

Causes of Language and Communication Impairments

In most cases, it is not possible to say with certainty what causes the language and communication impairments of any individual (just as it is not possible to explain normal language development). It is true that in some individuals there are obvious physical characteristics (such as a cleft palate or protruding tongue) that can explain some of the communication difficulties of that person. But, in most cases, the best we can do is to talk about factors that may *contribute* to language and communication disorders.

TABLE 6.2   Language and Communication of Individuals with Mental Retardation

Phonology and Morphology	Syntax	Semantics	Pragmatics
Development similar to non-mentally retarded, but delayed (Shriberg & Widder, 1990)	Sentence length similar to mental-age-matched controls (Lackner, 1968)	Problems understanding idiomatic expressions (Ezell & Goldstein, 1991)	Delays in understanding speech acts (Abbeduto, 1991)
Reduction of consonant clusters and final consonant deletion (Klink et al., 1986; Sommers et al., 1988)	More difficulty with advanced syntactic structures (Naremore & Dever, 1975; Kamhi & Johnson, 1982)	Delays in semantic development (Rosenberg, 1982)	Difficulty with speaker role (Longhurst, 1974)
Delays in morpho-logical development (Newfield & Schlanger, 1968		Vocabulary a relative strength (Chapman et al., 1991)	Turn taking intact (Tannock, 1988)
		More concrete concepts (Mac Millan, 1982)	

What are these contributing factors? We could have quite a long list, but we will limit our examination to three factors: cognitive functioning, specific language disorder, and input language.

Cognitive Functioning

Deficits in cognitive functioning are *the* defining feature of mental retardation. Cognitive abilities—as measured by intelligence tests—are the first criteria in determining whether an individual is cognitively disabled. There may be a temptation to assume a person having low measured intelligence is functioning low across the board. But, this is rarely the case. Each individual has a unique set of cognitive strengths and weaknesses. Likewise, the population called mentally retarded has general cognitive strengths and weaknesses that must be examined in some detail if we are to understand how deficiencies in cognitive functioning may contribute to difficulties with language and communication.

Let's look at three areas of cognitive functioning that have been researched extensively with regard to mental retardation: attention, organization, and memory (see Table 6.3 for a summary).

Children with mental retardation have been reported to have problems **discriminating** the important features of a task and attending to more than one dimension at a time (Zeaman & House, 1979). For example, if asked to sort objects on the basis of both size and color, most children with mental retardation would have difficulty. On the other hand, their ability to **sustain attention** has been found to be as good, or better than, mental-age-matched peers (Karrer, Nelson, & Galbraith, 1979).

TABLE 6.3   Research on the Cognitive Functioning of Persons with Mental Retardation

Attention	Organization	Memory	Generalization
Difficulty discriminating important features of task (Zeaman & House, 1979) Relatively good sustained attention (Karrer et al., 1979)	Ineffective techniques of organizing information (Spitz, 1966) Similar stages of development of organization (Stephens, 1972)	Long-term memory relatively intact (Belmont, 1966) Short-term memory problems (Ellis, 1970) Inefficient rehearsal strategies (Bray, 1979)	Difficulties in the ability to apply knowledge to new settings (Stephens, 1972)

Individuals with mental retardation have been described as having difficulty **organizing information** for recall (Spitz, 1966). This is an important skill. For example, if you were asked to remember the following list of items, you would probably use a *chunking* strategy to recall the list:

ball	apple	pear
orange	wrench	bike
hammer	doll	pliers

You would probably recognize that these items comprise three groups: toys, fruit, and tools. When asked to recall the items, you would probably report them in these three groups. Typically, children with mental retardation do not spontaneously recognize or use these groups for recall (Stephens, 1972).

Memory difficulties have long been associated with mental retardation. However, as we learn more about memory, we learn that people with mental retardation have both strengths and weaknesses in this domain. Long-term memory, for example, has been found to be relatively intact in most persons with mental retardation (Belmont, 1966). However, problems with short-term memory are frequently reported (Ellis, 1970). One explanation for the observed problems with short-term memory is that people with mental retardation have **inefficient rehearsal strategies** (Bray, 1979). In order to remember information, you have to store it. If you want to remember a telephone number for just a few seconds, it is usually enough to repeat the number over and over. But, if you want to remember the number for a few minutes or a few days or more, you need to store it in a way that is retrievable. For example, a phone number with the last four digits *1488* might be remembered by recalling *1492* (the year Columbus landed in the Americas) *minus 4* (1488). People with mental retardation tend to use rehearsal strategies that do not enhance their recall. They tend to persist with inefficient strategies (such as repetition) that do not always work.

Another specific cognitive impairment associated with mental retardation is **generalization** of information. Persons with mental retardation have often been described as having difficulty applying what they have learned previously to use in new settings, with different people, or in new ways (Stephens, 1972). Generalization is a critical skill for learning. If students do not know when and where to apply their skills, they have really learned nothing. Therefore, it is essential that students with mental retardation be taught in ways that will increase their likelihood of generalization.

How could the cognitive difficulties associated with mental retardation affect the acquisition of language and communication? Clearly, if someone has difficulty attending to a certain task—especially a complex task like social interaction—that person may have difficulty picking up pragmatic and, perhaps, syntactic aspects of language. Difficulties with organizing information may affect the child's ability to acquire new vocabulary, to differentiate new words from previously stored words, and to recall words when they are needed. Of course, memory impairments also have profound implications for language learning. To learn language, one must store and retrieve vast amounts of information. Syntactic rules, semantic rules, and vocabulary—all of these and more—have to be stored in a way that they are easily retrieved. Moreover, this has to be done instantaneously. Children with impairments in memory are likely to have a difficult time with the understanding and use of language.

For teachers, there are several implications that can be drawn from the research discussed. First, attention of the child to the task at hand is critical. It is important to **limit the task dimensions.** In other words, whenever possible only one aspect of a task (shape, size, color) should be varied, until the individual is ready to handle more. It is essential to **get and hold attention.** Using items that are familiar to the student, involving them in the lesson, and relating the lesson to their personal experience are ways to do this. Many children with mental retardation will need to have **organization cues** given to them. They will need to be told how and when to use these cues for learning. Finally, teachers need to **teach for generalization.** This means using a variety of materials and examples. It also means teaching in the natural environment—the place where the skill will be applied—whenever possible.

Specific Language Disorders

There is no doubt that most people with mental retardation have impairments of cognitive functioning. They also have problems in several areas of language development. Might we conclude, then, that the cognitive impairments cause the language disabilities? Might it be just as true to assert that the language impairments cause delays in cognitive development?

These are not easy questions to answer because language and cognition are interrelated in very complex ways. To try to answer these questions, researchers have compared the language of children with mental retardation to that of nondisabled children who are matched for mental age. If their language performance is similar, this suggests that language development is dependent on cognitive development. If, on the other hand, the language development of the subjects with mental retardation is less advanced than that of the nondisabled subjects, one could conclude that people with mental retardation have a specific language disorder that cannot be explained by cognitive delays alone.

Research on the relationship between cognition and language in persons with mental retardation has yielded inconsistent results. Our review of the research has revealed that delays in most aspects of language development are characteristic of children with mental retardation. For the most part, their language development is like that of younger children matched for mental age. However, there are exceptions to this (e.g., in pragmatics and syntax). When Kamhi and Johnston (1982) studied the language and cognitive abilities of children with mental retardation, children with language impairments, and normally developing children, they found that, for the most part, the language of the children with mental retardation was similar to that of the younger, nondisabled children matched for mental age. When there were deviations from the normal pattern, they were attributed to deficits in motivation and adaptive behavior. Abbeduto, Furman, and Davies (1989) studied the receptive language skills of school-age children with mental retardation. They found that mental age (MA) was a good predictor of the language performance of children at lower levels of mental age (MA = 5). However, mental age was *not* a good predictor for their subjects with higher mental age (7 and 9). They suggested that at least some of the language impairments of their higher MA group were the result of specific language deficits.

So, what can be said about the relationship between cognitive abilities and language in persons with mental retardation? Is there a specific language disorder that goes beyond what would be predicted by mental age alone? Well, yes and no. It appears that in younger children (MA < 5), there is a close connection between cognitive development and language development. It still is not possible to say with certainty which is the cause and which the effect, but there is a close relationship. For older individuals (MA > 7), there appear to be specific language deficiencies that cannot be explained by mental age alone. Problems relating to motivation, adaptive behavior, or a specific language disorder may explain the language impairments of these individuals.

What can teachers do with this information? First, the research suggests that although instruction in cognitive skills is important, such instruction by itself may not address some of the specific language impairments of children with mental retardation. Older children and adolescents, in particular, may need help with higher-order syntactic skills and with pragmatics. Second, because early intervention in language is so critical, the research provides a rationale for teachers and other education professionals to devote attention to the expressive and receptive language problems of children with mental retardation.

Input language

Parent-Child Interaction

In the search for causes of language and communication difficulties in mental retardation, another aspect is input language. We know from research on normal language development that children learn language by participating in communicative interactions with parents and other caregivers. We also know that parents alter their language to make it more compatible with their child's ability to comprehend. Some research has suggested that parents of children with mental retardation do not provide an effective language-learning environment for their children. For example, mothers of children with mental retardation have been found to use shorter, less complex sentences than do mothers of nondisabled children (Buium, Rynders, & Turnure, 1974). In addition, they tend to dominate interactions with their children by being more directive and by initiating more of the interactions with their children than do mothers of nondisabled children (Eheart, 1982). Mothers of children with mental retardation have also been reported to be less focused on their child's activities (Mahoney, Fors, & Wood, 1990).

The question here is why would parents of children with mental retardation intentionally (or unintentionally) provide their children with less than an optimal language-learning environment? The answer is, they do not. While it is undoubtedly true that communicative interaction between children with mental retardation and their parents is different from that between parents and their nondisabled children, this does not mean that the parents are doing something wrong. If children with mental retardation are developing language skills more slowly than normal, it should be no surprise to find that their parents are using simpler language. If children are slow to respond or are inattentive, it is not unlikely that parents will take a more directive role in the interaction.

In fact, mothers of children with mental retardation alter their linguistic input appropriately for the language-development level of their children (Rondal, 1978). As Owens (1993) noted, if mothers of children with mental retardation provided their children with language models similar to those provided by mothers of nondisabled children, these models would not be appropriate for the language learning needs of their children. On the other hand, parents of children with mental retardation must be careful not to overcompensate for their child's language impairments. They must work hard at giving their child the opportunity to initiate interaction and should be responsive to their child, even if they feel that the child may be acting inappropriately. It is often difficult to determine what children are trying to communicate until they are given a chance to do so.

Staff-Client Interaction

Individuals with mental retardation who live in institutions or in group settings in the community get much of their opportunity for communicative interaction from staff in those facilities. However, staff tend to communicate in ways that not only do not enhance interaction but actually discourage interaction. Studies have reported that staff tend to use a lot of *directives*—commands and directions that require little if any verbal response (Prior, Minnes, Coyne, Golding, Hendy, & McGillivray, 1979). When residents try to communicate, they are often ignored.

Part of the explanation for staff members' low rates of responsiveness may be that the residents' communicative attempts are unclear. Kuder and Bryen (1991) found that when residents clearly identified their communicative partner and used a conversational opener that encouraged a response, staff were highly responsive. They also found that staff and residents communicated more frequently in a structured classroom setting than they did in a less structured, residential environment.

The results from research on both parent-child and staff-resident interactions suggest that to conclude that parents or residential staff cause the language impairments experienced by individuals with mental retardation is too simple an explanation. More likely is that the language impairments themselves alter the interactions that individuals with mental retardation have with others. As a result, communicative interaction may become less frequent and less effective. There is a danger, however, that parents and staff may become so accustomed to a highly directive conversational role that they fail to give their children or residents the chance to communicate.

Conclusion

In the beginning of this section we noted the difficulty in finding a specific cause for the language impairments experienced by most persons with mental retardation. Indeed, our search for a cause has yielded some clues but no firm answers. Cognitive disabilities clearly play a role, but do not account for all of the language difficulties of people with mental retardation. Parents and other caregivers may talk differently to children with mental retardation, but it is likely that these differences are as much the *result* of language differences as the cause. Lack of motivation, adaptive behavior deficits, physical disabilities, and specific language impairments have also been proposed as the cause of the language deficiencies of individuals with mental retardation.

Approaches to Intervention

As we have seen, finding the cause of the language and communication disabilities of children with mental retardation is not always possible. Fortunately, it is not essential to know the cause of the problem in order to do something about it. This section presents some general principles for intervention with students with mental retardation, discussing two specific intervention approaches for language and communication impairments.

Instructional Principles

Owens (1993) suggested seven principles that teachers and other education professionals can use in developing intervention programs for individuals with mental retardation. These principles address some of the specific cognitive and language characteristics commonly found among students with mental retardation.

We know, for example, that many individuals with mental retardation have difficulty discriminating information. They have problems knowing what they are supposed to attend to. Teachers may address this problem by **highlighting new or relevant information.** New vocabulary words may be written in a different color, for example. In a conversational situation, the teacher could point out how people speak to children in different ways than they do to adults.

As discussed, another area of difficulty for many children with mental retardation is in organization of information for recall. Owens suggests that it may be helpful if teachers **preorganize information.** To get students to remember words, for example, the teacher may find it useful to group the words in ways that will enhance recall (all of the *toys* together). Of course, merely grouping the items together may not be enough. Students may have to be taught the category label and when to use it.

Since memory is problematic for most students with mental retardation, Owens suggests that teachers can help students enhance their recall by teaching them to use **effective rehearsal strategies.** We saw earlier in this chapter that different rehearsal strategies work for different situations. For students to remember for a long period of time, they may need to learn how to use a strategy to enhance their memory; for example, visual images or associating words that rhyme may enhance recall.

One of the most significant problems faced by teachers of students with mental retardation is helping them to generalize new learning. Owens offers two suggestions to help in this area: that teachers **use overlearning and repetition** and that teachers **train in the natural environment.** Not surprisingly, students who receive extra training and practice tend to retain more information. Moreover, a number of research studies have found that difficulties with generalization can be reduced if children are taught in the settings in which they will need the skill they are learning (e.g., Stowitschek, McConaughy, Peatross, Salzberg, & Lignngaris/ Kraft, 1988; Caro & Snell, 1989). If, for example, children learn to approach others by practicing this skill in the cafeteria, then it should be easier for them to ask someone in the cafeteria to share a table if they need to do so.

Owens further suggests that **training begin as early as possible** and that teachers **follow developmental guidelines.** Early training is especially critical for language, since these skills build on each other and there is a critical period for language learning. Developmental guidelines can be used to determine where to begin and how to sequence instruction. However, teachers who choose to follow developmental guidelines must be careful in making instructional decisions to also consider the child's environmental demands.

Specific Intervention Approaches

The instructional principles suggested by Owens can help teachers begin to plan for the needs of their students with mental retardation. These guidelines might be applied not just to language but to any domain of learning. A number of instructional methods have been developed to teach language and communication skills to students with mental retardation, especially those with more severe retardation. We will discuss two methods that demonstrate the range of available approaches.

The **interrupted behavior-chain strategy** (Goetz, Gee, & Sailor, 1985; Hunt, Goetz, Alwell, & Sailor, 1986) is an example of an *operant* (or behavioral) approach to the enhancement of communication skills in students with severe disabilities. Using this approach, a target skill is inserted in the middle of an established sequence of behaviors (washing dishes, brushing teeth, collecting school attendance slips). For example, the Hunt et al. study describes a student named Everett, a 7-year-old boy with severe mental retardation. The first step in this intervention was to identify sequences of behaviors that Everett could presently perform or were currently being taught. In Everett's case he was able to independently get a drink from the water fountain and get food from the refrigerator. He was being taught to start and listen to a record player and to play an arcade game. Then interruptions were inserted into these behavior sequences at particular points. For example, as he leaned down to take a drink, Everett would be asked *What do you want?* and then prompted to choose by pointing to the picture of the water fountain from among a group of four pictures. Using this approach, Everett increased his ability to identify the correct picture and learned to point to a picture to request water. The researchers suggested that interrupting a previously established chain of behavior may motivate students to learn the communication skill so they can continue with the activity.

The **mand-model procedure** was developed to teach students to use language to obtain items or to participate in social interactions. In this approach, the adult initiates the interaction using activities and objects that the student is using at the moment; the adult prompts a response by using a "mand" (a demand or request). Similar to the interrupted-chain strategy, this technique uses natural activities in the child's environment as the basis of instruction. However, modeling, rather than operant conditioning, is used to teach the language skill. Warren (1991) gives the following example:

Context: (The child is scooping rice with a spoon and pouring it into a bowl.)

Adult: Tell me what you are doing.

Child: Beans.

Adult: Well then say, "pour beans."

Child: Pour beans.

Adult: That's right, you're pouring beans into the pot.

In this example, the adult's *Tell me what you are doing* elicited a response. If the child had not responded, the adult could have told the child to say the name of the object. Since the child did respond, the adult modeled for the child a more adult form of responding. This technique helped children with significant language impairments increase their communication (Rogers-Warren & Warren, 1980).

These are only two of many examples of instructional techniques that have been developed to help enhance communication skills in children with mental retardation and significant language impairments. Both of these methods are designed to be used in natural settings where problems of generalization are better avoided.

Summary

In this chapter we have seen how changes in our understanding of mental retardation have evolved a new definition of persons with mental retardation. We have reviewed recent trends in residential and educational services. Then, in describing the specific language and communication characteristics of persons with mental retardation we noted that while delays in language development are often found in people with mental retardation, there appear to be some specific differences in their language abilities. We have examined possible causes of these language and communication impairments, including discussions of cognitive delay, specific language disorder, and deficiencies of input language. A discussion of intervention techniques revealed instructional methods that have been used to help individuals with mental retardation enhance their language and communication skills.

Review Questions

1. How does the 1992 definition of *mental retardation* differ from previous definitions?

2. How have residential and educational services for persons with mental retardation changed in the last ten years?

3. There has been considerable debate about the usefulness of teaching speech-production skills to children with mental retardation. List two arguments for and two arguments against speech instruction for this population.

4. Describe the syntactic skills of persons with mental retardation. Are they delayed, different, or both? Explain.

5. What does research on referential communication tell us about the communication skills of people with mental retardation?

6. What do we know about the conversational skills of people with mental retardation in regard to turn taking, conversational repairs, and topic management?

7. Discuss some of the implications of research on cognition for understanding the language development of individuals with mental retardation.

8. Describe the interaction between parents and their children with mental retardation. What could these parents do to enhance their child's language and communication skills?

Suggested Activities

1. Research on the communicative interaction between parents and their children with mental retardation has sometimes led to conflicting conclusions. Some researchers have concluded that parents of children with mental retardation do not provide their child with an appropriate language environment. Others have claimed that any differences in parent-child interaction may be the result of the adjustment of parents to their child's abil-

ities and needs. This debate suggests two essential questions that can be investigated in this activity:

– Does the language and other communication used by parents of children with mental retardation differ from that used by parents of nondisabled children?
– Do parents of children with mental retardation alter their language appropriately for the language level of the child?

To investigate these questions, find two parent-child dyads. The children should be between 18 months and 3 years of age, and one of them should be mentally disabled.

Ask the parents to play with their children using objects that are familiar to each child. It would be best to do this in the child's home. Record your observations of each parent-child interaction (on videotape, if possible), and compare the two parents on the following:

– Length of utterance
– Use of nonverbal communication
– Number of different words used
– Complexity of language (sentence structures used)
– Initiation of communication (whether child or parent)

2. We know from research on children with mental retardation that for them, comprehension of idiomatic expressions is often difficult. Try teaching such expressions to an individual with mental retardation. The student should have a mental age of at least 8 years.

Begin by asking the student to tell you what the following idiomatic expressions mean:

– Strike a bargain
– Hit the road
– Break a date
– Jump the gun

If the student has trouble explaining any of these expressions, explain the meaning and ask the child to try again. Once the student appears to have learned the expression, repeat the exercise a few days later to check retention.

References

Abbeduto, L. (1991). Development of verbal communication in persons with moderate to mild mental retardation. *International Review of Research in Mental Retardation, 17,* 91–115.

Abbeduto, L., Furman, L., & Davies, B. (1988). The development of speech act comprehension in mentally retarded individuals and nonretarded children. *Child Development, 59,* 1460–1472.

Abbeduto, L., Davies, B., Solesby, S., & Furman, L. (1991). Identifying the referents of spoken messages: Use of context and clarification requests by children with and without mental retardation. *American Journal on Mental Retardation, 95,* 551–562.

Abbeduto, L., & Rosenberg, S. (1980). The communicative competence of mildly retarded adults. *Applied Psycholinguistics, 1,* 405–426.

American Association on Mental Retardation. (1992). *Mental retardation: definition, classification, and systems of support* (9th ed.). Washington, DC: Author.

Bedrosian, J., & Prutting, C. (1978). Communicative performance of mentally retarded adults in four conversational settings. *Journal of Speech and Hearing Research, 21,* 79–95.

Belmont, J. (1966). Long-term memory in mental retardation. *International Review of Research in Mental Retardation, 1,* 219–255.

Bray, N. (1979). Strategy production in the retarded. In N. Ellis (Ed.), *Handbook of mental deficiency: Psychological theory and research* (pp. 699–726). Hillsdale, NJ: Erlbaum.

Buium, N., Rynders, J., & Turnure, J. (1974). Early maternal linguistic environment of normal and Down's syndrome language-learning children. *American Journal of Mental Deficiency, 79,* 52–58.

Caro, P., & Snell, M. (1989). Characteristics of teaching communication to people with moderate and severe disabilities. *Education and Training in Mental Retardation, 24,* 63–77.

Chapman, R., Schwartz, S., & Kay Raining-Bird, E. (1991). Language skills of children and adolescents with Down syndrome: I. Comprehension. *Journal of Speech and Hearing Research, 34,* 1106–1120.

Dunn, L. (1968). Special education for the mildly retarded—Is much of it justifiable? *Exceptional Children, 35,* 5–22.

Eheart, B. (1982). Mother-child interactions with nonretarded and mentally retarded preschoolers. *American Journal of Mental Deficiency, 87,* 20–25.

Ellis, N. (1970). Memory processes in retardates and normals. In N. Ellis (Ed.), *International review of research in mental retardation* (Vol. 4) (pp. 1–36). New York: Academic Press.

Epstein, M., Polloway, E., Patton, J., & Foley, R. (1989). Mild retardation: Student characteristics and services. *Education and Training in Mental Retardation, 24,* 7–16.

Ezell, H., & Goldstein, H. (1991). Comparison of idiom comprehension of normal children and children with mental retardation. *Journal of Speech and Hearing Research, 34,* 812–819.

Goetz, L., Gee, K., & Sailor, W. (1985). Using a behavior chain interruption strategy to teach communication skills to students with severe disabilities. *Journal of the Association for Persons with Severe Handicaps, 10,* 21–30.

Grossman, H. (1983). *Classification in mental retardation.* Washington, DC: American Association on Mental Deficiency.

Hunt, P., Goetz, L., Alwell, M., & Sailor, W. (1986). Using an interrupted behavior chain strategy to teach generalized communication responses. *Journal of the Association for Persons with Severe Handicaps, 11,* 196–204.

Kamhi, A., & Johnston, J. (1982). Towards an understanding of retarded children's linguistic deficiencies. *Journal of Speech and Hearing Research, 25,* 435–445.

Karrer, R., Nelson, M., & Galbraith, G. (1979). Psychophysiological research with the mentally retarded. In N. Ellis (Ed.), *International review of research in mental retardation* (Vol. 7). New York: Academic Press.

Kauffman, J. (1987). Research in special education: A commentary. *Remedial and Special Education, 85,* 57–62.

Klink, M., Gerstman, L., Raphael, L., Schlanger, B., & Newsome, L. (1986). Phonological process usage by young EMR children and nonretarded preschool children. *American Journal of Mental Deficiency, 91,* 190–195.

Kuder, S., & Bryen, D. (1991). Communicative performance of persons with mental retardation in an institutional setting. *Education and Training in Mental Retardation, 23,* 325–332.

Lackner, J. (1968). A developmental study of language behavior in retarded children. *Neuropsychologia, 6,* 301–320.

Long, S., & Long, S. (1994). Language and children with mental retardation. In V. Reed (Ed.), *Children with language disorders* (2nd ed., pp. 153–191). New York: Merrill.

Longhurst, T. (1974). Communication in retarded adolescents: Sex and intelligence level. *American Journal of Mental Deficiency, 78,* 607–618.

Loveland, K., Tunali, B., McEvoy, R., & Kelly, M. (1989). Referential communication and response adequacy in autism and Down's syndrome. *Applied Psycholinguistics, 10,* 301–313.

Mac Millan, D. (1982). *Mental Retardation in School and Society* (2nd ed.). Boston: Little, Brown.

Mahoney, G., Fors, S., & Wood, S. (1990). Maternal directive behavior revisited. *American Journal on Mental Retardation, 94,* 398–406.

Miller, J. (1988). The developmental asynchrony of language development in children with Down syndrome. In L. Nadel (Ed.), *The psychobiology of Down syndrome* (pp. 168–198). Cambridge, MA: MIT Press.

Naremore, R., & Dever, R. (1975). Language performance of educable mentally retarded and normal children at five age levels. *Journal of Speech and Hearing Research, 18*, 82–95.

Newfield, M., & Schlanger, B. (1968). The acquisition of English morphology in normal and educable mentally retarded children. *Journal of Speech and Hearing Research, 11*, 693–706.

Owens, R. (1993). Mental retardation: Difference and delay. In D. Bernstein and E. Morris (Eds.), *Language and communication disorders in children* (3rd ed., pp. 366–430). New York: Merrill.

Owens, R., & McDonald, J. (1982). Communicative uses of the early speech of nondelayed and Down syndrome children. *American Journal of Mental Deficiency, 86*, 503–510.

Prior, M., Minnes, P., Coyne, T., Golding, B., Hendy, J., & McGillivray, J. (1979). Verbal interactions between staff and residents in an institution for the mentally retarded. *Mental Retardation, 17*, 65–70.

Pruess, J., Vadasy, P., & Fewell, R. (1987). Language development in children with Down syndrome: An overview of recent research. *Education and Training in Mental Retardation, 22*, 44–55.

Robinson, E., & Whittaker, S. (1986). Learning about verbal referential communication in the early school years. In K. Durkin (Ed.), *Language development during the school years* (pp. 155–171). London: Croom Helm.

Rogers-Warren, A., & Warren, S. (1980). Mands for verbalization: Facilitating the display of newly-taught language. *Behavior Modification, 4*, 361–382.

Rondal, J. (1978). Maternal speech to normal and Down's syndrome children matched for mean length of utterance. In C. Meyers (Ed.), *Quality of life in severely and profoundly mentally retarded people*. Washington, DC: American Association on Mental Deficiency.

Rosenberg, S. (1982). The language of the mentally retarded: Development, processes, and intervention. In S. Rosenberg (Ed.), *Handbook of applied psycholinguistics: Major thrusts of research and theory* (pp. 329–392). Hillsdale, NJ: Erlbaum.

Scheerenberger, R. (1992). *Public residential facilities for persons with mental retardation: FY 1990–91*. Madison, WI: National Association of Superintendents of Public Residential Facilities for the Mentally Retarded.

Scherer, N., & Owings, N. (1984). Learning to be contingent: Retarded children's responses to their mother's requests. *Language and Speech, 27*, 255–267.

Shriberg, L. & Widder, C. (1990). Speech and prosody characteristics of adults with mental retardation. *Journal of Speech and Hearing Research, 33*, 637–653.

Skrtic, T. (1991). The special education paradox: Equity as a way to excellence. *Harvard Educational Review, 61*, 148–206.

Sommers, R., Patterson, J., & Wildgen, P. (1988). Phonology of Down syndrome speakers, ages 13–22. *Journal of Childhood Communication Disorders, 12*, 65–91.

Spitz, H. (1966). The role of input organization in the learning and memory of mental retardates. In N. Ellis (Ed.), *International review of research in mental retardation* (Vol. 2). New York: Academic Press.

Stephens, W. (1972). Equivalence formation by retarded and nonretarded children at different mental ages. *American Journal of Mental Deficiency, 77*, 311–313.

Stowitschek, J., McConaughy, E., Peatross, D., Salzberg, C., & Lignngaris/Kraft, B. (1988). Effects of group incidental training on the use of social amenities by adults with mental retardation in work settings. *Education and Training in Mental Retardation, 23*, 202–212.

Swetlik, B., & Brown, L. (1977). Teaching severely handicapped students to express selected first, second, and third person singular pronoun responses in answer to "who-doing" questions. In N. Haring & L. Brown (Eds.), *Teaching the severely handicapped* (Vol. II) (pp. 15–62). New York: Grune & Stratton.

Tannock, R. (1988). Mothers' directiveness in their interactions with their children with and without Down syndrome. *American Journal on Mental Retardation, 93*, 154–165.

Thomas, C., & Patton, J. (1994). Characteristics of individuals with milder forms of retardation. In M. Beirne-Smith, J. Patton, & R. Ittenbach (Eds.), *Mental retardation* (4th ed., pp. 204–240). New York: Merrill.

Warren, S. (1991). Enhancing communication and language development with milieu teaching procedures. In E. Cipani (Ed.), *A guide to developing language competence in preschool children with severe and moderate handicaps* (pp. 68–93). Springfield, IL: Charles Thomas.

Wolfensberger, W. (1972). *The principle of normalization in human services.* Toronto: National Institute on Mental Retardation.

Wyatt v. Stickney, 344 F. Supp. 387, 344 F. Supp. 373 (M.D. Ala. 1972), 334 F. Supp 1341, 325 F. Supp. 781 (M.D. Ala. 1971), 772 *aff'd* sub nom. Wyatt v. Aderholt, 503 F. 2d 1305 (5th Cir. 1974).

Zeaman, D., & House, B. (1979). A review of attention theory. In N. Ellis (Ed.), *Handbook of mental deficiency: Psychological theory and research* (2nd ed., pp. 63–120). Hillsdale, NJ: Erlbaum.

Chapter 7

Language and Students with Autism

Individuals with autism have significant problems in both cognitive and language development. In this chapter we will examine the syndrome of autism, including the characteristics, definition, and impairments of cognition and language that are usually associated with autism, also reviewing explanations of the cause of the disabilities associated with autism. We will examine some intervention approaches found effective with individuals with autism, as well as look at some new, controversial techniques.

After completing this chapter you should be able to:

1. List the characteristics that are shared by individuals with autism.
2. Explain how *autism* is defined.
3. Describe specific language and communication impairments that are associated with autism.
4. Explain what might cause the impairments of language and cognition associated with autism.
5. Describe intervention approaches that have been developed to help children with autism.

_____ **Case Studies** _____

Randy

At first Randy seemed to be an exceptionally "good" baby. She demanded little attention and seemed quite content to be left alone in her crib. She never cried. After initial appreciation of this behavior, the parents became concerned. Randy lay in the crib all day without uttering a whimper.

She remained aloof throughout early childhood, content to spin the wheels on a toy truck or twist a shoelace for hours at a time. Speech never developed. After a desperate search for an appropriate school program—and several disastrous trials in inappropriate programs—Randy was placed in a special program for autistic and severely impaired children at age 8. Here she was taught some signs and learned to communicate basic needs, although she rarely used signing to initiate interaction. When left with "free time" Randy continued to prefer her solitary, self-stimulatory activities, but with prompting, she could be engaged in more constructive pursuits.

At age 14, she moved into the residential component of the school program. At age 21, she continues to be involved in a day program of work activities including horticulture and wood shop. Randy functions in the severe range of mental retardation and still has little communicative ability beyond a few basic signs (adapted from Paul, 1987, p. 125).

Paul G.

Paul G. was referred in March 1941, at the age of 5 years, for psychometric assessment of what was thought to be severe intellectual defect. He had attended a private nursery school, where his incoherent speech, inability to conform, and reaction with temper outbursts to any interference created the impression of feeblemindedness.

Paul was a slender, well-built, attractive child, whose face looked intelligent and animated. He had good manual dexterity. He rarely responded to any form of address, even to the calling of his name. At one time he picked up a block from the floor on request. Once he copied a circle immediately after it had been drawn for him. But usually, when spoken to, he went on with whatever he was doing as if nothing had been said. Yet one never had the feeling that he was willingly disobedient or contrary. He was obviously so remote that the remarks did not reach him.

There was a marked contrast between his relations to people and to objects. Upon entering the room, he instantly went after objects and used them correctly. He was not destructive and treated the objects with care and even affection. He opened a box, took out a toy telephone, singing again and again: "He wants the telephone." He got hold of a pair of scissors and patiently and skillfully cut a sheet of paper into small bits, singing the phrase "Cutting paper," many times. While these utterances, made always with the same inflection, were clearly connected with his actions, he ejaculated others that could not be linked up with immediate situations.

There was, on his side, no affective tie to people. He behaved as if people as such did not matter or even exist. It made no difference whether one spoke to him in a friendly or a harsh way. He never looked up at people's faces. When he had any dealings with persons at all, he treated them, or rather parts of them, as if they were objects (adapted from Kanner, 1943).

Cases like those of Randy and Paul G. have fascinated both researchers and the general public. Researchers are intrigued by this mysterious disorder that defies their best efforts to find a cause and a treatment. The general public's interest in autism has been raised by depictions of those with the condition in films such as *Rain Man* and in books and appearances by authors like Barry Kauffman (1976; 1994)—the parent of a child with autism—and Donna Williams (1992)—a person with autism. What is it about autism that makes it so elusive and so fascinating?

Characteristics of Autistic Individuals

Part of the explanation for the intense interest in autism can be attributed to the unique characteristics associated with the syndrome. Some of the most frequently associated characteristics are discussed below. Of course, not all individuals with autism exhibit all of these characteristics.

Withdrawal from Interpersonal Contact

Withdrawal from contact with others is probably the most salient feature of autism. Young children with autism often are not responsive to parents and other caregivers. They may remain stiff when picked up and cuddled. In addition, children with autism fail to make eye contact with others. It sometimes seems as if they are "looking through" the other person. They rarely seek out others for comfort or reach out to others, seeking little or no social interaction (Rutter & Schopler, 1987).

Ritualistic Behavior

Children with autism are often described as engaging in *ritualistic* behaviors, such as spinning objects, twirling their fingers in front of their face, slapping their heads, flapping their hands, and the like. This behavior may be self-stimulating. Autistic children are not the only individuals with disabilities who engage in such behaviors, but the behaviors seem to be particularly characteristic of autism. In addition, individuals with autism often have a compelling desire for sameness and routine. They may become upset if something in their room is out of place or if their usual schedule is disrupted (Rutter & Schopler, 1987). If you saw *Rain Man*, you may remember the discomfort that Raymond—the individual with autism portrayed by Dustin Hoffman—experienced when he discovered that there was a book out of place in his room.

Cognitive Characteristics

Because most children with autism *look* normal and some possess unusual talents, at one time it was thought that intelligence in autistic children was normal or even above normal. But today researchers believe that children with autism have low, measured intelligence. A majority have IQ scores in the range of mental retardation (< 75). Although perhaps 20 to 25 percent score within the normal range of intelligence (75 to 120), the majority fall within an IQ range of about 35 to 70 (De Myer et al., 1974; Prior & Werry, 1986).

In addition to having lower IQ scores, children with autism often have significant impairments in specific cognitive abilities. Some of these problems appear to be developmental in nature. For example, the memory and discrimination problems often associated with autism are likely due to the slower cognitive development of children with autism (Prior & Werry, 1986). On the other hand, there are some cognitive impairments that seem specifically characteristic of autism. In a series of studies, Hermelin (1978) and Hermelin and O'Connor (1970) found that children with autism have special difficulty using meaning to solve problems and organizing information by rules and categories. For example, when asked to put together a jigsaw puzzle, children with autism may do as well when the pieces are face down as when the picture side is visible. They fail to use or extract meaning from this experience. Instead of using pictures or words to think, they try to retain information in a raw, unorganized state. This is not an effective way to think and remember. Ricks and Wing (1975) came to a similar conclusion in their description of the language problems of children with autism. Their research led them to conclude that children with autism have specific difficulty in forming language rules.

In contrast to the descriptions of cognitive difficulties in autism, there are reports that at least some individuals with autism have extraordinary abilities. They may have exceptional intact skills in one or more areas of functioning or have an extraordinary ability in a very narrowly defined area. There is a scene in *Rain Man* when the autistic character played by Dustin Hoffman is able to rapidly (and apparently accurately) count the number of toothpicks that spill from a box onto the floor. These abilities are sometimes called *splinter* skills because they are unrelated to other domains of learning and are generally not very useful (although Hoffman's character eventually was taught to apply his skills to counting cards in a casino). We should keep in mind that while the appearance of splinter skills is dramatic, it is not characteristic of most persons with autism.

Stimulus Selectivity and Sensitivity

Children with autism have been described as either *overselective* or *underselective* to environmental stimuli (Prior & Werry, 1986). When children are overselective, they focus on one characteristic to the exclusion of others. For example, they may focus on a smudge on a paper rather than on the print that they are supposed to be reading. Children with autism have often been reported to be inconsistent in their responses to environmental stimuli. For instance, at times they may be hypersensitive; parents have reported that their children can hear a fire engine down the street before anyone else can detect the sound. At other times, the same children may be remarkably unresponsive, and may not even flinch when a pan is dropped in the kitchen.

Language Impairments

There is no question that most children with autism have severe disorders in language and communication. Approximately half of the population have no functional spoken language (Rutter & Schopler, 1987). Language and communication difficulties are evident in young children with autism and persist through adulthood, even in adults with reasonably good language development (Baltaxe, 1977).

TABLE 7.1   Examples of Echolalia

Immediate Echolalia	Teacher says: "Gloria, what did you do last night?" Student responds: "What did you do last night?"
Delayed Echolalia	While working quietly at a desk, child suddenly shouts: "What's the matter with you? You can't do that."
Mitigated Echolalia	Teacher says: "So, what did you do last night?" Student responds: "Night."

There are significant delays in language development, but, even more important, there are some characteristic *differences* in language development in the autistic population.

Two specific language differences frequently associated with autism are **echolalia** and **pronoun reversal.** *Echolalia* may be defined as the meaningless repetition of speech produced by others (Prizant & Duchan, 1981). Long & Long (1994) identified three kinds of echolalia (see Table 7.1). **Immediate echolalia** occurs within a brief time period after the speaker talks. **Delayed echolalia** involves the repetition of words or phrases that may have been heard days, weeks, or even years previously. Sometimes echolalic individuals repeat back exactly what they hear, but often they change the structure of the original utterance. This is called **mitigated echolalia.** Although echolalia is found among many individuals with disabilities (and even at certain stages of normal language development), it occurs more frequently among individuals with autism (Cantwell, Baker, & Rutter, 1978) and persists for far longer than in normally developing children (Howlin, 1982).

The traditional view of echolalia has been that it indicates a lack of comprehension ability and is noncommunicative (Schreibman & Carr, 1978). Many language training programs have actively discouraged—and even punished—the use of echolalia by children with autism. However, in the past few years views about echolalia have changed. Today, many believe that echolalia actually serves an important communicative role for individuals with autism. Barry Prizant (1983), for example, holds the position that people with autism may use echolalia in an intentional way, to maintain social interaction. Prizant and Duchan (1981) went so far as to delineate seven communicative functions that echolalia may serve (see Table 7.2). Their research, as well as that by others, should remind us that we must look at the total context—not just at the spoken language produced—to fully understand what may be going on in an interaction.

Another language characteristic associated with autism is pronoun reversal. Many children with autism say *you* when referring to themselves, or *me* when referring to another person. At one time these errors were thought to indicate a problem with psychosocial development. That is, it was hypothesized that these errors indicated that autistic persons had no *sense of self.* Pronouns such as *you* or *I* had no meaning for them (Bettelheim, 1967). However, a number of alternative (and more likely) explanations for the pronoun reversals of individuals with autism have been suggested. These include:

TABLE 7.2   Seven Communicative Functions of Immediate Echolalia

Category	Description
Interactive	
Turn taking	Utterances used as turn fillers in an alternating verbal exchange
Declarative	Utterances labeling objects, actions, or location (accompanied by demonstrative gestures)
Yes answer	Utterances used to indicate affirmation of prior utterance
Request	Utterances used to request objects or others' actions. Usually involves mitigated echolalia
Noninteractive	
Nonfocused	Utterances produced with no apparent intent and often in states of high arousal (e.g., fear, pain)
Rehearsal	Utterances used as a processing aid, followed by utterance or action indicating comprehension of echoed utterance
Self-regulatory	Utterances which serve to regulate subject's own actions. Produced in synchrony with motor activity

Source: Adapted from B. Prizant & J. Duchan. (1981). The functions of immediate echolalia in autistic children. *Journal of Speech and Hearing Disorders, 46,* 241–249.

- Echolalia: Difficulty with pronoun usage may be the result of echolalia (Bartak & Rutter, 1976). If a parent says *What are you doing?* and the child responds *What are you doing?* the child has not only echoed the utterances but has also used an incorrect pronoun.
- Cognitive development: Words like *I* and *you* are **deictic** forms—that is, words that change their referent in relation to the context. A *ball* is always a *ball,* but sometimes *I* is *I* and sometimes *I* is *you,* depending on the context. This, cognitively, is a more complex notion and one that may be more difficult for children with cognitive difficulties (Tager-Flusberg, 1981).
- Lack of attention: Oshima-Takane and Benaroya (1989) have claimed that children with autism have trouble with pronouns, because the children fail to attend to pronoun usage by others. They found, however, that when autistic children were guided to attend to an adult model, they *could* learn to use pronouns correctly.

We do not have a firm understanding of why children with autism persist in making pronoun errors; however, the explanations listed above hold hope that this pronoun problem can be corrected with appropriate intervention.

Conclusion

As discussed, children with autism exhibit a variety of characteristics. Most have significant impairments in language and cognition, but some have intact or precocious skills. Often children with autism exhibit symptoms similar to those of children with other disabilities such as deafness, mental retardation, or emotional disorder. Since intervention approaches for these disorders may differ, defining autism and identifying children with the syndrome are key to successful intervention. In the next section we will see *autism* defined and some of the attempts to understand its cause.

Definition of Autism

At one time, autism was thought to be an early version of schizophrenia (Rutter & Schopler, 1987). In fact, the major journal in the field of autism—*The Journal of Autism and Developmental Disorders*—was at one time called *The Journal of Autism and Childhood Schizophrenia*. However, over the last 20 years there has been a growing recognition that autism and schizophrenia are two separate disorders (Rutter & Schopler, 1987). Although there is widespread agreement that autism is a distinct disorder, there remains considerable confusion about the term and its definition. It is not unusual to find children who are called *autisticlike* or *exhibiting autistic behaviors*. These descriptions reflect the difficulty of defining autism.

During the last 20 years or so there has been some progress made in narrowing and sharpening the definition of autism. Even the name (*Kanner's syndrome, infantile autism, autistic disorder*) has changed. One of the most widely used definitions is that contained in the *Diagnostic and Statistical Manual of Mental Disorders, Fourth Edition* (DSM-IV), published by the American Psychiatric Association (1994). In the DSM-IV, *autistic disorder* is considered one of a group of disorders called *pervasive developmental disorders*. In order to be diagnosed with autistic disorder, a child must exhibit at least six of the twelve symptoms included in the definition. These symptoms are distributed among three general categories:

1. Qualitative impairment in social interaction
2. Qualitative impairment in communication
3. Restricted repetitive and stereotyped patterns of behavior, interests, and activities

A child must have at least two symptoms from group 1, one from group 2, and one from 3 in order to be a candidate for the autistic disorder label. In addition, the onset of the disorder must occur during infancy or childhood (before 36 months of age).

Recently, in the Individuals with Disabilities Education Act (IDEA) the federal government recognized autism as a distinct disorder. The federal definition states that:

> *Autism means a developmental disability significantly affecting verbal and nonverbal communication and social interaction, generally evident before age three, that adversely affects educational performance. Characteristics of autism include—irregularities and impairments in communication, engagement in repetitive activities and stereotyped movements, resistance to environmental*

change or change in daily routines, and unusual responses to sensory experiences. (Department of Education, 1991, p. 41271)

The definitions contained in both the DSM-IV and the IDEA contain specific and easily recognizable symptoms. However, in practice, even highly skilled professionals have difficulty diagnosing autism. Frequently, children with autistic characteristics act like children with other disabilities. As we mentioned earlier, for many years autism was confused with schizophrenia. But, as Kauffman (1989) points out, schizophrenia is quite different from autism. Schizophrenia usually emerges in adolescence; autism emerges in early childhood. Individuals with schizophrenia often experience hallucinations and/or delusions. Children with autism do not. Schizophrenics may feel controlled by alien forces, whereas autistic children do not. Like autistic children, individuals with schizophrenia may withdraw from interaction, but when schizophrenics do interact, their behavior is described as "bizarre" or "inappropriate." People with schizophrenia may have difficulty expressing themselves, but do not have the degree of mutism and echolalia characteristic of autistic disorder. Finally, the stereotypic behaviors and desire for preservation of sameness commonly found among children with autism are not characteristic of schizophrenia. In summary, children with autism may be described as *withdrawn* from social interaction, while individuals with schizophrenia engage in unusual or bizarre interaction.

Sometimes autism is confused with other disabilities, such as pervasive language disorders or hearing impairments. However, as Bartak, Rutter, and Cox (1975) pointed out, unlike children with pervasive language disorders, children with autism fail to compensate for their deficits in spoken language by using gesture or other nonverbal means of expression. They also do not respond to communicative attempts by others. Additionally, children with autism have more severe cognitive and behavioral impairments than those found among children with pervasive language disorders. The same differences are found when comparing children with autism to deaf children. In addition, the sensory impairments of deaf children are stable, while those of children with autism fluctuate from one extreme to the other.

Causes of Autism

So much has been written about the causes of autism that it is difficult to condense the research into a few paragraphs—or even a few pages. Any discussion of the causes of autism must attempt to explain the myriad symptoms associated with the syndrome. This is no easy matter. Even if we cannot say for certain what causes autism, understanding what does *not* cause the disorder is important.

Early theories of autism focused on the family and family interaction as the likely cause of the syndrome. Kanner (1943) and later Bettelheim (1967) suggested that autism was caused by parents who were unusually rigid and emotionally cold. Kanner talked about the "refrigerator" parents who interacted with their children in a cold, aloof manner. This behavior by parents was thought to cause emotional deprivation in the child, which, in turn, caused the child to withdraw from human interaction. Although this psychoanalytic view of the cause of autism was widely accepted for many years, it is now rejected by most professionals. The reason is that controlled studies failed to find differences in either the personality traits of parents of children with autism or in the way they relate to their children (Prior & Werry, 1986). Although some differences have been found in interactions between parents and their autistic children, these can be attributed to the behavior of the autistic child rather than to psychopathology of the parent.

If parents do not cause autism, what does? More and more evidence points to a biological disorder underlying autism. However, the specific biological problem has been difficult to pinpoint. It has been suggested, for example, that damage to the brain-stem area of the brain may be the cause of the fluctuations in the processing of sensory information and the stereotypical behaviors found in autism (Tanguay & Edwards, 1982). Others have suggested that damage to the limbic system (Maurer & Damasio, 1982) or to a combination of cortical and subcortical regions (Fein, Pennington, Markowitz, Braverman, & Waterhouse, 1986) may cause the symptoms associated with autism. There has been a good deal of research on the role of biochemical differences in autistic individuals. Although this research has found several differences in the brain chemistry of autistic persons (e.g., De Myer, Hintgen, & Jackson, 1981), there remains no conclusive proof that all—or even most—individuals with autism have neurochemical differences. Researchers have also suggested that genetic factors (Folstein & Rutter, 1988) may cause autism.

Reviewing the research on the cause of autism, Folstein and Rutter (1988) reached two conclusions. First, there are many *etiologies* (causes) of autism. Second, the causes of autism are organic rather than psychosocial. Perhaps this is the most we can say at this point about the causes of autism. Although *many* causes have been found, no *single* cause has been (or is likely to be) found. It is quite possible that there are several subtypes of autism that will be found to have different causes and different treatments. Until research clarifies the situation, the role of educators must be to use the most effective techniques with all children with autism.

Language and Communication

The language development of children with learning disabilities and mental retardation is described, for the most part, as delayed rather than different. The same cannot be said about the language development of children with autism. As Michael Rutter (1978) put it, "It is well established that the problem is *not* just that autistic children use little speech but rather that their language, when it develops, is abnormal in many respects" (p. 86). We have already seen two ways in which the language development of children with autism differs from the norm—in their persistent use of echolalia and their tendency to confuse pronoun usage. Many children with autism do not develop spoken language at all (from 28–61%, depending on which studies are accepted). In this section, we will look at the development of language and communication in those autistic children who do develop spoken language.

Early Development

It is not easy to examine the early language development of children with autism because these children are often not identified as autistic until age 2 or 3. However, the studies that have been done suggest that right from the start, language development is a problem for children with autism. Of course, for many young children with autism, spoken language develops slowly, if at all. When language does develop, it is usually significantly delayed (Tager-Flusberg, 1981). But language development is more than delayed—it is different. For example, Wing (1971) asked parents of children with autism to complete a retrospective questionnaire about the development of their child. The parents reported that their children did not indicate that they wanted to be picked up, did not respond to their mother's voice, and did not point to objects. Bartak, Rutter, and Cox (1975) cited parent reports that babbling in their autistic children was absent or delayed.

Phonology

Studies of the speech production of children with autism have found that in those children who develop spoken language, the development of phonological rules follows the same course found in normally developing children. Bartolucci, Pierce, Streiner, and Eppel (1976) studied the phonological production of children with autism in comparison to children with mental retardation who were matched for mental age. They found that both groups used similar phonemes and made similar errors in the production of more advanced sounds and thereby concluded that verbal autistic children have a normal, but delayed, sequence of phonological development.

On the other hand, many observers have reported that children with autism have considerable trouble with **suprasegmental** features of sound production (stress and intonation). Children with autism have been described as speaking in a singsong pattern, having fluctuations in vocal intensity (too loud or too soft), and using intonations that are not appropriate to the meaning of the sentence (using a rising intonation for sentences that are not questions) (Goldfarb, Braunstein, & Lorge, 1956). Individuals with autism often lack expression in their voices and may speak in a monotone. It has been suggested that these problems are caused by an inability to process the suprasegmental features of speech (Fay & Schuler, 1980), but careful research has failed to confirm this hypothesis (Tager-Flusberg, 1981). However, it appears to be true that many individuals with autism have unusual vocal characteristics that cannot be explained by a lag in development.

Morphology and Syntax

As with phonological development, studies of the acquisition of morphological rules by children with autism have found some similarities to normally developing children and some differences. One study (Fein & Waterhouse, 1979) compared the acquisition of morphemes by children with autism to that development in schizophrenic and nondisabled children and found no significant differences in either the total number of morphemes used or in the frequency of morpheme usage. On the other hand, when Bartolucci, Pierce, and Streiner (1980) compared the use of morphemes by children with autism, children with mental retardation, and normally developing children, they found that the children with mental retardation and subjects with autism acquired morphemes in a different order than did normally developing children. In addition, there was a lag in the development of morpheme usage in both groups of children with disabilities. Bartolucci et al. (1980) suggested that the previously mentioned problems children with autism have with deictic terms (words that change their meaning with the context) may explain some of the differences in the morphological development. This problem is really more of a difficulty with the acquisition of semantic rather than morphological concepts.

In studies of their syntactic development, children with autism are generally seen as delayed and having particular problems using language in social situations. Cunningham (1968) observed the language development of a child with autism for 5 years (age 6–11). He found that the child's MLU gradually increased from 1.9 words to 3.0 words during the initial 6 months of observation but showed little progress after that. Cunningham noted that grammatical morphemes and *function words* (articles, auxiliaries) were often omitted by the child.

Bartak, Rutter, and Cox (1975) compared the syntactic development of children with autism and *dysphasia* (specific-language disorder). They found that although the children were similar in mean length of utterance, the children with autism performed much more poorly on tests of language comprehension. They also found that the language disorder of children with autism was more extensive, involving the use and understanding of gesture and written language, as well as spoken language. In a more detailed, follow-up study, Cantwell, Baker, and Rutter (1978) analyzed the tape-recorded language samples of some of the children from the original study. They found that the two groups were quite similar both in morphological rule usage and in development of syntactic rules. Where differences were found, they were in the *use* of language in social situations. The children with autism were described as using more "abnormal" speech and less "socialized" speech.

Pierce and Bartolucci (1977) compared the syntactic development of children with autism to that of children with mental retardation and normally developing children. In their sample they found that the syntactic development of ten children with autism lagged behind that of *both* the normally developing and mentally retarded subject groups. They described the language of the children with autism as less complex than that of the other children, even though children with autism used most of the same language structures. As did Cantwell et al. (1978), Pierce and Bartolucci concluded that children with autism seem to have particular difficulty *applying* syntactic rules in their language.

Finally, Helen Tager-Flusberg and her colleagues (Tager-Flusberg et al., 1990) compared the language development of a group of children with autism to that of children with Down syndrome. They found that for most of the children with autism, MLU increased over time and was a good indicator of level of language development. However, this was not true for one of the subjects. In addition, Tager-Flusberg et al. reported that the syntactic development of the children with autism followed a developmental course similar to that of both the normally developing and children with Down syndrome, although in children with autism, there appeared to be a leveling-out of their development at higher stages of MLU. But, once again there were exceptions; one child actually declined in syntactic development during the study.

Most of the research on the morphological and syntactic development of children with autism concludes that these domains of development are delayed. However, there also may be limits to this development (like those reported for some individuals with mental retardation). We should keep in mind that there is a great deal of variability in this population and some children may deviate from this pattern of delayed development. In addition, several studies have reported significant problems experienced by children with autism in *applying* linguistic rules in social situations.

Semantics

There is limited research on the semantic abilities of children with autism, but what there is suggests this is an area of significant difficulty for most individuals with autism. Difficulty with organizing information into categories and using this information for thinking and problem solving are types of semantic-skill difficulties that have long been associated with autism. Baltaxe and Simmons (1975) reported on a series of studies on the speech of higher-functioning adolescents with autism. They found that their autistic subjects, unlike individuals with Down syndrome, had most difficulty with semantic concepts. After reviewing research on the language difficulties of individuals with autism, Ricks and Wing (1975) concluded that the defining feature is difficulty in using symbols to form categories and abstractions. More recently, Brook and Bowler (1992) suggested that autism may be an example of a semantic-pragmatic language disorder.

All of the above *suggests* that semantic processing difficulties are an important feature of autism, but the evidence is largely circumstantial. A few studies, however, have begun to gather more direct evidence on the semantic abilities of children with autism and have reached some rather surprising conclusions. Tager-Flusberg (1985) directly examined the ability of children with autism to group information by conceptual categories. Children with autism and normally developing children matched for language development were asked to categorize pictures of objects into basic-level and superordinate categories. Tager-Flusberg found that the subjects with autism were no different from the nondisabled subjects in their categorization abilities. She concluded that the view of the world held by the subjects with autism that she tested was quite similar to that of the other children in the study. Similarly, Eskes, Bryson, and McCormick (1990) found that children with autism could comprehend both concrete and abstract words (such as *life* and *time*) much like children in a normally developing control group matched for reading ability.

The studies cited above suggest that the semantic functioning of children with autism may not be as deficient as previously thought. But this may not be entirely accurate. First, the autistic subjects in these studies were quite high functioning. In the Eskes et al. (1990) study, the mean nonverbal IQ of the subjects with autism was 88. Tager-Flusberg herself acknowledged that low-functioning children with autism have difficulty categorizing. Second, performance on laboratory tasks may not necessarily predict performance in the real world. In fact, Eskes et al. noted that several researchers have found that individuals with autism have particular difficulty *using* their knowledge in real situations. For example, they recall word lists organized by semantic category no better than lists that are randomly configured. Finally, we should keep in mind that the control groups in these studies were matched for language or reading age. As a result, the control subjects were much younger. Therefore, even for higher-functioning children with autism, semantic development is delayed.

Some studies have found that children with autism use more **idiosyncratic** language and **neologisms** in their language. Volden and Lord (1991) defined *idiosyncratic language* as "the use of conventional words or phrases in unusual ways to convey specific meanings" (p. 111). For example, a child with autism in their study said, "It makes me want to go as deep as economical with it," which was interpreted to mean *withdraw as much as possible. Neologisms* are nonstandard (or invented) words. Subjects with autism in the Volden and Lord study said "bloosers" for *bruises* and "bells" for *rings*. Volden and Lord compared the frequency of idiosyncratic language and neologisms in language samples from two groups of children with autism (IQ > 80 and IQ < 80) to the language of children with mental retardation and normally developing children matched for chronological age. They found that the children with autism made more semantic errors and produced far more neologisms than either of the comparison groups. Almost all of the children with autism produced unusual words or phrases, while few of the other subjects did so. This study suggests that individuals with autism may have difficulty using words correctly.

Although the research on the semantic skills of individuals with autism may seem to be confusing and inconsistent, one thing stands out. Individuals with autism have difficulty *using* semantic concepts in natural situations. As educators, we can help children with autism by modeling correct usage, by pointing out when a word is misused or when there is an opportunity to apply a semantic concept, and by teaching students to use semantic strategies for thinking and problem solving.

Pragmatics

One of the defining features of autism is withdrawal from social interaction. So, it should not be surprising to find that children with autism have significant impairments in the pragmatic aspects of language. In fact, children with autism have been described as rigid and socially inappropriate (Shapiro & Fish, 1969). Tiegerman (1993) listed the following specific pragmatics problems associated with autism:

TABLE 7.3   Examples of Pragmatic Impairments in Adults with Autism

Response does not address question

Experimenter:	Catherine is your . . .
Subject:	Sister.
E:	Sister, right. Is she younger than you or older than you?
S:	Catherine Smith.

Irrelevant response

E:	Is Jane married?
S:	No.
E.	Mhmm. She's got a friend and she lives in America?
S:	Museums all shut now.

Echolalia

E:	Where do Mummy and Daddy live?
S:	Mummy and Daddy live.

Source: M. Eales. (1993). Pragmatic impairments in adults with childhood diagnoses of autism or developmental receptive language disorder. *Journal of Autism and Developmental Disorders, 23,* 593–617.

- initiating and terminating interaction
- maintaining conversational topics
- functioning within speaker and listener roles
- using behavior for the purpose of communication

There is a good deal of research evidence to support the claim that individuals with autism have significant problems with pragmatics. Loveland, Landry, Hughes, Hall, and McEvoy (1988), for example, found that children with autism were very unresponsive to attempts by their parents to initiate communication. In addition, the children with autism rarely initiated communication spontaneously and also produced fewer communicative acts than did mental-age-matched children with language delays or normally developing children. Loveland et al. concluded that the pragmatic development of the children with autism in their study was below that of even the 2-year-old nondisabled children to whom they were being compared. Several studies (e.g., Baltaxe, 1977; Eales, 1993) have shown that the pragmatic problems associated with autism persist through adolescence, even in higher-IQ individuals (see Table 7.3 for examples).

It is possible that under certain circumstances individuals with autism communicate more than has generally been thought. Wetherby (1986) cites several pieces of research evidence to support this conclusion. For example, she notes that McHale, Simeonsson, Marcus, and Olley (1980) found that the communicative behavior of children with autism was greater with their teacher than with their classmates. Similarly, Bernard-Opitz (1982) observed a child with autism who interacted more with his mother and a clinician than he did with an unfamiliar adult. Wetherby and Prutting (1984) found that when both nonverbal and verbal means of communication were used, individuals with autism communicated as frequently as did nondisabled children matched for language ability, although they used fewer communicative acts.

TABLE 7.4   Language Development of Individuals with Autism

Phonology	Morphology	Syntax	Semantics	Pragmatics
Normal, but delayed development Impairments in suprasegmental features (stress and intonation) Fluctuations in vocal intensity Inappropriate intonation	Mixed findings Possible different order of development	Delays in nonverbal and written, as well as spoken, language Less complex language than those with mental retardation Difficulty using language	Problems using language to organize info Higher IQ may be intact Use more idiosyncratic language and neologism	Rigid, socially inappropriate Unresponsive Problems persist Speech-act development intact

Source: From American Psychiatric Association: *Diagnostic and Statistical Manual of Mental Disorders,* Fourth Edition. Washington DC, American Psychiatric Association, 1994. Reprinted by permission.

The research on pragmatic development in children with autism suggests that teachers and other education professionals can help these children with autism enhance their communication skills by interacting with them frequently, by being responsive to both verbal and nonverbal attempts to communicate, and by communicating with the children in comfortable, familiar contexts whenever possible.

Conclusion

Whenever we talk about children with autism, we must keep in mind the heterogeneous nature of the population. This may help explain some of the inconsistencies in the research on the language abilities of children with autism. Some aspects of language—such as phonology and syntax—seem relatively intact in the autistic population. There are delays, but for the most part, development progresses through the usual stages. Deficits in semantics and pragmatics are more significant. But, even in these domains, some individuals have relatively intact skills (see Table 7.4 for a summary).

Causes of Language and Communication Disorders in Autism

What causes the language impairments associated with autism? Answering this question is about as difficult as determining the cause of autism itself. But the search for the answer may help those working with children with autism focus their efforts on effective intervention approaches. Let's briefly examine a few of the hypotheses that have been suggested to explain the cause of the language and communications disorders of children with autism.

Parent-Child Interaction

As we know, one of the earliest theories on the cause of autism identified parents as the problem. Although research evidence has not generally supported this causal hypothesis, it is possible that deficiencies in parent-child interaction might have a negative effect on language development. In fact, the most problematic language domains for children with autism—semantics and pragmatics—are those that are most affected by parent-child interaction. Early research on the interaction between parents and their children with autism supported the conclusion that deficiencies in parent-child interaction caused (or at least contributed to) the language deficiencies of children with autism (Goldfarb, Goldfarb, & Scholl, 1966). However, later research failed to support this claim. In most studies, parents of children with autism have been found to interact with their children much like parents of other children with disabilities (Cantwell et al., 1977). In fact, the only differences that Cantwell et al. found were that mothers of children with autism used more affectionate remarks and more elaborations than did parents of children with dysphasia. Although parent-child interaction may differ in children with autism, this difference is more likely to be due to the behavior of the child than to that of the parent(s).

On the other hand, there is some research literature that reports language problems in parents of children with autism. For example, Landa, Folstein, and Isaacs (1991) found that parents of children with autism produced story narratives that were similar in length to those produced by other adults, but that a subgroup (34%) produced extremely poor stories. Landa et al. suggested that language difficulties may run in families who have children with autism. They believe that this language disorder is due to a genetic problem, however, not to deficient language interaction.

Teachers and other education professionals may help parents of children with autism enhance the quality of interaction with their children by suggesting ways parents might engage their child's attention, comment on what their child is doing, and learn how to interpret seemingly noncommunicative verbal and non-verbal behaviors. Knowing that some, but not all, parents of children with autism may themselves have language problems may help teachers be more alert to parents' needs.

Cognitive Impairments

Earlier in this chapter we reviewed some of the cognitive-impairment evidence associated with autism. Several of these problems (such as difficulty forming rules and problems organizing information) could have negative effects on language development. In addition, problems with perception and with the development of social play behavior may affect the development of language and communication. However, we know from research such as that by Wetherby and Gaines (1982) that cognitive problems alone do not account for the language impairments of children with autism.

Several cognitive-related theories have been suggested to explain the pervasive cognitive and language impairments of autism. Prizant (1983) suggested that individuals with autism may have a **gestalt processing style.** In other words, they take in information in large chunks, failing to analyze the information. As a result, they do not acquire the rules of language. As evidence, Prizant cites echolalia as an example of the memorization and repetition of whole chunks.

Wetherby and Prutting (1984) claimed that persons with autism have **asynchronous development.** In other words, the timing of their development is off. They claim that individuals with autism acquire the same skills as other children but do so out of the usual order. As a result, they are ahead on some things but behind on others.

Still another hypothesis explaining these cognitive and language impairments claims that individuals with autism lack a **theory of mind** (Baron-Cohen, Leslie, & Frith, 1985). The *theory of mind* hypothesis states that normally developing children possess an understanding of mental states in others; if this ability is impaired, children have difficulty understanding the behavior (including the communicative behavior) of other people. Research on the theory of mind does show difficulties experienced by children with autism. For example, Perner, Frith, Leslie, and Leekam (1989) found that children with autism had difficulty performing three tasks evaluating the understanding of mental states, tests that were within the ability of nondisabled children.

Clearly, teachers and others need to consider the possible effects that cognitive impairments could have on the language development of children with autism. These students may benefit from participation in a variety of classroom and community experiences. But even more important is that teachers understand *how* the child with autism has perceived these experiences, to know that their view may be quite different from what we *thought* they would experience. It may help for the teacher to recount what the group or individual did, to model analysis of new information, and to demonstrate how this information can be integrated with prior learning.

Neurological Causes

It is also possible that brain damage or dysfunction causes the specific language and communication disorders of autism. For example, damage to the brain-stem region could cause faulty processing of incoming perceptual information, whereas damage to the left hemisphere of the brain could cause specific language impairments. A neurochemical disorder could affect the functions of the brain that relate to producing spoken language. All of these are possible but, as we noted earlier, evidence for neurological causes of autism is not conclusive. In any case, if any or all of these neurological explanations turn out to be true, there is probably little that teachers of children with autism would do differently.

Intervention for Language and Communication Impairments

Because the language impairments of children with autism are so pervasive and have such devastating effects, many intervention approaches have been suggested, some of which do work. We will look at two approaches that have a proven record of success with children with autism: behavioral training and sign language instruction. We will then look at two other methods that are quite controversial: auditory training and facilitated communication.

Principles for Intervention

Wetherby (1986) suggested four principles for language intervention programs for children with autism, based on her review of the literature on autistic language and communication. First, **communicative intent** should be the critical focus of language intervention. Children with autism should be taught to express their needs through communication—spoken, gestural, or nonverbal (e.g., facial expressions). Second, language intervention programs should **diverge from the normal model and reflect the course of communicative development for the autistic child.** In other words, children with autism do not always follow a normal course of language development. Practitioners should be flexible enough to follow the lead of the individual child in developing instructional goals. A third suggestion by Wetherby was that clinicians **consider the developmental interplay between communicative means and communicative intentions.** New communicative functions (intentions) can be taught using more primitive communicative means (such as gesture). Similarly, in teaching a child to use a new means of expression (such as speech), it is probably best to start with communicative functions that the child has already mastered. Fourth, Wetherby suggested that clinicians consider the **social content** of language intervention. It is not enough to teach the child a discrete language skill. The social environment must be structured in such a way as to demand the use of this skill. It is essential that if children are taught to request, they have requesting (at lunch, for example) as part of their social environment. These principles should be useful guidelines for the design of language intervention programs for children with autism.

Behavioral Training

Behavioral approaches have been quite successful in enhancing the language and communication of children with autism. Such approaches use a **stimulus** to prompt a **response,** which is then **reinforced. Shaping** is used to mold the verbal behavior into the adult target form that is desired. A complete description of a behavioral approach to language instruction is available in Lovaas (1977). Lovaas gives the following example of a child being trained with a behavioral approach (p. 53):

> (E is the trainer; B is Billy, a child with autism.)
> (There is a breakfast tray (stimulus) between them.)

E: What do you want?

B: Egg.

E: No, what do you want? I . . .

B: I want . . . .

E: Egg (pause). O.K., what do you want?

E: No, what do you want? I . . .

B: I want egg.

E: Good boy (feeds Billy).

In several studies, Lovaas has documented his success using this type of approach with children with autism. For example, Lovaas has reported that children with autism who received early, intensive, behavioral intervention (including language) scored higher on tests of intelligence and were more successful in school than similar children who received less intensive intervention (Lovaas, 1987). A follow-up study several years later found that these differences continued to exist (McEachlin, Smith, & Lovaas, 1993).

Although behavior-intervention approaches to language instruction can work, they have limitations. The biggest concerns revolve around the generalizing of verbal behavior to natural, social situations. In other words, it is one thing to train a specific verbal behavior under a one-on-one clinical condition but something else to use that newly acquired skill to order a hamburger at McDonald's. Although Lovaas claims to be able to teach spontaneous verbalization, there is little data to support this claim.

Behavioral approaches to language instruction are most useful for training specific skill sequences (such as request routines or word endings). If using behavioral techniques, teachers should pay special attention to helping the child generalize newly acquired behavior and include practice in real social situations.

Sign-Language Training

Another effective approach to enhancing the language skills of children with autism is sign-language training. Sign language has several advantages over spoken language in training for children with autism. For one, signs can be kept in the air as long as necessary to get the child's attention, while words disappear quickly. A child's hands may be molded into the desired sign. It would be impossible (as well as dangerous) to try to mold a child's lips, teeth, and tongue to try to form words. Sign language also requires the use of motor skills that are usually intact (if not superior) in children with autism.

Studies of the use of sign-language training with children with autism have shown that it can be a useful way to enhance language and communication skills (Bonvillian & Nelson, 1976; Fulwiler & Fouts, 1976). Children who are nonverbal can acquire a reasonably large repertoire of signs. Even more encouraging are reports that spoken language may increase after sign-language training (Fulweiler & Fouts, 1976; Layton & Baker, 1981). In addition, some studies have reported that improvements in social and self-care skills follow the introduction of sign-language training (Konstantareas, Webster, & Oxman, 1979).

The limitations of sign-language training for children with autism should be obvious. Since there are relatively few persons who can sign, the potential number of communication partners for signers is limited. Additionally, children who use sign language as their primary means of communication will have a more difficult time being included in regular education and in community activities. However, sign-language training may be a good way to begin to build communication skills. Combining signing with spoken-language usage may be an effective way to enhance the communication skills of children with autism.

Auditory Training

Auditory problems are commonly found among children with autism and may, in part, account for some of the language problems associated with autism. Recently, Dr. Bernard Rimland has begun to investigate a controversial technique developed by Guy Berard, a French physician. This technique, known as *auditory integration training (AIT)*, entails 10 hours of listening to electronically modulated music over a 10-day period, using a variety of music (rock, pop, reggae), with high and low sound frequencies dampened on a near-random basis.

In the only study to date, Rimland and Edelson (1992) reported the use of auditory integration training with 17 subjects with autism. They found that children who received this therapy improved their behavior and reduced their auditory problems. Despite the results of this study, auditory integration training remains a controversial technique. There is still little research on AIT. Also, many of the clinical reports have claimed startling—almost unbelievable—improvements. Skeptics wonder how listening to music can cause such dramatic results. Clearly, auditory integration training deserves further investigation. If these early reports of success hold up, this training could be an important component of intervention for at least some children with autism.

Facilitated Communication

Facilitated communication (FC) is another new and very controversial intervention approach for children with autism. It is a technique for enhancing communication in persons having difficulty communicating in the usual ways—those with autism, mental retardation, and physical disabilities. The method is simple. A facilitator, using a special grip, holds the hand of the individual being facilitated. The facilitator is taught to provide resistance to the movement of the individual with whom he or she is working. The facilitator may place a hand over that of the other person or simply provide a light touch at the elbow or shoulder. It is hypothesized that this touch steadies the person with autism and allows them to better focus their motor movements.

From the beginning, the technique has engendered both great excitement and profound skepticism. A 1990 article by Douglas Biklen in the *Harvard Educational Review* sparked a debate that continues to this day. There were many spectacular and controversial early claims about facilitated communication. For example, there were claims that all (or almost all) children with autism who were exposed to FC were able to produce written communication. In one study (Biklen & Schubert, 1991), it was reported that following the implementation of FC, 20 of 21 subjects were able to type words. Individuals previously thought to have autism and mental retardation were suddenly able to demonstrate unexpected levels of literacy (Biklen, 1990). Students who had previously been in special schools were now attending regular high school classes and were excelling. Some were going to college.

A number of research studies published since 1992 have raised significant concerns about the effectiveness of facilitated communication. Most of the studies have found that under clinical conditions, when the facilitator was "blind" to the stimulus item, the subject was unable to produce independent communication (e.g., Wheeler, Jacobson, Paglieri, & Schwartz, 1993; Eberlin, McConnachie, Ibel, & Volpe, 1993; Regal, Rooney, & Wandas, 1994). Instead, the communication appeared to be influenced, even guided, by the facilitator. This influence, while apparently unintended, nevertheless was real and pervasive. Study after study has found that when the facilitator did not know the content of the information to which the subject had been exposed, the subject was unable to identify the information being facilitated.

Because of concerns regarding claims regarding facilitated communication, the American Speech-Language-Hearing Association (ASHA) (1994) issued a position statement on facilitated communication that reads in part:

> *When information available to facilitators is controlled and objective evaluation methods are used, peer-reviewed studies and clinical assessments find no conclusive evidence that facilitated messages can be reliably attributed to people with disabilities. Rather, most messages originate with the facilitator. Moreover, Facilitated Communication may have negative consequences if it precludes the use of effective and appropriate treatment, supplants other forms of communication, and/or leads to false or unsubstantiated allegations of abuse or mistreatment.*
>
> *It is the position of the American Speech-Language-Hearing Association (ASHA) that the scientific validity and reliability of Facilitated Communication have not been demonstrated to date. Information obtained through or based on Facilitated Communication should not form the sole basis for making diagnostic or treatment decisions.*

Recent research on facilitated communication has suggested that the initial claims for FC may have been overstated and that, in fact, there is little evidence that most persons with autism and other disabilities can produce independent communication through facilitated communication. On the other hand, there are questions about the validity of the research techniques used to evaluate FC. It is also possible that even if the initial claims for FC turn out to be untrue, the technique may help some students focus their attention and reduce off-task behaviors.

Those choosing to use facilitated communication should be very cautious, following ethical standards of practice, including informing participants and their families of potential risks and benefits. Facilitated communication should be used in conjunction with other validated methods of communication enhancement such as behavioral intervention or sign-language training, thus assuring students would be given the best possible opportunity to develop their communication abilities.

Summary

In this chapter we have seen that autism is a complex and still somewhat mysterious disorder. There are a variety of characteristics associated with autism, but severe impairments in socialization and in language appear to be most important. Many individuals with autism develop little or no spoken language. When language does develop, there are often oddities such as echolalia and pronoun reversal. Although phonological and syntactic development is relatively normal, significant impairments in the development of semantics and pragmatics are often found in persons with autism. It is very difficult to teach children with autism. However, the use of behavioral techniques and sign-language training have met with some success. New and controversial techniques such as auditory training and facilitated communication hold great promise but require more research before being used extensively.

Review Questions

1. List and briefly describe three characteristics associated with autism.

2. It has been said that some children with autism have stimulus overselectivity. What is this? How would a child with stimulus overselectivity act?

3. How could echolalia be considered functional?

4. Why do most experts on autism reject the theory that parents cause autism?

5. Describe three ways in which the early language development of children with autism differs from that of normally developing children.

6. Some researchers have found children with autism to have relatively good semantic skills, while others have found their semantic skills deficient. How can these apparent inconsistencies be explained?

7. Prizant claims that children with autism have a gestalt processing style. What evidence supports such a conclusion?

8. List two advantages and two disadvantages in using the behavioral approach to language intervention for children with autism.

9. Why has sign-language training been successful for some children with autism? Consider the characteristics associated with autism in answering this question.

Suggested Activities

1. Pronoun reversal is often considered characteristic of the language of children with autism. Yet, pronoun reversal theory is controversial. Part of the controversy is whether the problem is one of language or whether difficulty using pronouns reflects the cognitive problems associated with autism.

If you have access to an individual with autism, try to evaluate that person's ability to use and understand pronouns. You might try the following techniques:

Method: Assemble a number of pictures that show individual people and animals performing actions. These pictures should include boys and girls, men and women, and cats and dogs. If possible, include among these pictures photos of the subject with autism, as well as pictures of yourself.

Ask the subject to point to the correct picture as you say a sentence. Then, say sentences that describe the picture (e.g., *He is going to school; She is playing ball*). Be sure to include pronouns such as *he, she, her, his, I,* and *you.* Also, include other words, such as *the boy, the dog,* and so on.

Evaluation: How does the subject perform when pronouns are used? How about when other words *(boy, girl)* are used? Is there any difference in the response for people, as compared to animals? What do the results indicate about the ability of persons with autism to use pronouns?

Alternative: If you do not have access to an individual with autism, try this with a younger (4–5-year-old) and an older (7–8-year-old) child.

2. There have been a number of popular books written about autism—describing experiences both of parents of autistic children, as well autistic persons themselves. Read one of these books and discuss its author's experiences.

3. Visit a school or clinical program for persons with autism. If possible, observe teachers or clinicians working with autistic individuals. What kinds of intervention procedures are being used? What kind of results are being achieved?

References

American Psychiatric Association. (1994). *Diagnostic and statistical manual of mental disorders* (4th ed.). Washington, DC: American Psychiatric Association.

American Speech-Language-Hearing Association. (1994). Position statement on facilitated communication.

Baltaxe, C. (1977). Pragmatic deficits in the language of autistic adolescents. *Journal of Pediatric Psychology, 2,* 176–180.

Baltaxe, C., & Simmons, J. (1975). Language in childhood psychosis: A review. *Journal of Speech and Hearing Disorders, 40,* 439–458.

Baron-Cohen, S., Leslie, A., & Frith, U. (1985). Does the autistic child have a "theory of mind"? *Cognition, 21,* 37–46.

Bartak, L., & Rutter, M. (1976). Differences between mentally retarded and normally intelligent autistic children. *Journal of Autism and Childhood Schizophrenia, 6,* 109–120.

Bartak, L., Rutter, M., & Cox, A. (1975). A comparative study of infantile autism and specific developmental receptive language disorder. I. The children. *British Journal of Psychiatry, 126,* 127–145.

Bartolucci, G., Pierce, S., Streiner, D., & Eppel, P. (1976). Phonological investigation of verbal autistic and mentally retarded subjects. *Journal of Autism and Childhood Schizophrenia, 6,* 303–316.

Bartolucci, G., Pierce, S., & Streiner, D. (1980). Cross-sectional studies of grammatical morphemes in autistic and mentally retarded children. *Journal of Autism and Developmental Disorders, 10,* 39–50.

Bernard-Opitz, V. (1982). Pragmatic analysis of the communicative behavior of an autistic child. *Journal of Speech and Hearing Disorders, 47,* 99–109.

Bettelheim, B. (1967). *The empty fortress—Infantile autism and the birth of the self.* New York: Free Press.

Biklen, D. (1990). Communication unbound: Autism and praxis. *Harvard Educational Review, 60,* 291–314.

Biklen, D., & Schubert, A. (1991). New words: The communication of students with autism. *Remedial and Special Education, 12,* 46–57.

Bonvillian, J., & Nelson, K. (1976). Sign language acquisition in a mute autistic boy. *Journal of Speech and Hearing Disorders, 41,* 339–347.

Brook, S., & Bowler, D. (1992). Autism by another name? Semantic and pragmatic impairments in children. *Journal of Autism and Developmental Disorders, 22,* 61–81.

Cantwell, D., Baker, L., & Rutter, M. (1977). Families of autistic and dysphasic children. II. Mothers' speech to the children. *Journal of Autism and Developmental Disorders, 7,* 313–327.

Cantwell, D., Baker, L., & Rutter, M. (1978). A comparative study of infantile autism and specific developmental receptive language disorder IV. Analysis of syntax and language function. *Journal of Child Psychology and Psychiatry, 19,* 351–362.

Cunningham, M. (1968). A comparison of the language of psychotic and nonpsychotic children who are mentally retarded. *Journal of Psychiatry, 9,* 229–244.

De Myer, M., Barton, S., Alpern, G., Kimberlin, C., Allen, J., Yang, E., & Steele, R. (1974). The measured intelligence of autistic children. *Journal of Autism and Childhood Schizophrenia, 4,* 42–60.

De Myer, M., Hintgen, J., & Jackson, R. (1981). Infantile autism reviewed: A decade of research. *Schizophrenia Bulletin, 7,* 388-451.

Department of Education. (1991, August 19). Notice of proposed rule-making. *Federal Register, 56 (160),* 41271.

Eales, M. (1993). Pragmatic impairments in adults with childhood diagnoses of autism or developmental receptive language disorder. *Journal of Autism and Developmental Disorders, 23,* 593–617.

Eberlin, M., McConnachie, G., Ibel, S., & Volpe, L. (1993). Facilitated communication: A failure to replicate the phenomenon. *Journal of Autism and Developmental Disorders, 23,* 507–530.

Eskes, G., Bryson, S., & McCormick, T. (1990). Comprehension of concrete and abstract words in autistic children. *Journal of Autism and Developmental Disorders, 20,* 61–73.

Fay, W., & Schuler, A. (1980). *Emerging language in autistic children.* Baltimore: University Park Press.

Fein, D., Pennington, B., Markowitz, P., Braverman, M., & Waterhouse, L. (1986). Toward a neuropsychological model of infantile autism: Are the social deficits primary? *Journal of the American Academy of Child Psychiatry, 25,* 198–212.

Fein, D., & Waterhouse, L. (1979, February). Autism is not a disorder of language. Paper presented at the New England Child Language Association, Boston, MA.

Folstein, S., & Rutter, M. (1988). Autism: Familial aggregation and genetic implications. *Journal of Autism and Developmental Disorders, 18,* 3–30.

Fulwiler, R., & Fouts, R. (1976). Acquisition of American sign language by a noncommunicating autistic child. *Journal of Autism and Developmental Disorders, 6,* 43–51.

Goldfarb, W., Braunstein, P., & Lorge, I. (1956). A study of speech patterns in a group of schizophrenic children. *American Journal of Orthopsychiatry, 26,* 544–555.

Goldfarb, W., Goldfarb, N., & Scholl, M. (1966). The speech of mothers of schizophrenic children. *American Journal of Psychiatry, 122,* 1220–1227.

Hermelin, B. (1978). Images and language. In M. Rutter & E. Schopler (Eds.), *Autism: A reappraisal of concepts and treatment* (pp. 141–154). New York: Plenum Press.

Hermelin, B., & O'Connor, N. (1970). *Psychological experiments with autistic children.* London: Pergamon Press.

Howlin, P. (1982). Echolalic and spontaneous phrase speech in autistic children. *Journal of Child Psychology and Psychiatry, 23,* 281–293.

Kanner, L. (1943). Autistic disturbances of affective contact. *Nervous Child, 2,* 217–250.

Kauffman, J. (1989). *Characteristics of behavior disorders of children and youth.* Columbus, OH: Merrill.

Kaufman, B. (1976). *Son rise.* New York: Harper & Row.

Kaufman, B. (1994). *Son rise: The miracle continues.* Tiburon, CA: H.J. Kramer.

Konstantareas, M. (1985). Review of evidence on the relevance of sign language in early communication training of autistic children. *Australian Journal of Human Communication Disorders, 13,* 81–101.

Konstantareas, M., Webster, C., & Oxman, J. (1979). Manual language acquisition and its influence on other areas of functioning in four autistic and autistic-like children. *Journal of Child Psychology and Psychiatry, 20,* 337–350.

Landa, R., Folstein, S., & Isaacs, C. (1991). Spontaneous narrative-discourse performance of parents of autistic individuals. *Journal of Speech and Hearing Research, 34,* 1339–1345.

Layton, T., & Baker, P. (1981). Description of semantic-syntactic relations in an autistic child. *Journal of Autism and Developmental Disorders, 11,* 385–399.

Long, S. H. & Long, S. T. (1994). Language and children with autism. In V. Reed (Ed.), *An introduction to children with language disorders* (pp. 385–411). New York: Macmillan.

Lovaas, O. (1977). *The autistic child.* New York: Irvington Publishers.

Lovaas, O. (1987). Behavioral treatment and normal educational and intellectual functioning in young autistic children. *Journal of Consulting and Clinical Psychology, 55,* 3–9.

Loveland, K., Landry, S., Hughes, S., Hall, S., & McEvoy, R. (1988). Speech acts and pragmatic deficits of autism. *Journal of Speech and Hearing Research, 31,* 593–604.

Maurer, R., & Damasio, A. (1982). Childhood autism from the point of view of behavioral neurology. *Journal of Autism and Developmental Disorders, 12,* 195–205.

McEachlin, J., Smith, T., & Lovaas, O. (1993). Long-term outcome for children with autism who received early intensive behavioral treatment. *American Journal on Mental Retardation, 97,* 359–372.

McHale, S., Simeonsson, R., Marcus, L., & Olley, J. (1980). The social and symbolic quality of autistic children's communication. *Journal of Autism and Developmental Disorders, 10,* 299–310.

Oshima-Takane, Y., & Benaroya, S. (1989). An alternative view of pronominal errors in autistic children. *Journal of Autism and Developmental Disorders, 19,* 73–85.

Paul, R. (1987). Natural history. In D. Cohen & A. Donnellan (Eds.), *Handbook of autism and pervasive developmental disorders* (pp. 121–130). New York: Wiley.

Perner, J., Frith, U., Leslie, A., & Leekam, S. (1989). Exploration of the autistic child's theory of mind: Knowledge, belief, and communication. *Child Development, 60,* 689–700.

Pierce, S., & Bartolucci, G. (1977). A syntactic investigation of verbal autistic, mentally retarded, and normal children. *Journal of Autism and Childhood Schizophrenia, 7,* 121–134.

Prior, M., & Werry, J. (1986). Autism, schizophrenia, and allied disorders. In H. Quay & J. Werry (Eds.), *Psychopathological disorders of childhood* (pp. 156–210)). New York, Wiley.

Prizant, B. (1983). Language acquisition and communicative behavior in autism: Toward an understanding of the "whole" of it. *Journal of Speech and Hearing Disorders, 48,* 296–307.

Prizant, B., & Duchan, J. (1981). The functions of immediate echolalia in autistic children. *Journal of Speech and Hearing Disorders, 46,* 241–249.

Regal, R., Rooney, J., & Wandas, T. (1994). Facilitated communication: An experimental evaluation. *Journal of Autism and Developmental Disorders, 24,* 345–355.

Ricks, D., & Wing, L. (1975). Language, communication, and the use of symbols in normal and autistic children. *Journal of Autism and Childhood Schizophrenia, 5,* 191–221.

Rimland, B., & Edelson, S. (1992, June). Auditory integration training in autism: A pilot study. *Autism Research Institute Publication 112.*

Rutter, M. (1978). Language disorder and infantile autism. In M. Rutter & E. Schopler (Eds.), *Autism: A reappraisal of concepts and treatment* (pp. 85–104). New York: Plenum.

Rutter, M., & Schopler, E. (1987). Autism and pervasive developmental disorders: Concepts and diagnostic issues. *Journal of Autism and Developmental Disorders, 17,* 159–186.

Schreibman, L., & Carr, E. (1978). Elimination of echolalic responding to questions through training of a generalized verbal response. *Journal of Applied Behavior Analysis, 11,* 453–464.

Shapiro, T., & Fish, B. (1969). A method to study language deviation as an aspect of ego organization in young schizophrenic children. *Journal of American Academy of Child Psychiatry, 8,* 36–56.

Tager-Flusberg, H. (1981). On the nature of linguistic functioning in early infantile autism. *Journal of Autism and Developmental Disorders, 11,* 45–56.

Tager-Flusberg, H. (1985). Basic level and superordinate level categorization by autistic, mentally retarded, and normal children. *Journal of Experimental Child Psychology, 40,* 450–469.

Tager-Flusberg, H., Calkins, S., Nolin, T., Baumberger, T., Anderson, M., & Chadwick-Dias, A. (1990). A longitudinal study of language acquisition in autistic and Down syndrome children. *Journal of Autism and Developmental Disorders, 20,* 1–21.

Tanguay, P., & Edwards, R. (1982). Electrophysiological studies of autism: The whisper of the bang. *Journal of Autism and Developmental Disorders, 12,* 177–184.

Tiegerman, E. (1993). Autism: Learning to communicate. In D. Bernstein & E. Tiegerman (Eds.), *Language and communication disorders in children* (pp. 432–481). New York: Macmillan.

Volden, J., & Lord, C. (1991). Neologisms and idiosyncratic language in autistic speakers. *Journal of Autism and Developmental Disorders, 21,* 109–130.

Wetherby, A. (1986). Ontogeny of communicative functions in autism. *Journal of Autism and Developmental Disorders, 16,* 295–316.

Wetherby, A., & Gaines, B. (1982). Cognition and language development in autism. *Journal of Speech and Hearing Disorders, 47,* 63–70.

Wetherby, A., & Prutting, C. (1984). Profiles of communicative and cognitive-social abilities in autistic children. *Journal of Speech and Hearing Research, 27,* 364–377.

Wheeler, D., Jacobson, J., Paglieri, R., & Schwartz, A. (1993). An experimental assessment of facilitated communication. *Mental Retardation, 31,* 49–60.

Williams, D. (1992). *Nobody nowhere.* New York: Times Books.

Wing. L. (1971). Perceptual and language development in autistic children: A comparative study. In M. Rutter (Ed.), *Infantile autism: Concepts, characteristics, and treatment* (pp. 27–45). London: Churchill.

$$Chapter \quad 8$$

Language and Students with Hearing Impairment

Children with hearing impairments challenge us to consider both theoretical and applied questions about language and hearing. At the theoretical level, questions about the role of language input in language development and about the relationship between language and thought can be examined. At the applied level, there has been an ongoing debate about the best way to teach children with significant hearing impairments, about the effects of hearing disorders on academic and social growth, and about the extent to which children with hearing disabilities can (and should) be integrated into regular education classes.

This chapter examines these questions and others on language and hearing impairments and provides definitions and classifications of hearing impairments. The impact of hearing impairments on language and cognitive development and on academic and social performance is also examined. The chapter also includes instructional methods that have been used effectively with children with hearing impairments.

After completing this chapter, you should be able to:

1. Describe how hearing impairments have been defined and classified.
2. Describe the impact of hearing impairments on:

    - cognitive development
    - language development
    - educational performance
    - social interaction

3. List the advantages and disadvantages of various intervention techniques for children with hearing impairments.
4. Discuss the impact of otitis media on language development and school performance.

_____ **Case Study** _____

Student: John A.   Grade: 3
Sex: Male   Age: 9:5

Reason for Referral

John presently attends a special class for children with hearing impairments. Since he has made good progress in the development of communication skills, he is being considered as a candidate for inclusion in a regular education classroom.

Background Information

John is the second child of Mr. and Mrs. A. At birth, John was small, weighing 5 pounds, 2 ounces. John spent two days in an intensive care nursery, but his parents were told that he would probably have no long-term problems. Mrs. A. reports that John was often sick, running high fevers several times. Following one of John's more severe bouts of fever and illness at age 3, Mrs. A. began to notice some changes in his behavior. It seemed as if he sometimes did not hear things. He was slow to respond or did not respond at all. His speech, which had begun to develop, became harder to understand and did not develop as quickly as that of other children.

When John was 4 years old, he was taken for a speech and hearing examination. The results indicated that John had both a moderate, high frequency hearing loss and receptive aphasia. It was suggested that John use a hearing aid and begin speech therapy; however, John did not begin to use a hearing aid until entering school at the age of 6 because his parents were concerned about social rejection.

School Background

John's educational difficulties began in kindergarten. His teacher observed that he was often slow in following directions. When told to line up, for example, John seemed to move slowly, as if he did not know what to do. Although he excelled at physical games, he was shy and other children teased him. At the end of kindergarten, John was placed in a class for hearing-impaired children, because of his difficulty communicating with others and his slow development in reading.

John has made considerable progress in this class: His speech has become more intelligible. He has adapted to his hearing aid and can generally understand the teacher. Though he excels in math, John continues to lag behind in reading and writing. He has several friends among his hearing-impaired peers but has few friends outside the classroom.

Test Results

Audiology
John was recently given an audiological exam. He had a 50-decibel (dB) hearing loss in the right ear and a 60-dB loss in the left ear. These results suggests that he has a moderate hearing disability.

Speech
John's test results from the Goldman-Fristoe Test of Articulation indicated an overall percentile rank of 20. John had difficulty producing several consonant sounds in initial and medial positions, and he also had difficulty with consonant blends.

Aptitude

John took the WISC-III (a test of intelligence), achieving a verbal-scale score of 75 and a performance score of 105. Though he did not do well on the information and vocabulary subtests, he did perform well on the block-design and object-assembly tests. These results indicate that John has measured intelligence in the average range, with performance scores significantly higher than verbal scores.

Achievement

The *Peabody Individual Achievement Test (PIAT)* was administered, and John achieved the following results:

	Standard Score	Percentile Rank
Mathematics:	112	52
Reading recognition:	83	13
Reading comprehension:	84	14
Spelling:	70	2
General information:	99	35

The results of the PIAT indicate that John has academic achievement significantly below the norm in reading and in spelling. His achievement level in mathematics indicates an area of relative strength.

Conclusion

John is a 9-year-old boy with a moderate hearing impairment. His excellent progress in a self-contained class suggests that he may be a good candidate for inclusion in a regular education classroom.

Children with hearing impairments run the gamut from those with mild impairments to the profoundly deaf. They may have a disability that fluctuates, is stable, or gets progressively worse or which may be either hard to identify in the classroom or easily recognizable. With this much variation in the population with hearing impairments, it is essential that teachers have a clear definition of hearing impairment.

Defining Hearing Impairment

One way to define hearing impairment is by considering the **functional impact** of the disability, in other words, the effect of the disability on the individual. The Conference of Executives of American Schools for the Deaf (CEAD) adopted the following definitions to classify persons with hearing impairments:

- **Hearing impairment.** This generic term indicates a hearing disability that can range from mild to profound. It includes the subsets of deaf and hard-of-hearing.

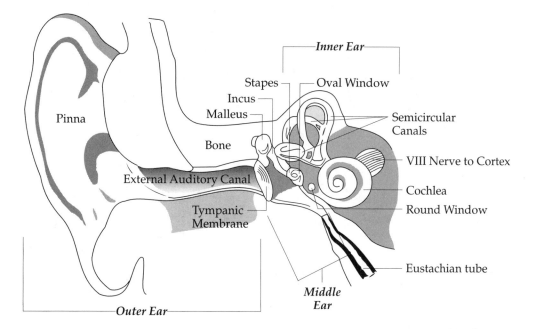

FIGURE 8.1   The Human Ear

Source: From *Exceptional Children and Youths,* 6th ed., by Haring/McCormick, © 1982. Adapted by permission of Prentice-Hall, Inc., Upper Saddle River, NJ.

- **Deaf.** A person who is deaf is one whose hearing disability precludes successful processing of linguistic information through audition, with or without a hearing aid.
- **Hard-of-Hearing.** A hard-of-hearing person has residual hearing sufficient for successful processing of linguistic information through audition, generally with the use of a hearing aid.

The most important distinction made by these definitions involves the ability to process language. Children who are deaf are *unable* to use hearing to process language. Hard-of-hearing children *can* process spoken language, although they may experience delays and differences in development.

Another approach to the classification and definition of hearing impairments is by the **type of hearing loss.** There are three types of hearing impairments (Diefendorf, Leverett, & Miller, 1994). **Conductive hearing loss** is caused by a problem with transmission of sound from the outer to the middle ear (see Figure 8.1). This hearing loss is usually mild to moderate. The most common cause of conductive hearing loss is **otitis media (middle-ear infection).** Conductive hearing losses are usually treatable but, if left untreated, may cause significant problems. **Sensorineural hearing loss** results from damage to structures that transmit sound from the ear to the brain and often involves auditory nerve damage. This condition usually results in moderate to severe hearing losses, and it is usually

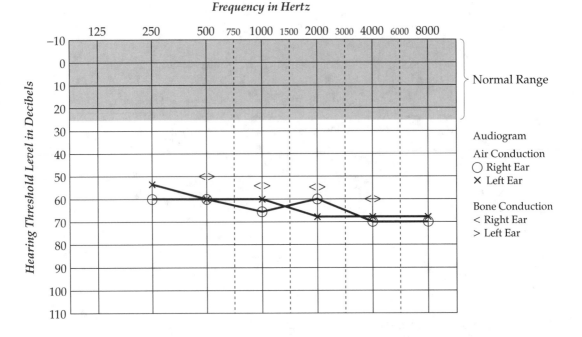

FIGURE 8.2 Audiogram Depicting a Bilateral Sensorineural Hearing Loss

Source: From *Exceptional Children and Youths,* 6th ed., by Haring/McCormick, © 1982. Adapted by permission of Prentice-Hall, Inc., Upper Saddle River, NJ.

not reversible. **Central hearing loss** is caused by damage to the brain resulting from many factors, including tumors, disease, or stroke. Central hearing losses are often difficult to identify because a child may seem to hear normally but may have problems in interpretation and integration of acoustic information.

The most commonly used approach to the classification of hearing impairments is to find the **degree of hearing loss.** With this approach, hearing impairments are classified according to the results of audiometric testing. The speech-language clinician evaluates the child's hearing by determining how loud a sound or word must be in order for the child to recognize it. The results are recorded on an **audiogram** (see Figure 8.2). The audiogram shows the hearing threshold (the point at which the child can identify sounds) and the pitch frequencies of those sounds.

When the results for several different types of audiometric testing are averaged, that average indicates how seriously the child's hearing is impaired. Knowing the child's level of hearing impairment allows for predictions about that child's ability to learn and interact in the classroom (see Table 8.1). For example, children with **mild hearing loss** (15–30 dB) have minimal difficulty hearing, though they may have some problems hearing faint speech. However, these children may have some articulation difficulties, language delays, and difficulty with

TABLE 8.1   Levels of Hearing Impairment

Classification	Hearing Threshold Level	Impact	Intervention
Mild	15–30 dB	Minimal difficulty hearing Some articulation problems Possible reading/writing delays	Preferential seating Visual cues
Moderate	31–60 dB	Delays in speech and language Difficulty hearing with background interference	Amplification Speech/language instruction
Severe	61–90 dB	Considerable difficulty with normal speech Significant delays in speech/ language Abnormal voice quality	May benefit from amplification Speech reading or sign language
Profound	91+ dB	Little residual hearing Reliance on visual/tactile cues	Manual communication or total communication

Source: Adapted from S. Shaw. (1994). Language and hearing-impaired children. *An introduction to children with language disorders.* New York: Macmillan.

reading and writing. It is important that teachers learn to recognize those with mild hearing disorders, since relatively simple interventions (such as preferential seating and the use of visual cues) may help these children.

Children with **moderate hearing loss** (31–60 dB) have more significant hearing and speech disorders. Many of these children experience significant delays in speech and language development, and they may have difficulty hearing in noisy environments or when speech is not directed at them. Children with moderate hearing losses may benefit from hearing aids and intensive speech and language instruction.

Children with **severe hearing loss** (61–90 dB) have considerable difficulty hearing normal speech and frequently have significant delays in speech and language development. Many have abnormal voice quality as well. Children with severe hearing losses will usually require some sort of amplification system. Therefore, early identification and intervention is important so these children can learn to utilize their residual hearing.

Children with **profound hearing loss** (91+ dB) can hear little if anything. They learn to rely heavily on visual and tactile cues, and amplification is usually of little help to them. These children are most likely to benefit from training in the use of a manual communication system (Shaw, 1994).

In addition to the degree of hearing loss, several other factors should be considered to understand the effects of a hearing impairment on a particular child. The **age of onset** of the disability is critical. Children who acquire hearing disabilities after the initial stages of language learning usually have less impairment than children whose disability is present at birth. **Age of identification of the**

hearing loss is also very important. Children who are identified early and who receive appropriate intervention services are usually able to progress more quickly than children who are not identified early. **Stability of the hearing loss** should also be considered. Children with fluctuating or progressive hearing losses may require different types of intervention than children with stable hearing losses.

Cognitive Characteristics

Moores (1987) described three stages in the development of understanding of the cognitive abilities of persons who are deaf. In the first stage, which lasted from the beginning of the 20th century until the 1950s, the prevailing notion was that persons who were deaf had deficient intellectual abilities. The development of intelligence testing in the early part of the twentieth century confirmed the assumptions about the intellectual abilities of deaf persons. Although there were inconsistencies in the findings, most researchers concluded that persons who were deaf functioned below the norm on most tests of cognitive skills (Pinter, Eisenson, & Stanton, 1941).

During the second stage of research on the cognitive development of the deaf, Myklebust (1960) examined the research on the intellectual functioning of people who are deaf and reached a different conclusion. He believed that persons who were deaf were not intellectually inferior to hearing persons but that they thought in qualitatively *different* ways. He claimed that deafness caused differences in perception that, in turn, caused persons with hearing loss to think in a more concrete manner. Myklebust's work strongly influenced educational practices for children with deafness. There was more emphasis on using concrete materials and examples and less emphasis on having these children use abstract thinking.

Since the 1960s there has been increasing evidence that persons with hearing loss are neither intellectually inferior nor do they think in different ways. As part of this third stage of research, psychometric testing has been reevaluated and reinterpreted, with the result that most researchers believe that the intellectual abilities of persons who are deaf cover the same range as those of the hearing population. For example, when Vernon (1967) reviewed a number of studies on the intellectual functioning of persons with deafness, he found that in a majority of the studies the deaf subjects equaled or exceeded the performance of hearing subjects. In those cases where the performance of persons who are deaf has been found to be below the norm, the results may have been invalidated by the testing procedures. In such cases, even when nonverbal tests were used, directions were often given via spoken language or test items may have assumed prior experience with spoken language.

Research other than psychometric-testing results has supported the conclusion that the cognitive abilities of persons who are deaf are similar to those of the hearing population. In a series of studies, Hans Furth and his colleague (Furth, 1973; Furth & Youniss, 1971) evaluated the ability of deaf children to perform Piagetian tasks. They found that children with hearing loss progressed through the same stages of development at about the same times as those Piaget had found in hearing children. However, they also found that development lagged at the latter stages of concrete operations and in formal operations. If true, these delays may be the result of the lack of spoken language or less opportunity to engage in abstract thinking.

So, what can we conclude about the cognitive abilities of persons who are deaf? It is likely that their intellectual abilities are similar to those found in the hearing population, that is, with some persons with hearing loss having higher-than-average intellectual skills, most falling around the norm, and a few ranging below normal (assuming no other disabilities are involved). There may be some delays in the development of higher-order thinking skills, delays which could result from a lack of spoken language or a lack of opportunity to engage in challenging problem-solving tasks.

Language Characteristics

Impairments in language are the most important consequence of deafness. But there is a great deal of variability in the hearing impaired population and a wide range of language abilities and disabilities. In this section we will review some of the research on the language development and language characteristics of hearing-impaired persons. We will look at spoken language first, then at manual language development. Finally, we will look at several factors that may help to explain the language impairments associated with significant hearing loss.

Spoken Language

The development of spoken language is usually delayed in children who are deaf. Some children fail to develop spoken language at all. Even children with relatively mild hearing impairments often experience delays in some aspects of language development.

Phonology and Speech

Most of the research on the phonological abilities of children who are deaf has focused on their ability to *produce* language sounds. For the most part, researchers have found that speech production is delayed in these children but is not qualitatively different. Horton (1974) pointed out that although the very early vocalizations of hearing-impaired and hearing babies are similar, by the time they reach the babbling stage (approximately 4 months) there is a significant change. This change is not in the quality of the babble produced but rather in the amount. At this critical stage of early language development, the vocalizations of babies who are deaf tend to decrease while those of hearing babies increase.

Studies of older children have also found delays in the development of speech production. Children who are deaf or hard of hearing have been found to make more phonological errors and substitutions than do hearing children (Markides, 1970; Smith, 1975). However, researchers have also found that children who are deaf develop the same phonological rules as do hearing children. These rules may develop more slowly, but when they do emerge they are similar to those used by hearing children (Oller, Jensen, & Lafayette, 1978).

It is important for hearing-impaired children to acquire phonological rules but even more important that these children be understood. Most people find the speech of children with significant hearing impairments difficult to understand. Intelligibility seems to be related to the degree of hearing impairment; that is, children with more serious impairments generally are more difficult to understand. However, several factors may affect the child's ability to be understood, one of the most important being the experience of the listener. Several studies have found that those listeners more experienced in interacting with persons who are deaf are better able to understand such speakers (McGarr, 1983; Monsen, 1983). Other factors that affect speech intelligibility are the context of the conversation and the ability of the listener to see the face of the speaker (Monsen, 1983).

The research on the speech capabilities of children who are deaf or hard of hearing suggests that these children will have significant delays in speech development. These delays often result in speech that is difficult to understand, thus creating significant problems in the classroom. But, the research has also suggested that teachers and others who work with these children can help them to be better understood through seating them so they can be seen and by having listeners use context clues as an aid to understanding.

Morphology and Syntax
Word parts such as prefixes and suffixes are a rather subtle aspect of language and are sometimes hard to acquire—even for children without disabilities. In English, word parts are often unstressed, a situation making it all the more difficult for children with hearing disabilities to acquire these structures. Children with hearing impairments, not surprisingly have been found to be delayed in their acquisition of morphological rules. This is true of both children with profound hearing impairments (Russell, Power, & Quigley, 1976) as well as individuals with less serious difficulties (Brown, 1984). Although researchers have generally found that children who are deaf follow the same sequence of morphological development as do hearing children, their delays in development can be up to 6 years or more.

There has been a good deal of research on the syntactic skills of persons who are deaf. Most of these studies have found that these children experience significant delays, relative to hearing children. For example, Schirmer (1985) examined the spontaneous spoken language of 20 children between the ages of 3 and 5 with severe to profound hearing-impairments. The children were videotaped during a 1-hour play session. Analysis of their spoken-language production indicated that the children with hearing impairments were developing a syntactic-rule system similar to that of hearing children, but with significant delays.

Some researchers have concluded that these delays are so great that some syntactic structures fail to develop at all. In their summary of a series of studies of the syntactic development of persons who are deaf, Quigley, Power, and Steinkamp (1977) reported that many of the syntactic structures usually acquired by hearing children between the ages of 10 and 18 had not been acquired by most 18-year-old

TABLE 8.2   Syntactic Structures of Deaf Students

Structural Environment	Description of Structure	Example Sentences
Conjunction	Marking only first verb	Beth threw the ball and Jean catch it.
Complementation	Extra *for* Infinitive in place of gerund	For to play baseball is fun. John goes to fish.
Question formation	Incorrect inversion	Who TV watched?
Relativization	Object-subject deletion	The dog chased the girl had on a red dress.

Source: Adapted from S. Quigley, D. Power, & M. Steinkamp. (1977). *Volta Review, 79,* 73–84.

persons who are deaf. Quigley et al. also noted that persons who are deaf produce unique syntactic structures that are rarely if ever produced by hearing subjects. For example, they place the negative marker *(no)* outside the sentence, as in, *Beth made candy no* (for other examples, see Table 8.2). These structures appear to be rule based, since they are used consistently. Quigley et al. suggested adapting reading materials for those who are deaf to include these unique syntactic structures, to facilitate their reading. This would be a difficult and time-consuming task. Alternatively, teachers who are aware that hearing-impaired children may produce unusual syntactic structures can be alert for these constructions and can point out to the children how their language differs from that of standard English.

So, are children who are deaf *delayed* in their development of syntax or is their language *different* from the norm? This is not an easy question to answer. One reason is that researchers have used different methods to study the language development of persons who are deaf. Schirmer's study examined spontaneous spoken language. The Quigley et al. studies gave deaf children a paper-and-pencil test of syntactic skills. Still other studies have analyzed written language samples. Despite these methodology limitations, teachers and other educators can expect that most children with serious hearing impairments will be delayed in their development of syntax. Some structures may not develop at all, while some structures may be unique to children with hearing impairments.

Semantic and Pragmatic Development
Research on the emergence of semantic and pragmatic functions in young children with hearing impairment has typically found that pragmatic functions are more fully developed. Skarakis and Prutting (1977), for example, studied the spoken language of four children with hearing impairments (2–4 years old) who were being taught to use spoken language. They found their subjects using the same semantic and pragmatic functions as younger, hearing children. However, some higher-order semantic functions were not used by the children with hearing impairment. Similarly, in their study of 12 children with severe and profound hearing impairments, Curtiss, Prutting, and Lowell (1979) found that pragmatic development was very similar to that of hearing children, while semantic devel-

opment lagged far behind. Curtiss et al. attribute their results to the fact that their subjects were primarily using gesture to communicate. They note that it is very difficult to use gestures to express semantic notions.

Studies directly examining the development of semantic skills in children with hearing impairment have also generally found significant delays and difficulties with receptive vocabulary (Davis, Elfenbein, Schum, & Bentler, 1986), with expressive vocabulary (Easterbrooks, 1987), and with the use of abstract language (Moeller, Osberger, & Morford, 1983). What causes these difficulties is not known. They may result from the fact that many children who are deaf have not had the range of experiences available to hearing children and that their educational programs have failed to challenge them with language activities and reading materials that enhance semantic skills. Regardless, semantic development appears to be a particular problem for children with serious hearing impairments and should be a focus of instruction.

We have already seen that some studies have found that pragmatic development is relatively intact in young children who are deaf. Although the emergence of pragmatic functions may be delayed, the sequence of development is similar to that of hearing children. In a recent study, Nicolas, Geers, and Kozak (1994) looked at the use of communicative functions by young (2-year-old) children with hearing impairments compared to two control groups—one matched for chronological age, the other matched for language ability. The researchers found that the children with hearing impairments lagged well behind their same-age hearing peers but were actually ahead of the language-age-matched group. In other words, although they were delayed in the development of communicative functions, children with hearing impairments were ahead of where they should be for their level of language development. The authors suggested that these results may have been due to the fact that the subjects with hearing impairments participated in an educational program that emphasized communicative interaction.

What about later pragmatic development? There is really very little research on this. One reason is that many persons who are deaf develop little, if any, spoken language. Therefore, they have little opportunity to develop the elusive rules of pragmatics.

This brief review of the spoken-language development of persons who are deaf suggests that significant delays, as well as some language differences, can be expected. There may be several causes of these language impairments. Obviously, the major factor is the hearing impairment itself. With limited opportunity to participate in oral-verbal conversations, children who are deaf do not have the same chance to learn the rules of language. This just seems like common sense. However, the relation between hearing impairments and language development may not be so simple. Some studies (e.g., Davis et al., 1986) have failed to find a clear link between the degree of hearing loss and language and cognitive impairments, while others (e.g., Davis, Shepard, Stelmachowica, & George, 1981) *have* reported such a link. Davis et al. (1986) suggest that factors such as parents' efforts, educational programming, and individual differences intrinsic to the child may have significant effects on the language and cognitive development of a child with hearing impairments.

Manual Language

So far we have focused on the development of spoken language in children who are deaf. But some would argue that this focus is entirely wrong, that manual communication (i.e., sign language), not spoken language, is the natural language of those who are deaf. To understand the language development of children who are deaf, the argument goes, look at their development of manual language.

Support for the claim that manual language is the natural language of those who are deaf comes from studies of early communication such as that of Goldin-Meadow and Feldman (1977), who videotaped interaction between hearing parents and their children with hearing impairment. The parents were selected for the study because they had decided that their child should not acquire a manual sign language. Therefore, the children were attending an educational program that emphasized spoken language. Yet, when the children were observed interacting with their parents, the researchers found something quite amazing. These children had acquired a number of gestures that could be called signs. They used these gestures consistently and even combined them into "multiword" phrases. Even more surprising was the discovery that the parents themselves, who were opponents of manual language, were unknowingly communicating via sign language. Through careful analysis of their videotapes, Goldin-Meadow and Feldman concluded that the children had developed the signs on their own, while their parents had unconsciously acquired signing from their children. So, it appears that even if they are not encouraged to develop manual language, children who are deaf will develop it anyway.

Researchers who have looked at manual-language development in children who are deaf have found the development following a course similar to that found in hearing children as they acquire a spoken language (Bonvillian, Nelson, & Charrow, 1976; Klima & Bellugi, 1979). Children who are deaf begin with a form of signed "babble," progress to a single "word" stage, then on to the use of multi-sign phrases. This is important information because it suggests that language development itself is not impaired in children who are deaf, but rather, the development of *spoken* language is delayed.

It is interesting that a number of studies have found that the English-language development of children who are deaf whose parents are deaf is superior to that of deaf children of hearing parents (e.g., Bonvillian, Charrow, & Nelson, 1973; Brasel & Quigley, 1977). It may be that parents who are deaf are more accepting of their deaf child or that early exposure to a manual language sets the stage for acquiring a second (English) language. Geers and Schick (1988) suggest that the *type* of language used by parents (manual or English) is not as important as the opportunity to receive language stimulation. This is an important point for teachers who work with children who are deaf. If Geers and Schick are right, giving children who are deaf the opportunity to engage in language interaction—whether with spoken or manual language—may be most important.

Research on the language development of children who are deaf has led to several important findings. First, spoken-language delays and even some language *differences* are characteristic of most children who are deaf. However, these delays are *not* found when manual-language development is observed. Therefore, while hearing impairment is clearly an important contributing factor to impairments in spoken-language development, teachers must recognize other contributing factors (such as parental input and educational programming) as important, as well. Perhaps the most important consideration is that language needs *stimulation.* When children are exposed to a rich language environment and given the opportunity to interact, they are more likely to develop language skills.

Educational Performance

Since cognitive ability and language development (with the exception of spoken language) is intact in most children with hearing impairments, there is no reason to expect that their educational performance should be below normal. Yet, study after study has found the academic achievement of children who are deaf to be below that of hearing children. In one of the most comprehensive studies, Gentile (1972) reported the results of standardized testing of 16,908 students who were deaf. Gentile found that the academic achievement of these students was generally below that of hearing children and that the gap increased with age. At age 8, the children who were deaf were only slightly behind their hearing peers in paragraph comprehension and in arithmetic computation. But by age 11 the gap had widened to about 3 years for paragraph comprehension and 2 years for math computation. The average level of math-computation achievement for 17-year-olds was 6 years below the norm, while their average for paragraph comprehension was 8 years below. Other studies (e.g., Davis et al., 1981; Davis et al., 1986; Phelps & Branyan, 1990) have found that the educational performance of students with moderate to severe hearing impairments is below that of hearing students, especially in reading and language arts.

Reading

The reading achievement of students who are deaf is an area of particular concern. Most of the studies cited above found significantly poorer performance on reading tests than on math tests. Reading comprehension seems to be a particular problem. In fact one study (Trybus & Karchmer, 1977) reported that more than half of a sample of 20-year-old persons with hearing loss had a median reading comprehension grade level of 4.5. They also found that the average gain in reading scores was only .3 grade equivalents per year at all age levels for students who were deaf. Because of findings such as these, reading was identified as a major area of concern by the Commission on Education of the Deaf (COED) in their report to the president and Congress in 1988.

Geers and Moog (1989) reported the results of a study of the reading achievement of children with hearing impairments who were educated in a program emphasizing the development of spoken language. In contrast to the general finding that reading is significantly impaired in students who are deaf, their study showed the mean reading level of these 16- and 17-year-old students was at grade

8. Moreover, some 30 percent of the sample had reading skills at or above the tenth-grade level. The authors claimed that development of residual hearing was the primary factor that accounted for these favorable results, but they acknowledged that other factors (such as the high nonverbal intelligence of their students and parents' high socioeconomic status) may have also contributed to the results.

Writing

Writing is another area of concern for students who are deaf. Difficulties in written language are well documented (see Moores, 1987; Yoshinaga-Itano, 1986; Quigley & Paul, 1990). Typically, the writing of students who are deaf is shorter and less complex than that of hearing students. In addition these students make more errors in their writing, errors that include using unnecessary words, omitting essential words, substituting the wrong word, and using incorrect word order (Quigley & Paul, 1990). According to Quigley and Paul (1990), there is no evidence that the written language of students with hearing impairments has improved significantly in the last several decades.

What accounts for the poor educational performance of these students? One factor that has been suggested is the severity of the hearing impairment itself. For example, the Davis et al. (1981) study mentioned previously examined the standardized test scores for academic achievement, as well as intelligence and language development, of more than a thousand children whose hearing impairments ranged from mild to severe. The authors found that the academic achievement of children with mild hearing impairments did not differ significantly from the norm. However, children with more severe hearing impairments (greater than 50 dB) exhibited significant achievement problems that increased with age. However, when Davis et al. (1986) did a more intensive study of the academic achievement of 40 children who differed in the severity of their hearing impairments, they found that the degree of hearing impairment had little to do with the test results. All of their subjects tested below the norm of hearing children on tests of vocabulary and reading but scored close to the norm for math achievement. Degree of hearing impairment was not highly related to academic achievement, although there was a great deal of variation in academic performance among the individuals in their study. The authors concluded that even minimal hearing loss can cause difficulty with academic achievement.

If the degree of hearing impairment is not the critical factor in explaining the academic-achievement difficulties of students with hearing impairments, what is? Two factors appear to be critical, the first of which is language ability. In the Davis et al. (1986) study, the best predictor of academic achievement was verbal IQ score. Students with higher verbal IQ tended to do better on academic tasks. It is interesting to note that in this study, the degree of hearing impairment was not significantly related to verbal IQ. In other words, degree of hearing impairment alone does not explain language development. Other factors, such as early and consistent exposure to language and the type of language training the child has received, are also important. The second critical factor that might help in understanding the achievement difficulties of children with hearing impairments is the educational program. La Sasso (1983) and Wilbur (1977) have suggested that deficiencies in educational programs for persons who are deaf may be an important contributor to the academic difficulties of these students. Moores (1992) has pointed out that children who are deaf spend less time than hearing children do on academic subject matter. He cautions that magic solutions to this problem are not likely. The answer, he says, is that "teachers and children must work harder on academic tasks" (p. 3).

Research on the academic achievement of students who are deaf can be viewed in two ways. The pessimistic view is that despite years of effort, the academic achievement of these students has not significantly improved. Children who are deaf still struggle with reading and writing, and the gap between their performance and that of hearing children generally widens with time. The optimistic view is that the factors that appear to cause these academic deficiencies also appear to be subject to remediation. Early intervention, consistent language development, and appropriate educational programs can make a difference. In the next section we will take a look at some of the educational interventions that have been developed for children with hearing impairments.

Educational Programs

Although there is general agreement that appropriate educational intervention is essential for children who are deaf, there continues to be a lack of consensus as to what constitutes an appropriate education. For decades there has been a raging debate over the best way to enhance language development. Now there is a new debate about where children who are deaf should be educated. In this section we will examine three aspects of educational programming for these children: language instruction, technological innovations, and educational placement.

Language Instruction—The Great Debate

In her review of the history of U.S. educational programs for persons who are deaf, Lou (1988) divided the history into four periods. In the first period (1817–1860) manual-language programs were established. In 1815 Thomas Gallaudet had traveled to Europe to learn about the instructional methods developed there for persons who are deaf. It was his intention to visit both programs emphasizing the development of spoken language and those employing sign language. But, denied access to oral schools, he observed only French schools that emphasized sign language. When he returned to the United States he established the American School for the Deaf in Hartford, Connecticut. This school became the model for education for people who are deaf in the United States. Since there was no instruction in spoken language, there was complete reliance on sign language for communication. In the first half of the nineteenth century, a significant proportion of the teachers at this and other such schools were themselves deaf.

By the middle part of the century, however, there was a growing interest in the oral approach to language development for people with hearing impairments.

According to Lou, among the causes of this interest were reports by Horace Mann about the wonderful results European schools for people who are deaf were achieving with the oral approach. By 1867 the first schools emphasizing the oral approach were established in the United States. Meanwhile, even advocates of the manual approach, such as Edward M. Gallaudet (the son of Thomas Gallaudet), were suggesting that oral methods of instruction, such as lipreading and articulation instruction, should be included in the curriculums of manual-based schools. Another strong and influential supporter of the oral-instruction approach was Alexander Graham Bell. Bell opposed any use of sign language, believing that use of it interfered with the development of spoken language.

By the end of the nineteenth century the "oralists" had won. Both in the United States and around the world, oral programs predominated. For this reason, Lou called the period from 1900 to 1960, "the period of oral domination" (p. 86). More and more schools for people who were deaf used spoken English as the basis of instruction in their programs. Most schools discouraged students from using manual language. Some even punished students who dared to communicate through sign language. Gallaudet, who had earlier sought to include oral instruction in manual training programs, now argued for the need to retain sign language. One of the unfortunate side effects of the dominance of oral programs was the parallel reduction in the number of teachers who were deaf. In fact, discrimination against these teachers grew to the point where in the 1920s Gallaudet College actively discouraged students who were deaf from pursuing teaching careers.

Since 1960 the tide has again turned away from oral only programs. Now many educators advocate programs that include both oral and manual methods for teaching persons who are deaf. This new approach, called *total communication,* is actually not that dissimilar to what E. M. Gallaudet was suggesting in the latter part of the nineteenth century. Two developments have contributed to the ascendancy of total communication as the preferred language-instruction method for persons who are deaf. First, American Sign Language (ASL) has become accepted as a language in its own right. Today, most linguists acknowledge that although ASL has a syntactic structure all its own, it is a viable language. With the acceptance of ASL has come a recognition by many that manual language is the natural language of individuals who are deaf. The second development contributing to the rising acceptance of total communication results from research in the 1960s and 1970s reporting that children who were deaf who had parents who were deaf outperformed children who were deaf with hearing parents on academic tasks (e.g., Stevenson, 1964; Brasel & Quigley, 1977). The implication is that children who acquire manual language as their first language have a better chance for academic success.

Today, all three approaches coexist in the education of children who are deaf—oral, manual, and total communication. The goal of oral approaches is to help the students become integrated into hearing society through development of skills in understanding and using spoken language. Oral programs use methods such as speech reading (lipreading), auditory training, and speech and language training to reach these goals, with mixed results. While some programs claim to

TABLE 8.3   Types of Sign Language

Sign System	Description	Advantages/Disadvantages
Seeing Essential English (SEE)	Uses ASL signs and invented signs with English syntactic structure	Uses some ASL signs English syntax should make transition to English easier
Signing Exact English (SEE II)	Modification of SEE I Closer to ASL Uses English syntax	Easier for ASL users
Signed English	Uses ASL signs in English word order	Even closer to ASL Still based in English syntax
American Sign Language (ASL)	Unique syntax Uses both abstract and iconic signs	"Natural" language of deaf persons Syntax differs from English

have high rates of success, many graduates have a difficult time using spoken language. Methods such as speech reading take a long time to learn and are limited in their usefulness.

The goal of manual programs is to enable children who are deaf to develop a first language as quickly as possible. Manual programs use either American Sign Language (ASL) or a manual language based on English syntax such as Seeing Essential English (SEE I) or Signing Exact English (SEE II) (see Table 8.3). The idea with SEE I and SEE II is that the children with hearing impairments will make more academic progress if they are exposed to a manual-language system that is based on the same syntactic structure as English. Many advocates argue, however, that ASL should be the mode of instruction, since it is the natural language of the deaf; English, if introduced at all, should be used as a second language.

Today, many education programs for persons who are deaf follow a total-communication approach. Quigley and Paul (1990) have defined total communication as "the philosophy or system which permits any and all methods of communication to be used with deaf children" (p. 25). In actuality, total-communication programs usually combine spoken-language instruction with manual communication. Two examples of total-communication methods are *cued speech* and the *Rochester method*. With cued speech, hand signals are used near the face to differentiate speech sounds that look alike in speech reading. The Rochester method combines finger spelling with speech. Total communication approaches can use any combination of spoken and signed language to enhance students' learning. While the logic behind total communication seems appealing, some have argued that total communication approaches can slow down the natural language development of deaf children.

The debate about the best approach to teaching children who are deaf is likely to go on for some time. At this point there is no one approach that addresses all of the problems faced by persons with hearing loss (see Table 8.4). However, total communication has emerged recently as the preferred approach to instruction

TABLE 8.4   Intervention Approaches for Persons Who Are Deaf

Program Type	Goals	Methods	Outcomes
Oral/aural	Development of spoken language Integration into hearing society	Amplification Speech reading Instruction in English Speech therapy	Generally poor intelligibility Reading may be better
Manual communication	Development of a first language Integration into deaf culture	ASL or other sign-language system	Good manual language development Generally poor academic outcomes
Total communication	Develop social, language, and academic skills	Uses both sign- and spoken-language development	Generally fair academic outcomes Some spoken-language development

because it combines the development of a first manual language with the instruction in spoken English that is essential for the development of reading and writing skills.

Technological Aids

Advances in technology hold promise for individuals with hearing impairments. In the past 20 years there have been remarkable advances in hearing aid technology. New developments in digital technology may mean that we are on the threshold of even greater advances. It is important for teachers and other education professionals to understand how to make the best use of these technological advances.

Amplification Devices

There are many types of amplification devices (hearing aids) in use today. No matter what their shape or where they are worn, all amplification devices work in essentially the same way. A microphone picks up sound and converts it to electrical energy. An amplifier boosts the electrical signal, which is transferred to a receiver that converts the electrical signal back into sound waves. A battery supplies the electrical energy needed to power the components.

Behind-the-ear hearing aids are the most common type for children. It is essential that the hearing aid, which is shaped to fit behind the ear, be fitted properly to avoid feedback of sound. Because of this the aid must be resized as the child grows. **In-the-ear** hearing aids are becoming increasingly popular. Although they are small and inconspicuous, they are powerful devices that can provide good sound amplification. However, they may not always be a good choice for young children because they have to be repaired and resized frequently. **Cochlear implants** are one of those recent innovations that hold great promise for individuals with hearing impairments. Cochlear implants work by directly stimulating the auditory nerve fibers, unlike conventional hearing aids, that merely amplify sound. A microphone is contained within a wearable speech processor that filters out background noise while enhancing speech signals. These signals are transferred to a receiver implanted in the mastoid bone behind the ear and then to electrodes that have been implanted into the **cochlea** (inner ear) which, in turn, delivers the sound to the auditory nerve. Some individuals with hearing impairments who have not previously benefited from hearing aids report that their hearing is significantly enhanced with cochlear implants. **FM radio hearing aids** are group amplification devices that permit a teacher's voice to be amplified for a group of students with hearing impairments. With this system, the teacher wears a microphone that transmits on an FM radio frequency being received in an earphone worn by the child. The FM system allows the teacher to move freely around the room and reduces background interference.

Amplification devices can increase the loudness of the sound heard by individuals with hearing impairments. In some cases these devices can also screen out nonspeech signals, thus reducing background interference. However, there are limitations to hearing aids. One problem is that hearing aids do not correct the problem of speech distortion. As Van Tasell (1993) noted, hearing aids may actually increase the amount of speech distortion. A problem specific to children is the need to refit the hearing aid as the child grows. In addition, when batteries grow weak and the devices need to be repaired, children may go for days or weeks hearing a weak or nonexistent signal. Some individuals, especially those with more serious hearing impairments, may have hearing that is little improved by amplification. Teachers who work with children who wear amplification devices should check to see that the device is being worn properly and that it is still operational.

Placement Issues

Where should children with hearing impairments be educated? In separate schools—as has been the case for most children with hearing impairments for most of the history of education? In separate programs within public schools? Or should children with hearing impairments be *included* in regular education classes? While the intellectual debate about inclusion for all children with disabilities has become increasingly strident, the issue is of more than theoretical importance when it comes to the population with hearing impairments. Indeed, the question of inclusion goes to the heart of the debate about the culture and education of persons who are deaf, a topic that has been an underlying theme for many years in the community of persons who are deaf.

The question is at once simple and quite complex. Should the goal of education for students with hearing impairments be to *integrate* them into hearing society to the maximum extent possible, or should the goal be to prepare children who are deaf to be contributing members of their own culture? Advocates of such a culture argue that most persons who are deaf can never be fully integrated and successful in a hearing society. Therefore, children who are deaf will do best when

---

BOX 8.1   Shelley: A Story about Inclusion

With a 95 percent hearing loss in each ear, she'd been diagnosed as "profoundly deaf" shortly after birth. So she had received therapy and special education from infancy on. With the support of two hearing parents, Shelley learned American Sign Language as a toddler and also had considerable therapy in lipreading and speech.

When Cathey Humble, a third-grade teacher, found out that Shelley would be entering her classroom she admitted that she experienced a brief period of panic. "Will I be able to meet this child's needs?" she wondered.

Mrs. Humble made sure that Shelley was seated so that she could always see what was going on in the classroom. She made sure that she faced the class, not the blackboard, when she gave directions. She learned to use more charts and pictures than she had been accustomed to using. She discovered captioned films and used these in a number of lessons.

Mrs. Humble found that, not only did Shelley do well in her classroom, but children who had learning problems began to do better as well. The children in the class accepted Shelley's deafness and included her as a classmate.

Source: Excerpt reprinted with permission from the September issue of *Learning,* 1989, Copyright The Education Center®, 1607 Battleground Ave., Greensboro, NC 27408.

taught by teachers like themselves, and using sign language in programs that respect the beauty of their particular culture. At its most extreme, this culture movement rejects the whole notion of deafness as a disability. Proponents of the movement argue that deafness is a disability only for those who attempt to learn spoken language. Otherwise, deafness is simply a difference (Solomon, 1994).

On the other hand, advocates for inclusion argue that *all* children, including those with hearing impairments, have the right to be included in regular education programs. Improved amplification technologies, increased use of computers, and other educational innovations increase the likelihood of success for students who are deaf, and by including these children in regular education classes, the argument goes, the stigma of disability will be reduced, educational expectations will increase, and children with hearing impairments will have increased opportunities for socialization (see Box 8.1). Stinson and Lang (1994) cautioned that although these goals may be appealing, research has not generally found that the social development of children who are deaf is improved by placing them in regular education classrooms.

As with all students with disabilities, it is not easy to find a solution to the question of what constitutes the *best* educational placement. Part of the answer lies in what the goals are. If integration into hearing society is expected, then inclusion, with appropriate support, would seem to be the best route. Alternatively, if the goal is integration into a culture for individuals who are deaf, then special programs will be necessary. Perhaps these programs could be offered in regular education settings to give both hearing-impaired and hearing children the maximum opportunity to get to know each other.

Otitis Media

We have seen that moderate to severe hearing disabilities interfere with the ability to understand and use spoken language. But what about milder hearing impairments? Do they also interfere with language development? This is the question posed by the occurrence of *otitis media,* commonly known as middle-ear infection.

Parents of young children sometimes experience being awakened in the middle of the night by howling children who are holding their ears. These children may have otitis media, one of the most common childhood illnesses. By 3 years of age about two-thirds of all children have experienced at least one bout of otitis media. During the worst phase of the infection, children experience pain, fever, and fluid in their ears *(effusion)* (Teele, Klein, & Rosner, 1980). However, some children do not exhibit these outward signs of otitis media at all.

During episodes of otitis media there may be a slight loss in hearing ability. This is of no great concern except when the child experiences frequent and long-lasting bouts of otitis media or when the infection goes untreated. Then the child may be at risk for more serious impairments. Since these fluctuating hearing losses occur just at the time when children are beginning to acquire language, there is concern about the effect of chronic, persistent otitis media on language development.

The research on the short-term effects of otitis media on the developing child has been mixed. Some studies (e.g., Wallace, Gravel, McCarten, & Ruben, 1988) have reported that children with otitis media experience delays in the development of expressive language. These delays, if they exist, may be caused by the hearing impairment that results from otitis media (Friel-Patti & Finitzo, 1990). Other studies have failed to find a relationship between otitis media and the development of language in the young child (e.g., Paul, Lynn, & Lohr-Flanders, 1993; Grievink, Peters, van Bron, & Schilder, 1993).

While the debate continues on the short-term effects of otitis media on language development, we should still be concerned about the possible long-term effects of persistent bouts of otitis media. Some studies that failed to find a relationship between otitis media and language development at an early age did find that as the children got older, their language development lagged (Roberts, Burchinal, Boch, Footo, & Henderson, 1988). Other research suggests that children with early chronic otitis media are at higher risk for learning disabilities and behavior disorders (Silva, Chalmers, & Stewart, 1986; Reichman & Healey, 1983).

The best advice for parents is to have their child examined by a physician if they suspect their child may be having ear infections. Otitis media can often be treated with drug therapies, but when this approach is not successful, surgery may be necessary. Teachers of younger children can help by looking for the symptoms of otitis media—frequent colds, fluid from the ears, unusual crankiness, and/or difficulty hearing. Teachers of older children should be aware that a history of chronic and persistent otitis media may be related to later problems with language-related activities, such as reading and writing. These children may benefit from additional practice on phonological analysis.

Summary

This chapter examined two major questions regarding hearing impairment: What is the impact of hearing impairment on language development, and what is the best way to help children with hearing impairments? As we have seen, hearing impairments can have significant effects on spoken-language development. Even so, the ability to develop a language (including sign language) remains intact. Despite intact cognitive abilities, children with hearing impairments frequently have a difficult time acquiring written language skills.

We have seen that there is a good deal of disagreement about the best way to teach children with hearing impairments. Advocates of the oral approach stress the need for children who are deaf to become integrated into a hearing society. Proponents of the use of sign language claim that this is the "natural" language of individuals who are deaf. Current instructional practices attempt to combine elements of both approaches.

Review Questions

1. Briefly describe the difference between the terms *deaf* and *hard of hearing*.

2. Fill in the blank with the correct type of hearing impairment:

   _____ results from damage to structures that transmit sound from the ear to the brain.

   _____ is caused by damage to the brain.

   _____ is caused by problems with transmission of sound from the outer to the middle ear.

3. Contrast the educational adjustments and strategies that would be needed for a child with a mild versus a severe hearing impairment.

4. In addition to degree of hearing loss, what other factors should be considered in determining the impact of a hearing impairment?

5. What conclusions can be drawn about the cognitive abilities of persons who are deaf?

6. While some researchers have argued that the syntactic development of persons who are deaf is delayed, others have claimed that it is different from the norm. Briefly review the evidence in support of each of these positions.

7. What evidence is there that sign language is the "natural'" language of persons who are deaf?

8. What factors might explain the generally poor academic outcomes of persons with hearing impairments?

9. Compare and contrast the goals, methods, and outcomes of both the oral and manual approaches to the education of individuals who are deaf.

10. Why should parents and teachers be concerned about otitis media?

Suggested Activities

1. There have been a number of popular books written about persons who are deaf. Two examples are *Train Go Sorry: Inside a Deaf World* by Leah Cohen (1994, Boston: Houghton-Mifflin) and *When the Mind Hears: A History of the Deaf* by Harlan Lane (1984, New York: Random House).

Read a book on this subject, and prepare a report that describes the experience of deafness.

2. Arrange to attend a cultural activity sponsored by, or largely attended by, persons who are deaf. This might be a theater play, a social event, or some other activity.

Report on your feelings about your participation in this activity. Did you understand what was going on? Did you feel left out?

3. Try to simulate the experience of deafness with one of the following activities:

- Turn off the sound as you watch television. How much can you understand about what is going on? How does your viewing differ from when you can hear the sound?
- Try lipreading. Put earplugs in your ears, and see how well you can read the lips of those around you. What problems do you encounter in doing this?

References

Bonvillian, J., Charrow, V., & Nelson, K. (1973). Psycholinguistic and educational implications of deafness. *Human Development, 16,* 321–345.

Bonvillian, J., Nelson, K. & Charrow, V. (1976). Language and language-related skills in deaf and hearing children. *Sign Language Studies, 12,* 211–250.

Brasel, K., & Quigley, S. (1977). The influence of certain language and communication environments in early childhood on the development of language in deaf individuals. *Journal of Speech and Hearing Research, 20,* 95–107.

Brown, J. (1984). Examination of grammatical morphemes in the language of hard-of-hearing children. *Volta Review, 86,* 229–238.

Curtiss, S., Prutting, C., & Lowell, E. (1979). Pragmatic and semantic development in young children with impaired hearing. *Journal of Speech and Hearing Research, 22,* 534–552.

Davis, J., Elfenbein, J., Schum, R., & Bentler, R. (1986). Effects of mild and moderate hearing impairments on language, educational, and psychosocial behavior of children. *Journal of Speech and Hearing Disorders, 51,* 53–62.

Davis, J., Shepard, N., Stelmachowicz, P., & Gorga, M. (1981). Characteristics of hearing-impaired children in the public schools: Part II—Psychoeducational data. *Journal of Speech and Hearing Disorders, 46,* 130–137.

Diefendorf, A., Leverett, R., & Miller, S. (1994). Hearing impairment. In S. Adler & D. King (Eds.), *Oral communication problems in children and adolescents* (pp. 141–164). Needham Heights, MA: Allyn and Bacon.

Easterbrooks, S. (1987). Speech/language assessment and intervention with school-age hearing-impaired children. In J. Alpiner & P. McCarthy (Eds.), *Rehabilitative audiology: Children and adults* (pp. 188–240). Baltimore: Williams and Wilkins.

Friel-Patti, S., & Finitzo, T. (1990). Language learning in a prospective study of otitis media with effusion in the first two years of life. *Journal of Speech and Hearing Research, 33,* 188–194.

Furth, H. (1973). *Deafness and learning: A psychosocial approach.* Belmont CA: Wadsworth.

Furth, H., & Youniss, J. (1971). Formal operations and language: A comparison of deaf and hearing adolescents. *International Journal of Psychology, 6,* 49–64.

Geers, A,. & Moog, J. (1989). Factors predictive of the development of literacy in profoundly hearing-impaired adolescents. *Volta Review, 91,* 69–86.

Geers, A., & Schick, B. (1988). Acquisition of spoken and signed English by hearing-impaired children of hearing-impaired or hearing parents. *Journal of Speech and Hearing Disorders, 53,* 136–143.

Gentile, A. (1972). *Academic achievement test results of a national testing program for hearing-impaired students: 1971.* Annual Survey of Hearing-Impaired Children and Youth. Gallaudet College Office of Demographic Studies, Ser. D, No. 9, 1972.

Goldin-Meadow, S., & Feldman, H. (1977). The development of language-like communication without a language model. *Science, 197,* 401–403.

Grievink, E., Peters, S., van Bron, W., & Schilder, A. (1993). The effects of early bilateral otitis media with effusion on language ability: A prospective cohort study. *Journal of Speech and Hearing Research, 36,* 1004–1012.

Horton, K. (1974). Infant intervention and language learning. In R. Schiefelbusch and L. Lloyd (Eds.), *Language perspectives-Acquisition, retardation, and intervention* (pp. 469–491). Baltimore: University Park.

Klima, E., & Bellugi, U. (1979). *The signs of language.* Cambridge, MA: Harvard University Press.

La Sasso, C. (1983). Reading comprehension of deaf readers: The impact of too many or too few questions. *American Annals of the Deaf, 138,* 435–441.

Lou, M. (1988). The history of language use in the education of the deaf in the United States. In M. Strong (Ed.), *Language learning and deafness,* (pp. 79–98). New York: Cambridge University Press.

Lowenbraun, S., & Thompson, M. D. (1994). Hearing impairments. In N. Haring, L. McCormick, and T. Haring (Eds.), *Exceptional children and youth* (pp. 381–410). New York: Merrill.

Markides, A. (1970). The speech of deaf and partially-hearing children with special reference to factors affecting intelligibility. *British Journal of Disorders of Communication, 5,* 126–140.

McGarr, N. (1983). The intelligibility of deaf speech to experienced and inexperienced listeners. *Journal of Speech and Hearing Research, 26,* 451–458.

Moeller, M., Osberger, M., & Morford, J. (1987). Speech-language assessment and intervention with preschool hearing-impaired children. In J. Alpiner & P. McCarthy (Eds.), *Rehabilitative audiology: Children and adults* (pp. 163–187). Baltimore: Williams and Wilkins.

Monsen, R. (1983). The oral speech intelligibility of hearing-impaired talkers. *Journal of Speech and Hearing Disorders, 48,* 286–296.

Moores, D. (1987). *Educating the deaf: Psychology, principles, and practices* (3rd ed.). Boston: Houghton-Mifflin.

Moores, D. (1992). Take longer steps faster, work more hours harder. *American Annals of the Deaf, 137,* 3.

Myklebust, H. (1960). *The psychology of deafness.* New York: Grune & Stratton.

Nicholas, J., Geers, A., & Kozak, V. (1994). Development of communicative function in young hearing-impaired and normally hearing children. *Volta Review, 96,* 113–135.

Oller, D., Jensen, H., & LaFayette, R. (1978). The relatedness of phonological processes of a hearing-impaired child. *Journal of Communication Disorders, 11,* 97–105.

Paul, R., Lynn, T., & Lohr-Flanders, M. (1993). History of middle ear involvement and speech/language development in late talkers. *Journal of Speech and Hearing Research, 36,* 1055–1062.

Phelps, L., & Branyan, B. (1990). Academic achievement and nonverbal intelligence in public school hearing-impaired children. *Psychology in the Schools, 27,* 210–217.

Pinter, R., Eisenson, J., & Stanton, M. (1941). *The psychology of the physically handicapped.* New York: Crofts and Company.

Quigley, S., & Paul, P. (1990). *Language and deafness.* San Diego, CA: Singular Publishing Group.

Quigley, S., Power, D., & Steinkamp, M. (1977). The language structure of deaf children. *Volta Review, 79,* 73–84.

Reichman, J., & Healey, W. (1983). Learning disabilities and conductive hearing loss involving otitis media. *Journal of Learning Disabilities, 16,* 272–278.

Roberts, J., Burchinal, M., Koch, M., Footo, M., & Henderson, F. (1988). Otitis media in early childhood and its relationship to later phonological development. *Journal of Speech and Hearing Disorders, 53,* 416–424.

Russell, W., Power, D., & Quigley, S. (1976). *Linguistics and deaf children.* Washington, DC: Alexander Graham Bell Association for the Deaf.

Schirmer, B. (1985). An analysis of the language of young hearing-impaired children in terms of syntax, semantics, and use. *American Annals of the Deaf, 130,* 15–19.

Shaw, S. (1994). Language and hearing-impaired children. In V. Reed (Ed.), *An introduction to children with language disorders.* New York: Macmillan.

Silva, P., Chalmers, D., & Stewart, I. (1986). Some audiological, psychological, educational and behavioral characteristics of children with bilateral otitis media with effusion: A longitudinal study. *Journal of Learning Disabilities, 19,* 165–169.

Skarakis, E., & Prutting, C. (1977). Early communication: Semantic functions and communicative intentions in the communication of the pre-school child with impaired hearing. *American Annals of the Deaf, 122,* 383–391.

Smith, C. (1975). Residual hearing and speech production in deaf children. *Journal of Speech and Hearing Research, 18,* 795–811.

Solomon, A. (1994). Defiantly deaf. *New York Times Magazine,* August 28, p. 38.

Stevenson, E. (1964). A study of the educational achievement of deaf children of deaf parents. *California News.* Berkeley: California School for the Deaf.

Stinson, M., & Lang, H. (1994). Full inclusion: A path for integration or isolation? *American Annals of the Deaf, 139,* 156–159.

Teele, D., Klein, J., & Rosner, B. (1980). Epidemiology of otitis media in children. *Annals of Otology, Rhinology, and Laryngology, 89,* 5–6.

Trybus, R., & Karchmer, M. (1977). School achievement scores of hearing impaired children: National data on achievement status and growth patterns. *American Annals of the Deaf, 122,* 62–69.

Van Tasell, D. (1993). Hearing loss, speech, and hearing aids. *Journal of Speech and Hearing Research, 36,* 228–244.

Vernon, M. (1967). Relationship of language to the thinking process. *Archives of General Psychiatry, 16,* 325–333.

Wallace, I., Gravel, J., McCarton, C., & Ruben, R. (1988). Otitis media and language development at 1 year of age. *Journal of Speech and Hearing Disorders, 53,* 245–251.

Wilbur, R. (1977). An explanation of deaf children's difficulty with certain syntactic structures of English. *Volta Review, 79,* 85–91.

Yoshinaga-Itano, C. (1986). Beyond the sentence level: What's in a hearing-impaired child's story? *Topics in Language Disorders, 6,* 71–83.

Chapter 9

Language and Students with Physical Disabilities

This chapter examines the impact of a variety of physical disabilities, including blindness, neuromotor disorders, and brain injury, on language acquisition and development. Although the conditions discussed in this chapter are quite different from each other, they have several factors in common. First is the fact that language difficulties can also exist in all these conditions, even though the physical aspects of the disabilities are most apparent and may be of primary importance. Second, in many cases intervention includes some type of augmentative communication device or system. Third, children with these physical disabilities are rapidly being included in the mainstream of education, making it even more critical that they have good language and communication skills.

By the end of this chapter you should be able to:

1. Discuss the impact of blindness, neuromotor disorders, and brain injury on language.
2. Describe the language characteristics of children with visual impairments, neuromotor disorders, and brain injury.
3. List factors that determine the impact of physical disabilities on language development and use.
4. Describe intervention strategies that have been found to be effective to help children with physical disabilities enhance their language and communication skills.

_____ **Case Studies** _____

"Joey Was Blind"

Joey came to school ready to learn. "Hi, Ms. Thom!" he called out as he arrived on the first day. "What's the plan for today?" His enthusiasm and eagerness swept over me.

Of course, I had a plan. Knowing that Joey would be in my class, I'd discussed his needs with his kindergarten and 1st-grade teachers over the summer. I ordered all his text-books in braille from the Commission for the Blind. My main concern, besides adapting my teaching style to meet Joey's special needs, was to give him every chance to build on the independence he'd already achieved.

Joey didn't need much help getting around. He could recognize every wall in the school by touch. And before school started, I'd given him a guided tour of the classroom so he could become familiar with the setup.

But I still had to be conscientious about giving Joey specific instructions. For instance, if I wanted him to get a book from a shelf, I had to give clear directions: "Take two steps forward, turn right, then go three more steps." I learned to describe items without focus-ing on their color or pattern.

Knowing that Joey used his hands as his eyes, I made every subject concrete in some way. This wasn't too difficult: Manipulatives and hands-on projects are standard fare in 2nd grade anyway. For science we planted seeds and tracked their growth. For math we used geometric shapes made of clay. For writing, Joey used his brailler (braille typewriter), which always sat on the right-hand corner of his desk. His aide then transcribed his work.

Joey could even play catch with the other children. His special ball had a beeper in it.

I wanted Joey to be able to work independently of his tutor and aide when he couldn't do what the other kids were doing. So I prepared cassette tapes with instructions for enrichment projects that he could do.

When I saw that Joey had to depend on his aide to read him my comments on his papers and show him his mistakes, I made some changes in the way I provided him with feedback. I learned how to use his brailler so he didn't have to rely on anyone to read the notes I wrote him. Also, I began putting pieces of masking tape over errors in his brailled work so he could make corrections without help. With a fruit-scented marker, I put stars on his tests so he would know without being told that he'd done well.

Throughout the year, Joey struggled with spatial concepts but distinguished himself in reading and writing. And his positive attitude continued to impress me. He believed that if he worked hard, he'd do well. And he did.

Alfonso: A Child with Cerebral Palsy

Alfonso is a 12-year-old student with cerebral palsy. When he was born, he suffered *anox-ia*, or lack of oxygen, for several minutes in a protracted labor. Although his intellect is unimpaired, Alfonso's motor and speech abilities were affected. He cannot walk or control many fine motor activities, and he requires assistance with self-care activities such as dress-ing and feeding. His writing with a pencil or pen results in scribbles and much frustration for Alfonso. His speech is intelligible only to family, teachers, and others who have known him for at least several months.

After being carefully assessed, Alfonso was provided with an augmentative commu-nication device called a Light Talker. This device is programmed with words and phrases customized to Alfonso's school and home environment. There are switches attached both to the lapboard on Alfonso's wheelchair and near the side of his face. Alfonso presses the switches with his hand or head to direct the scanning mode of the Light Talker and select what he wants to say. Then he activates the "voice." One of the greatest benefits of a syn-thesized voice for Alfonso is his ability to talk with friends during recess.

Technology also assists Alfonso in his schoolwork. An adaptation on his computer allows Alfonso to access word processing programs with his switch devices. Because of this technology, when other students turn in written assignments, so can Alfonso.

Alfonso attends a class where there is a reverse mainstreaming program: Students from an adjacent third-fourth grade class join Alfonso's class each day for activities that include reading, spelling, writing, and readers' theater. Alfonso will soon leave this class and move to an integrated fifth-grade classroom. Though excited by this prospect, Alfonso is a little frightened, too.

Ethan—A Child with Traumatic Brain Injury

Ethan was 7 years old when he was hit by a car while riding his bicycle without a helmet. Minutes after the accident, medics arrived and found Ethan with an abnormal flexion motor response and no verbal or eye opening responses. A cranial CT scan showed a large subdural hematoma over the left frontal, temporal, and parietal lobes. Ethan was taken to the operating room for removal of the hematoma and placement of an intercranial pressure monitor.

Ethan remained in a coma for 10 weeks. He then began to respond to the command *move your hand* by moving his left hand. He also followed objects placed in his field of vision, but he did not speak. He was transferred to the neurorehabilitation service, where twice daily he received physical, occupational, and speech therapy. Gradually, over the next 12 weeks, his motor control improved, although he had spasticity on the right side of his body. He began to walk with a leg brace and was able to independently complete self-care activities. Communication remained a major problem, as both expressive and receptive difficulties were evident. Cognitive testing revealed persisting problems, with scores on both verbal and performance subtests falling more than two standard deviations below the norms.

Ethan was discharged and enrolled in an outpatient rehabilitation program, where he received physical and occupational therapy weekly and speech-language therapy three times weekly. Three months later he returned to school, entering a self-contained communication-disability class with added physical and occupational therapy. At a 1 year follow-up, both his expressive and receptive language skills had significantly improved. His IEP for the next school year included continued placement in his communication-disability class, with mainstreaming in a third-grade class for 20 percent of the day and continued physical and occupational therapies.

Visual Impairment and Language

You were probably not surprised to know that hearing impairments can have a significant impact on language learning. After all, language is usually relayed by speech and, therefore, relies on hearing. But what about visual impairments?

What effect, if any, do impairments of vision have on language development? Is it possible that language abilities are actually *enhanced* in those who have visual impairments? There is a widespread belief that individuals with visual impairments develop heightened sensory abilities that enable them to compensate for their vision disability (Erin, 1990). Conversely, is it possible that visual impairments *interfere* with language development—causing delays and even developmental differences?

Defining Visual Impairment

Before examining the evidence on the language abilities of individuals with visual impairments, we first need to define this population. This is not such an easy task. Dekker and Koole (1992) note that the population with visual impairments is often divided into the **low vision** and **blind,** but there is a good deal of disagreement as to just how to measure vision. They go on to report that there are as many as 65 definitions of blindness in the professional literature. While disagreement among professionals about the best way to define visual impairments is likely to continue, the Individuals with Disabilities Education Act (IDEA) defines **visually handicapped** as "a visual impairment which, even with correction, adversely affects educational performance." For educational purposes, however, a child who learns primarily through tactile or auditory input is considered blind. For legal purposes, a person considered to be blind must have visual acuity of 20/200 or less in the better eye, after correction. A child is generally considered to be low vision if the child can benefit from the use of optical aids and environmental and instructional modifications (e.g., preferential seating or enlarged print) in order to learn.

Early Development

Studies of the early development of children who are blind have generally found that the timing and sequence of their language development is very much like that of sighted children, but there are some qualitative developmental differences. For example, Bigelow (1987) studied the emergence of the first 50 words in three congenitally blind children (age 9–21 months). She found that the timing and growth of these first words was quite similar to that of sighted children. In addition, Bigelow found that blind children tend to talk about the same kinds of things as sighted children. They use nouns and verbs that reflect their personal experiences. However, the specific referents named by blind children often differed from those reported in studies of sighted children. Not surprisingly, blind children tended to use words that described objects that could be heard (*piano, drum, bird*) or actually experienced (*dirt, powder*).

Other studies have discovered additional differences in the early language acquisition of blind children. Andersen, Dunlea, and Kekelis (1984) found that the children with visual impairments they studied rarely used overextensions or idiosyncratic forms of language. As children learn new words, it is not uncommon for them to incorrectly extend these words to other similar items *(overextension)* or to make up words *(idiosyncratic)*. Yet, Andersen et al. did not find this same phenomenon in their subjects. They suggested that blind children were learning words as a whole—via imitation—not experimenting with words, as do sighted children. The result, they claim, is that blind children "have less understanding of words as symbolic vehicles and are slower to form hypotheses about word meaning than sighted children" (p. 661).

The early experiences of blind children may influence the subtle inconsistencies in their language development. For example, while the motor development of blind children in the first few months of life is similar to that of sighted infants, later motor development of blind children tends to be delayed. Also, blind children are often slower to crawl and walk. Though there may be many reasons for these delays, including lack of visual stimulation and parental overprotectiveness, whatever the reasons, less movement means less opportunity to explore and experience the world. Limited experience may, in turn, lead to delays in the development of some cognitive concepts.

Bigelow (1990) examined the development of cognition and language in three children with vision loss. Mothers kept a record of the first 50 words spoken by their children, and the children were tested on ten tasks that measure aspects of the development of object permanence. Bigelow found that the beginning of word usage and the rate of word acquisition by the three subjects were quite similar to those of sighted children. However, there were some differences in the development of object permanence. One child who was not totally blind showed no differences from the development of sighted children, but two other children, both of whom were totally blind, were delayed in their object permanence development. Bigelow suggested that blind children may have more difficulty *decentering*—that is, taking the perspective of another person. Consequently, it takes them longer to develop *object permanence*—the understanding that things that are not present are not gone forever. Understanding delays in object-permanence development may help us understand why at least some blind children talk primarily about present objects and events rather than those in the past and future.

In addition to some motor and cognitive differences, some researchers have reported that interaction between blind children and their parents differs from that observed between parents and their sighted children (Kekelis & Andersen, 1984; Urwin, 1984). This should come as no surprise. After all, many of the early communicative exchanges between infants and their care givers are visual—baby looks at mom, mom smiles, baby gurgles. The baby who is blind lacks an important means of initiating interaction, while the mother is deprived of the subtle cues provided by her baby's eye contact. Blind infants *do* attempt to communicate, but their cues are often hard to discern and parents must be on the lookout for subtle hints that the baby wants to communicate. It is interesting to note that research has found that blind children whose parents were more responsive to them had better pragmatic language skills (Dote-Kwan & Hughes, 1994).

In their study, Kekelis and Andersen (1984) reported specific differences in the way that parents talk to their young blind children. For example, they found that parents of blind children used more commands and more requests for action,

TABLE 9.1   **Summary of Studies of the Early Language Development of Children with Visual Impairments**

Study	Subjects	Results
Bigelow (1987)	3 congenitally blind children (9 mo.–21 mo.)	Timing and growth rate of first words similar to sighted Types of words similar to sighted but specific referents differed Words used for objects that can be heard and touched
Andersen, Dunlea, & Kekelis (1984)	6 young children (9–40 mos.) with varying degrees of blindness	Rarely used overextensions and idiosyncratic words Seemed to be learning words by imitation
Bigelow (1990)	3 young children with visual impairments (9–26 mos.)	Delays in object permanence for the two blind children No delays for child with visual impairment
Kekelis & Andersen (1984)	6 children (12–36 mos.) Varying degrees of blindness	Parents of blind children were highly directive and initiated more topics

while parents of sighted children used more requests for information. Also, parents of blind children tended to label the objects with which their children interacted *(That's your belly)* while parents of sighted children provided richer, more detailed information about the objects. These differences, while subtle, may help account for the differences in early language development often found in blind children.

There appear to be some subtle, but significant, differences in the early language development of blind children (see Table 9.1 for a summary of the research). While the timing and sequence of their development is similar to that of sighted children, there are some qualitative differences. For example, children with significant visual impairments are more likely to talk about things they have *heard* and *touched*, they tend to learn words as a whole, and they appear to have delays in the development of object permanence—especially in children with more serious visual impairments. These differences in language development may be the result of more limited opportunities to experience the world and/or to deficient parent-child interaction. The good news is that these are factors that teachers and other education professionals can address in the classroom. Later, we will discuss some ways to increase the world experiences and communicative interactions of children with visual impairments.

Language Characteristics

Like other children with disabilities, children with visual impairments are a heterogeneous group. Many factors other than their disability affect their learning, including home environment, educational history, and opportunities for learning;

however, it is possible to make some generalizations about the language development of children with visual impairments.

Syntax

Generally, researchers have found few differences between blind and sighted persons in their development of syntax. Utterance length, a measure of syntactic development, has been found to be the same (Landau & Gleitman, 1985) or slightly shorter in blind children when compared to sighted children. (Erin, 1990). However, blind children use fewer different sentence types and tend to use a few types repeatedly (Erin, 1990).

Semantics

Earlier we reviewed research by Andersen and her colleagues and by Bigelow which found that the early semantic development of blind children differs in subtle ways from that of sighted children. Blind children talk about different things. They talk more about items that are immediately present in their environment and less about the past and the future. Erin (1990) reported that the children with visual loss in her study used imaginative play less frequently. One specific problem that has been frequently reported is in pronoun usage (Fraiberg, 1977; Erin, 1990). Blind children often confuse *I* and *You*.

For many years it was claimed that blind children developed *verbalisms* (Cutsforth, 1951), that is, they used words without understanding the word's meanings. When blind children used words such as *white* or *black* it was thought that they could not possibly understand these words, that they must just be parroting what they had previously heard. However, more recent research has found that although blind children may develop idiosyncratic meanings, their word usage is much like that of sighted children (Civelli, 1983). Although there may be some specific differences between blind and sighted children in their semantic development, these differences appear to be subtle and limited in scope.

Pragmatics

There has not been a great deal of research on the pragmatic language of blind persons, but what there is again suggests some subtle differences. For example, the research literature reports the use of idiosyncratic gestures (Fraiberg, 1977) and changes in body posture (Urwin, 1984) that may cause the listener to misinterpret what a person with visual impairment is trying to communicate. Parke, Shallcross, and Anderson (1980) also found some subtle differences in nonverbal communication when they compared the videotaped interactions of 30 blind children and a similar number of sighted children. Specifically, they found that many of the blind children smiled constantly (and inappropriately), nodded less frequently to signal understanding, and raised their eyebrows inappropriately. Any one of these behaviors might seem trivial in itself, but any taken together could cause some misunderstanding of communicative intent. Differences in vocal quality have been found as well. Children who are blind often speak in a loud, strident voice (perhaps because they are not sure of the distance between them and the speaker) and show less awareness of the need to adapt their speech to the

TABLE 9.2   Summary of Language Development of Children with Visual Impairments

Syntax	Utterance length same or slightly shorter (Landau & Gleitman, 1985; Erin, 1990)
	Fewer sentence types used (Erin, 1990)
Semantics	Less imaginative play used (Erin, 1990)
	Confusion of pronouns (Fraiberg, 1977; Erin, 1990)
	Idiosyncratic meanings used (Civelli, 1983)
Pragmatics	Idiosyncratic gestures (Fraiberg, 1977)
	Misleading body postures (Urwin, 1984)
	Inappropriate and less frequent nonverbal cues (Park, Shallcross, & Anderson, 1980)
	Less awareness of need to adjust speech to needs of listener (Freeman & Blockberger, 1987; Erin, 1990)

needs of the listener (Freeman & Blockberger, 1987; Erin, 1990) (see Table 9.2 for a summary of the research).

The effects of visual impairments on language, as we have seen, tend to be subtle but widespread. In particular, there are delays in the development of some semantic concepts (pronouns and words that require vision) and in several aspects of pragmatics. These language differences may have an impact on the academic and social development of children with visual impairment.

Implications for Teaching

Since there is a good deal of variation in the language and communication skills of children with visual impairments, teachers and other education professionals should be careful to observe and assess individual children. Do they have delays in development? Are essential vocabulary words missing? Do they have difficulty conveying their messages and understanding what others say? Freeman and Blockberger (1987) caution that some language differences may reflect an adaptation to blindness. Sometimes language differences may be caused by other disabilities the child may have, in addition to impairment of vision. When intervention is necessary, they suggest that strategies should focus on:

- helping the child to compensate for lack of visual stimulation through use of other sources of information
- helping parents learn how to interact with their blind child
- altering those behaviors which interfere with successful communication

Our review of the language problems associated with visual impairments suggests that the following areas may be appropriate targets for intervention:

- vocabulary development
- use of nonverbal communication
- voice modulation
- varying language for different communication situations
- pronoun usage

TABLE 9.3 Suggestions for Enhancing Interaction with Blind Children

- Use rich detail and variation in language input.
- In speaking, be responsive to the child's own interests.
- Present communication in a natural manner.
- Expand the child's messages. (If the child says, *Blanket*, the parent may respond, *Here's your blanket. It's soft, isn't it.*)
- Create a stimulating environment with items that appeal to the child's interests.
- Include the child in everyday routines.
- Inform the child about what other people are doing.

Source: Adapted from L. Kekelis and E. Andersen. (1984). Family communication styles and language development. *Journal of Visual Impairment and Blindness, 78,* 54–65.

One of the best ways to enhance language skills is to engage the child in communicative exchanges. Kekelis and Andersen (1984) provide suggestions that parents can use to enhance their interaction with their blind children (see Table 9.3). These suggestions would be useful for teachers to consider as well.

If teachers and parents create a stimulating environment where there is plenty of opportunity for learning about the world and for communicative interaction, it is likely that most children with visual impairment will develop good language skills. They may continue to have specific problems with words that rely on visual input (e.g., colors) and with nonverbal communication, but these difficulties should be minimized by effective teaching.

Effects of Motor Impairments on Language

Children with motor impairments such as cerebral palsy, muscular dystrophy, and spina bifida face a number of serious challenges. Their primary difficulties are in the areas of motor development and movement. Until recently these problems usually resulted in social isolation and significantly reduced opportunities for life experiences. However, with new technologies and new attitudes toward individuals with physical challenges, the emphasis today is on including these persons in society to the maximum extent possible. An increasing number of children with motor impairments are likely to be found in both regular and special education classes. With higher expectations and greater inclusion comes the need for enhanced language and communication skills.

Cerebral Palsy

Cerebral palsy is the most common motor impairment (Best, Bigge, & Sirvis, 1994), occurring in approximately 3 of every 1000 births (Bigge, 1991). It is a disorder of movement and posture, caused by damage to the brain. This damage often takes place during the birth process, but it may also be caused by trauma during prenatal development or by brain injury during early childhood. Cerebral palsy is a *nonprogressive* disorder; that is, the damage to the brain does not get

TABLE 9.4 Subtypes of Cerebral Palsy

Subtype	Characteristic
Hypertonia (spasticity)	Significant limitations to range of motion Muscles contracted Movements slow and jerky
Athetoid (extrapyramidal)	Involuntary movement of limbs Lack head control Flail arms and legs Writhing (coreoathetoid) movement
Ataxic	Difficulty with balance Overshoot when reaching for object
Rigidity	Simultaneous contraction of all muscle groups—extreme form of spasticity
Mixed	Combination of two or more types

Sources: Adapted from: E. Bleck. (1982). Cerebral palsy. In E. Bleck & D. Nagel (Eds.), *Physically handicapped children: A medical atlas for teachers* (pp. 59–132). Orlando, FL; Grune & Stratton.
J. Bigge. (1991). *Teaching individuals with physical and multilple disabilities.* New York: Macmillan.
E. McDonald. (1987). *Treating cerebral palsy.* Austin, TX: Pro-Ed.

worse over time. However, the associated motor problems may worsen if they are left untreated (Bleck, 1982).

Cerebral palsy can be divided into several subtypes according to two criteria: type of movement disorder and part of the body affected. Five types of movement disorders are commonly recognized. **Hypertonia** *(spasticity)* is characterized by significant limitations in the individual's range of motion. Muscle tone is increased and the muscles contract. Movement may be slow and jerky. Significant problems with posture can develop in this type of cerebral palsy. In **athetoid** *(extrapyramidal)* cerebral palsy, the limbs have involuntary movements. Individuals with athetoid cerebral palsy seem to have little control over their movements. They may lack head control, flail out their arms or legs when they try to move, or may have writhing (choreoathetoid) movements. Individuals with **Ataxic** cerebral palsy have difficulty balancing. When reaching for an object they may overshoot their target. Bleck (1982) described the walk of children with ataxic cerebral palsy as like that of a "sailor on a rolling ship at sea, with feet apart, trunk weaving" (p. 65). **Rigidity** is an extreme form of spasticity in which there is a simultaneous contraction of all muscle groups. Movement is very limited. Ataxia and rigidity are relatively rare disorders. Often several types of movement disorders may be identified in a single individual. This is known as **mixed** cerebral palsy (Bleck, 1982; Bigge, 1991; McDonald, 1987) (see Table 9.4).

Disabilities other than serious motor impairments may also be associated with cerebral palsy. According to Cruickshank (1976), between 50 and 75 percent of individuals with cerebral palsy have intellectual impairments. However, individuals with serious motor impairments are often difficult to test, and their intellectual abilities may be underestimated. Other disabilities associated with cerebral palsy include hearing loss, seizures, and visual impairments.

Speech and Language Impairments

Since speech production involves the precise control and coordination of a variety of muscle groups, it is not surprising that speech impairments are very common among children with cerebral palsy. One author estimates the incidence of speech problems at 48 to 49 percent of that population (Bleck, 1982). Persons with cerebral palsy may slur their words, sound like they are stuttering, speak in a monotone or a whisper, or speak in a slow, laborious manner (Meacham, 1986).

What is the impact of these serious speech disorders on *speech comprehension* and language development in persons with cerebral palsy? This question was posed by Bishop, Brown, and Robson (1990). In a series of studies, they examined the ability of 48 individuals with cerebral palsy to discriminate sounds and understand language. Half of their sample exhibited serious speech-production difficulties. The other half had no serious speech problems. They found that the group with speech impairments had considerable difficulty with a phoneme discrimination task that used nonwords, but did much better when real words were used. The group with speech impairments did poorly on a test of receptive vocabulary. However, there was no difference between the two groups on their syntactic development. After doing further testing, the authors concluded that individuals with cerebral palsy and speech impairments have more difficulty retaining meaningless strings of sounds in memory. The authors suggest that this problem may be the result of lack of opportunity to use spoken speech sounds. This may not seem like a significant problem, but Bishop et al. point out that this is the process children use when they are learning new words. At first these strings of sounds are meaningless. Only later do they become meaningful words. Difficulty retaining sounds in memory may slow down vocabulary acquisition.

On the other hand, the results of the research reported by Bishop et al. (1990) also indicate that despite limited opportunities to use language, individuals with cerebral palsy who also have significant speech impairments can develop structural aspects of language (e.g., syntax) much like other persons. This suggests that *language* may be intact for these individuals. Yet many, if not most, children with cerebral palsy appear to lag behind their nondisabled peers in language development. There are several reasons why this may occur. Most significantly, cerebral palsy is often associated with other disabilities. As we pointed out earlier, it is not unusual to find children with cerebral palsy who also have hearing or vision problems or who have intellectual impairments. We know that all of these conditions can adversely affect language.

Another factor in understanding the apparent language impairments of children with cerebral palsy is the way in which they are tested. Many tests of language require children to perform a motor movement. For example, the *Peabody Picture Vocabulary Test* requires a pointing response to a verbal command. Others tests ask parents or care givers to rate the observed performance of the child. Of course, these sorts of procedures may tell nothing about language comprehension. Cauley, Golinkoff, Hirsh-Pasek, and Gordon (1989) reported on a procedure they developed to more accurately assess the language skills of children with motor disorders. Children were shown two different pictures on screens simultaneously as a target word was spoken. An observer recorded which screen the child looked at in response to the word by noting the child's eye fixation. The results suggested that children with motor impairments seemed to be able to respond to this sort of testing. This kind of procedure may enable researchers to more accurately assess the language development of children with motor disorders.

Because of the variety of problems associated with cerebral palsy and the difficulties in testing children with motor disorders, it is difficult to be specific about the language development of children with cerebral palsy. Research mentioned previously suggests that many experience significant delays in language but that in some, language is intact. However, unless there is specific brain damage in regions of the brain that process language, there is no reason to expect that most children with cerebral palsy will have serious language deficits.

Other Neuromotor Disorders

Other neuromotor disorders, such as spina bifida and muscular dystrophy, can also affect language acquisition and development. *Spina bifida* refers to a group of conditions in which a portion of the spinal cord is not completely enclosed by the vertebrae in the spinal column. In some cases part of the spinal cord protrudes. In the most serious form of the disorder, *myelomeningocele,* damage to the spinal cord can cause sensory and motor losses. In addition, in about 80 percent of the cases, fluid accumulates in the brain, causing the condition known as *hydrocephalus.* If not treated quickly, hydrocephalus can cause mental retardation. Surgery can often correct the spinal cord abnormality in spina bifida, but some sensory and motor disabilities can remain (Bigge, 1991). *Muscular dystrophy* is a progressive disorder that produces weakness in muscles. Over time, the muscles waste away and children become unable to walk and talk. There are several forms of muscular dystrophy. The most common is Duchenne type which affects about one in 3500 children, mostly males, and begins in early childhood. Children may have problems with balance and in climbing stairs and eventually lose the ability to walk and sit up as muscle weakness spreads and muscles deteriorate. Children with muscular dystrophy usually live only into adolescence or early adulthood (Bigge, 1991).

Impairments in language and communication, in addition to the very serious motor problems, are also associated with spina bifida and muscular dystrophy. For example, children with spina bifida who also have hydrocephalus are frequently reported to have problems with semantic and pragmatic usage. One example of these problems is the "cocktail chatter" phenomenon. As reported by Tew (1979), this difficulty in pragmatics is characterized by chatty conversations that remain at a superficial level. On the other hand, studies have generally found that syntactic development is relatively intact. In a recent study, Byrne, Abbeduto, and Brooks (1990) attacked some of the long-held beliefs about the language disabilities of children with spina bifida and hydrocephalus (SBH). They pointed out that in most of the previous studies, the subjects with SBH also had mental retardation. Therefore, it was impossible to determine whether the language deficits were the result of SBH or mental retardation. They examined the language of seven SBH children who had IQ scores in the normal range and compared them to nondisabled children of the same chronological age. They found very few differences between the groups of children in their use of language. They found that their SBH sample of children responded appropriately to questions and stayed on task. Their language production was equal in sophistication to that of the nondisabled children. Byrne et al. concluded that the language deficiencies previously reported in the SBH population are likely the result of mental retardation, not spina bifida or hydrocephalus. Therefore, teachers and other education professionals should be careful about jumping to conclusions regarding intelligence or language abilities of children with one of these conditions (spina bifida or hydrocephalus). With newer surgical procedures and early intervention, many of these children can function quite normally.

Language and cognitive abilities can also be affected by Duchenne muscular dystrophy. Typically, researchers have found that measured intelligence is lower in children with muscular dystrophy, with language skills being especially low in younger children (Karagan & Zellweger, 1978). Dorman, Hurley, and D'Avignon (1988) reported mean IQ scores of about 87, with verbal scores lower than performance. In a more intensive analysis of 15 cases, Dorman et al. found that children with Duchenne muscular dystrophy can exhibit a wide discrepancy in their abilities. They found that six of their fifteen cases had very low measured intelligence and significant problems in reading, writing, and spelling, functioning much like children with severe dyslexia. The other children had performance levels similar to those found in nondisabled children. The implication of this research is that Duchenne muscular dystrophy may manifest itself in different ways. In some cases, language-based abilities are significantly impacted but in other cases remain intact. With time, however, most children with this disorder have increasing difficulty communicating because of the deterioration of muscles involved in speech production.

Implications for Intervention

Typically, intervention for individuals with motor disorders has focused on speech therapy. For children with cerebral palsy, speech therapy often focuses on developing the muscles used in eating and swallowing. Most children with neuromotor disorders at some point will need help with breathing, vocal production, and articulation. While speech therapy is important and should not be ignored as part of an instructional program, it can often be very slow to produce results and frustrating for both the child and the therapist.

In addition to their receiving speech therapy, children with motor impairments should be given numerous opportunities to engage in literacy-based activities and to communicate with a variety of people. Literacy-based activities may include listening to stories, watching movies or videotapes of stories, and using computer word processing programs that permit the user to write with a minimum of motor movement. It is essential that children with neuromotor disorders be involved in as many communicative interactions as possible. Teachers can facilitate these interactions through appropriate positioning. McDonald (1987) suggests that children with neuromotor disabilities be positioned so that they can see, feel, or hear the communication. If necessary, a mirror can be used so the child can read the facial expressions of communication partners, or others can see the child's face. In addition, by providing appropriate play materials, the teacher can also increase the possibilities for communicative interaction. In any case, it is essential that teachers encourage children with neuromotor disabilities to communicate with others and that the teachers themselves engage the children in communicative exchanges whenever possible.

For many children with neuromotor disorders, the use of augmentative communication devices will be an important option. When properly designed and used effectively, these devices can open up new worlds of communication to children who were previously unable to communicate. Chapter 13 provides more information about augmentative communication devices, but most important to this discussion is that the user be taught and encouraged to *use* the device for communication. Too often the child with an augmentative communication device sits idly in a classroom until called upon to respond. Children who use such devices must continually be encouraged to use the device to initiate interaction and to respond appropriately.

Brain Injury and Language

Traumatic brain injury is the leading cause of death and disability in children and adolescents in the United States (National Information Center for Children and Youth with Disabilities, 1993). Each year approximately 1 in 25 children receives medical attention because of a head injury. While most of these injuries are minor and leave no lasting problems, some result in significant impairments in motor, cognitive, and language functioning. Approximately 150,000 children a year suffer traumatic brain injuries, with the rate for boys almost double that for girls (Michaud & Duhaime, 1992).

The Individuals with Disabilities Education Act (IDEA) includes traumatic brain injury (TBI) as a separate category of disability. It is defined as:

> *An acquired injury to the brain caused by an external physical force, resulting in total or partial functional disability or psychosocial impairment, or both, that adversely affect a child's educational performance. The term applies to open and closed head injuries resulting in impairments in one or more areas, such as: cognition; language; memory; attention; reasoning; abstract thinking; judgment; problem-solving; sensory, perceptual, and motor abilities; psychosocial behavior; physical functions; information processing; and speech. The term does not apply to brain injuries that are congenital or degenerative, or brain injuries induced by birth trauma. (U.S. Federal Register, 57[189], September 29, 1992, p. 44802)*

As the IDEA definition indicates, there are two types of head injuries. *Open-head injury* (also known as *localized)* is characterized by a visible injury, often a gunshot wound. The brain damage is usually confined to one portion of the brain. *Closed-head injury* is caused by a rapid acceleration and deceleration of the head, during which the brain bounces around inside the skull. Closed-head brain damage is most often cased by automobile accidents, but can also be caused by falls and sports injuries (National Head Injury Foundation, 1989). This is the type of injury suffered by Ethan, the boy in the case study, while he was riding his bicycle.

Head injuries can cause a variety of problems, depending on the location and severity of the injury and the age of the victim. Symptoms can include:

- **Physical impairments:** speech, vision, hearing, and other sensory impairments; headaches, problems with coordination; spasticity and/or paralysis.
- **Cognitive impairments:** memory difficulties; slowness in thinking; problems concentrating; problems with perception and attention; problems planning and sequencing.
- **Behavior and personality problems:** fatigue; mood swings; anxiety; depression; difficulty with emotional control (National Head Injury Foundation, 1989; Telzrow, 1987).

In most cases, children with head injuries show improvement over time, but there may be lasting effects that can have an impact on classroom performance.

Language Characteristics

If a head injury affects the left hemisphere of the brain, there is likely to be an effect on language functioning. Children who lose language functioning as a result of brain injury are said to have *acquired aphasia*. In other words, they have lost some language functions that they had acquired earlier. Language difficulties resulting from traumatic brain injury can involve expressive language, receptive language, or both (Michaud & Duhaime, 1992). Some children with brain injury experience significant language losses, while others show little, if any, impairment (Cooper & Flowers, 1987).

There has been a big (and ongoing) debate among researchers about the effects of brain injury on language and about recovery of language skills. Briefly, the debate centers on the issues of *laterality* and *plasticity*. Lenneberg (1967), among others, argued that cerebral dominance was not established at birth but developed over time. He argued that children are better able to recover their language abilities after damage to the brain because uninjured areas of the brain take over the function of the damaged area (plasticity). While it is true that children seem more capable of recovery of function than adults, more recent research (e.g., Kinsbourne & Hiscock, 1977) has suggested that cerebral dominance is largely established at birth.

Whatever the reason, children with brain injuries do frequently show marked improvements in their language abilities (Satz & Bullard-Bates, 1981). Campbell and Dollaghan (1990) investigated the phenomenon of language recovery by evaluating the language abilities of nine brain-injured children during the 13 months following their injuries. When first tested, the brain-injured children scored far below a group of nondisabled children matched for age and gender on all measures of expressive language. However, by the end of the 13-month period, the groups differed on only one measure—total number of utterances. There were, however, big differences in the language recovery of each of the brain-injured children. Two of the children showed no significant expressive language problems, even at the first session. Two other children eventually caught up to the nondisabled children their own age. But five of the brain-injured children never fully recovered their language skills, although they did show improvements. The results of this study show just how difficult it is to make generalizations about the recovery of children with brain injuries.

Specific Language Disorders

Though there is variability among brain-injured children, there are certain kinds of language impairments that are more common in this population. For example, Ewing-Cobbs, Fletcher, Landry, and Levin (1985) found that most of a group of children with moderate to severe closed-head injury had little trouble understanding individual words, but many had difficulty understanding syntactically complex sentences. In their study of 15 children with acquired aphasia, Cooper and Flowers (1987) found that the greatest language deficiencies were in naming pictures, understanding paragraphs, and making word associations. They noted that no one pattern of language problems characterized their subjects, but that difficulties in later developing syntactic and metalinguistic abilities were most likely to occur. Reading and writing can also be impaired in children with brain injury.

Teachers can expect children with brain injuries to have a variety of language impairments. Some may have no obvious problems; others have subtle language impairments that may only show up in conversation or in reading and writing; still others may have significant difficulties, with word retrieval, speech fluency, and syntactic skills affected.

Intervention

The best intervention for head injury is prevention. Most head trauma is preventable. Use of seat belts, bicycle helmets, and appropriate sports equipment can reduce the incidence of head injury, as can efforts to reduce drunk driving and child abuse. Despite efforts aimed at prevention and education about brain injuries, they continue to occur at high rates.

With the high frequency of brain trauma and the trend to inclusion of children with disabilities in regular education settings, most teachers are likely to have a brain-injured child in their classroom at some time. A child's returning to school following a head injury can be very difficult for the child, as well as the teacher. As Douglas Harrington (1990) put it, "The dilemma of returning to school after a traumatic brain injury is that life is just not the same" (p. 479). There can be changes in thinking, in behavior, in language, and in academic skills such as reading and writing. The child may have physical problems such as headaches and difficulty staying alert.

Telzrow (1987) has suggested ten elements that should be part of an educational program for children with traumatic brain injury. These include:

- **Maximally controlled environment:** The child should begin in a self-contained classroom, becoming gradually integrated into other school activities.
- **Low pupil-teacher ratio:** It may be necessary to provide a classroom aide or other assistant to work with the child.
- **Intensive and repetitive instruction:** The brain-injured child often needs more time to learn. Reducing nonacademic activities and lengthening the school year can provide more learning time.
- **Emphasis on process:** The child may need to be helped in learning *how* to learn. Instruction should include help in sustaining attention and on memory.
- **Behavioral programming:** Instructional strategies that use task analysis and careful measurement of progress have been found successful.
- **Integrated instructional therapies:** Integrate allied therapies such as speech and physical therapy into the student's primary instructional setting to facilitate generalization and transfer of skills.
- **Simulation experiences:** Use simulations to enable the child to transfer skills to a new setting.
- **Cuing, fading, and shadowing:** Students may require cues to respond, which should be faded as soon as possible. When shadowing, the teacher closely monitors the child attempting a new task or moving to a new environment.
- **Readjustment counseling:** This may help the child adjust to their new environment and abilities.
- **Home-school liaison:** It is essential to build and maintain a strong link between parents and the school.

For brain-injured children with language impairments, a range of services and methods may be necessary. Some will need speech and language therapy; some others may need more help than most children do when learning (or relearning) to read and write; still others will need augmentative communication devices to enable them to communicate effectively. Teachers can help by responding to the child and being alert to the child's language abilities. In some cases, teachers may need to adjust their language so the children can better understand directions and assignments. In addition, it may help to put the children in many situations where there are opportunities to interact with other children.

Teachers and other education professionals who work with children with traumatic brain injury must be prepared for just about anything. These children may have few problems or many disabilities. They may readily adjust to their disabilities, or be emotionally upset. Parents may be overly protective of their child or deny that there are any problems. If teachers are aware of the range of needs and abilities that brain injured children may bring to the classroom, they can better help these children reach their learning potential.

Summary

Language impairments do not generally come to mind when we think about children with physical disabilities such as blindness, neuromotor disorders, and brain injury. Yet, difficulties with language are associated with each of these disorders. It is important that teachers and other education professionals understand the impact of physical disabilities on language, especially since so many children with these disabilities are being integrated into regular education settings. Impairments of vision and mobility are certainly important and have an impact on instruction, but recognition of their associated speech and language impairments can also be critical to the academic and social success of children with physical disabilities.

Review Questions

1. Contrast the vision abilities and the implications for teaching of blind children with those of children with low vision.

2. What sorts of words would young blind children be likely to have difficulty learning and using appropriately? Give some examples.

3. List three of the specific differences in language that have been found in persons with significant vision impairments.

4. Give three suggestions that teachers could use in the classroom to enhance the language of children with severe visual impairments.

5. Which neuromotor disorder is degenerative in nature—cerebral palsy or muscular dystrophy?

6. What did Bishop et al. (1990) discover about the ability of individuals with cerebral palsy to understand language?

7. Why are tests of the language and cognitive abilities of children with cerebral palsy sometimes inaccurate?

8. Explain the "cocktail chatter" phenomenon.

9. What has recent research indicated about the language development of children with spina bifida and hydrocephalus?

10. Give three suggestions that teachers could use to enhance the language and communication of children with neuromotor disorders.

11. What is acquired aphasia?

12. What are some of the problems faced by children with traumatic brain injury as they return to school?

Suggested Activities

1. Reread the case study of Joey—the child with a severe visual impairment who is included in a regular education classroom. Analyze the case carefully and respond to the following questions:

 – What did Joey's teacher do to accommodate Joey's visual impairment?
 – What could the teacher do to help Joey become a more independent learner?
 – What could be done to help Joey build good relationships with his peers?

2. One of the ongoing debates about the language of children with visual impairments has been about their understanding of words that would seem to need vision to be understood. Some have claimed that these words can have no meaning, while others have argued that individuals with severe visual impairments develop unique meanings for such words. For example, how can you understand the idea of *clouds* or *colors* without having vision?

If you have access to a child with a vision disability, you could test the child's understanding of the words below. How does the child understand these words? What do they mean to her/him? Do the child's definitions seem to be an imitation of those of adults, or are they different from the standard definition?

Word List:	mountain	yellow	cloud
	ocean	sun	

3. If you have access to a person with a neuromotor impairment who also has significant difficulty with speech, you could evaluate this person's ability to *comprehend* language.

You will need some pictures of action sequences (these could be pictures from books or magazines or be drawlings or photographs). Next, develop a list of sentences describing the pictures, for example, *The girl is hitting the baseball.*

Place three pictures in front of the person. Read a sentence that describes one of the pictures, and ask the person to touch or point to the picture that shows the action described by the sentence. If the subject can neither touch or point, you could point to each picture, in order, until the subject indicates the correct picture.

What do the results indicate about the ability of persons with neuromotor disorders to understand language?

4. There has been a great deal of debate about cerebral dominance and language. Part of the debate focuses on the question of whether cerebral dominance is established at birth or develops over the first few years of life.

Research this question and write a brief (three to five page) paper presenting evidence for and against each position. Try to come to a conclusion about this question.

References

Andersen, E., Dunlea, A., & Kekelis, L. (1984). Blind children's language: Resolving some differences. *Journal of Child Language, 11,* 645–664.

Best, S., Bigge, J., & Sirvis, B. (1994). Physical and health impairments. In N. Haring, L. McCormick, & T. Haring (Eds.), *Exceptional children and youth* (pp. 300–341). New York: Macmillan.

Bigelow, A. (1987). Early words of blind children. *Journal of Child Language, 14,* 47–56.

Bigelow, A. (1990). Relationship between the development of language and thought in young blind children. *Journal of Visual Impairment and Blindness, 84,* 414–419.

Bigge, J. (1991). *Teaching individuals with physical and multiple disabilities.* New York: Macmillan.

Bishop, D., Brown, B., & Robson, J. (1990). The relationship between phoneme discrimination, speech production, and language comprehension in cerebral-palsied individuals.

Journal of Speech and Hearing Research, 33, 210–219.

Bleck, E. (1982). Cerebral palsy. In E. Bleck & D. Nagel (Eds.), *Physically handicapped children: A medical atlas for teachers* (pp. 59–132). Orlando, FL: Grune & Stratton.

Byrne, K., Abbeduto, L., & Brooks, P. (1990). The language of children with spina bifida and hydrocephalus: Meeting task demands and mastering syntax. *Journal of Speech and Hearing Disorders, 55,* 118–123.

Campbell, T., & Dollaghan, C. (1990). Expressive language recovery in severely brain-injured children and adolescents. *Journal of Speech and Hearing Disorders, 55,* 567–581.

Cauley, K., Golinkoff, R., Hirsk-Pasek, K., & Gordon, L. (1989). Revealing hidden competencies: A new method for studying language comprehension in children with motor impairments. *American Journal of Mental Retardation, 94,* 55–63.

Civelli, E. (1983). Verbalism in young blind children. *Journal of Visual Impairment and Blindness, 77,* 61–63.

Cooper, J., & Flowers, C. (1987). Children with a history of acquired aphasia: Residual language and academic impairments. *Journal of Speech and Hearing Disorders, 52,* 251–262.

Cruickshank, W. (1976). The problem and its scope. In W. Cruickshank (Ed.), *Cerebral palsy: A developmental disability.* Syracuse, NY: Syracuse University Press.

Cutsforth, T. (1951). The blind in school and society: A psychological study. American Foundation for the Blind.

Dekker, R., & Koole, F. (1992). Visually impaired children's visual characteristics and language. *Developmental Medicine and Child Neurology, 34,* 123–133.

Dorman, C., Hurley, A., & D'Avignon, J. (1988). Language and learning disorders of older boys with Duchenne muscular dystrophy. *Developmental Medicine and Child Neurology, 30,* 316–327.

Dote-Kwan, J., & Hughes, M. (1994). The home environments of young blind children. *Journal of Visual Impairment and Blindness, 88,* 31–42.

Erin, J. (1990). Language samples from visually impaired four-and five-year olds. *Journal of*

Childhood Communication Disorders, 13, 181–191.

Ewing-Cobbs, L., Fletcher, J., Landry, S., & Levin, H. (1985). Language disorders after pediatric head injury. In J. Darby (Ed.), *Speech and language evaluation in neurology: Childhood disorders.* Orlando, FL: Grune & Stratton.

Fraiberg, S. (1977). *Insights from the blind.* London: Souvenir Press.

Freeman, R., & Blockberger, S. (1987). Language development and sensory disorder: Visual and hearing impairments. In W. Yule & M. Rutter (Eds.), *Language development and disorders* (pp. 234–247). Philadelphia: J. B. Lippincott.

Haring, N., McCormick, L., & Haring, T. (1994). *Exceptional children and youth.* New York: Merrill.

Harrington, D. (1990). Educational strategies. In M. Rosenthal, E. Griffith, M. Bond, & J. Miller (Eds.), *Rehabilitation of the adult and child with traumatic brain injury* (pp. 476–493). Philadelphia: F. A. Davis and Co.

Karagan, N., & Zellweger, H. (1978). Early verbal disability in children with Duchenne muscular dystrophy. *Journal of Nervous and Mental Disease, 168,* 419–423.

Kekelis, L., & Andersen, E. (1984). Family communication styles and language development. *Journal of Visual Impairment and Blindness, 78,* 54–65.

Kinsbourne, M., & Hiscock, M. (1977). Does cerebral dominance develop? In S. Segalowitz & F. Gruber (Eds.), *Language development and neurological theory.* New York: Academic Press.

Landau, B., & Gleitman, L. (1985). *Language and experience: Evidence from the blind child.* Cambridge, MA: Harvard University Press.

Lenneberg, E. (1967). *Biological foundations of language.* New York: Wiley.

McDonald, E. (1987). *Treating cerebral palsy.* Austin, TX: Pro-Ed.

Meacham, M. (1986). *Cerebral palsy.* Austin, TX: Pro-Ed.

Michaud, L., & Duhaime, A. (1992). Traumatic brain injury. In M. Batshaw, & Y. Perret (Eds.), *Children with disabilities: A medical primer* (pp. 525–546). Baltimore: Brooks Publishing Co.

National Head Injury Foundation. (1989). Basic questions about head injury and disability.

National Information Center for Children and Youth with Disabilities. (1993). Traumatic brain injury. Fact sheet number 18. Washington, DC: NICHCY.

Parke, K., Shallcross, R., & Anderson, R. (1980). Differences in coverbal behavior between blind and sighted persons during dyadic communication. *Visual impairment and blindness, 74,* 142–146.

Satz, P., & Bullard-Bates, C. (1981). Acquired aphasia in children. In M. Sarno (Ed.), *Acquired aphasia.* New York: Academic Press.

Telzrow, C. (1987). Management of academic and educational problems in head injury. *Journal of Learning Disabilities, 20,* 536–545.

Tew, B. (1979). The "cocktail party syndrome" in children with hydrocephalus and spina bifida. *British Journal of Disorders of Communication, 14,* 89–101.

Urwin, C. (1984). Language for absent things: Learning from visually handicapped children. *Topics in Language Disorders, 4,* 24–37.

Part III

Language and Communication in the Classroom

Our interest in language development in nondisabled children as well as in children with disabilities is more than theoretical. We are interested in how this information can be applied to identifying and helping children with language difficulties. In the next five chapters we will examine current techniques for the identification of language difficulties in school-age children as well as methods for enhancing their language skills.

The emphasis throughout this section is on assessment and instructional procedures that are directly applicable to the classroom. There is increasing evidence that, when language skills are taught in settings where they are likely to be needed, there is a greater chance that they will be learned and used. Consequently, the emphasis in these chapters is on methods of assessment and instruction that can be used in classrooms. Usually it is the classroom teacher (regular and/or special education) who has the greatest opportunity to work with the child with language difficulties.

Included in this part is a chapter on language and culture (Chapter 14). It is essential that teachers understand the difference between a language difference and a language disorder. Additionally, it is important to understand the differences in language usage that children who speak a language other than English or a variant of "standard" English bring to the classroom.

Chapter 10

Assessing Language and Communication

Language assessment can serve several purposes. It can help determine what difficulties a child may have, what aspects of language are involved, and the degree of delay or the severity of the child's development problems. Assessment can help focus intervention, by identifying objectives for intervention and even indicating approaches that might be most successful, and it can even, at times, reveal the underlying causes of speech, language, or communication difficulty.

Unfortunately, assessment is also sometimes seen as a burdensome chore and a waste of time. Federal and state mandates require that particular areas be tested and even, to some extent, dictate the types of assessment procedures that must be used. Assessment is sometimes viewed as a necessary evil—a way to comply with IEP requirements or to enable a child to receive services.

The goal of this chapter is to point out positive assessment practices. Specifically, the goal is to describe those assessment procedures that can reveal the most information about the language and communication of children with disabilities. While assessment may be necessary to comply with legal mandates, it should also be useful. It should help teachers and other education professionals make instructional decisions and evaluate the outcomes of instruction.

After completion of this chapter you should be able to:

1. Define *assessment* and discuss how it differs from *testing*.
2. List the purposes of language assessment.
3. List what should be included in a comprehensive assessment of language.
4. List some formal tests for assessing language skills.
5. Describe some informal techniques for language assessment.
6. Explain how to gather and analyze a language sample.
7. Describe some informal techniques for assessing specific language skills.

Understanding Assessment

Defining Assessment

Assessment, testing, and *diagnosis*—these are terms that are frequently used in educational settings. They appear in reports, are used in parent-teacher conferences, and are frequently a part of informal discussions among teachers. Sometimes these terms are not used with a great deal of precision. Although they are related, the terms assessment, testing, and diagnosis have quite different technical meanings. In order to avoid confusion, it may be useful to review these meanings.

Assessment is the most inclusive of the terms listed above. *Assessment* has been defined by Salvia and Ysseldyke (1995) as "the process of collecting data for the purpose of making decisions about students" (p. 5). Assessment may include testing, but other procedures—such as interviews, observations, and work samples—may be included, as well. As the definition indicates, assessment should be thought of as a process rather than a product. It is an information-gathering process that should reveal findings essential for making instructional decisions.

Salvia and Ysseldyke (1995) define *testing* as "administering a particular set of questions to an individual or group of individuals in order to obtain a score" (p. 5). The score is the product of that testing procedure. The term *diagnosis* has two meanings. When used within a medical model, diagnosis suggests the search for the underlying cause of a problem. Cohen, Swerdlik, and Smith (1992) define diagnosis as "the act or process of identifying or determining the nature of a disease through examination" (p. 346). However, the search for an underlying cause is often a fruitless task for educators, in that often it is not possible to discover the underlying cause and, even if the cause is identified there is usually nothing educators can do about it. However, diagnosis is also used in another way. When educators talk about diagnostic tests, they are referring to instruments that can give specific information about a skill area, such as reading or spoken language.

We will use the term *assessment* to refer to the process of gathering and evaluating information to help educators better understand individual children and their instructional needs. We will limit the use of the term *testing* to the actual procedures for gathering information.

Purposes of Assessment

We alluded to some of the purposes of assessment at the beginning of this chapter. Assessment can help identify children with disabilities, provide specific information about an individual child, or yield clues about the effectiveness of the educational program. McLoughlin and Lewis (1994) list five purposes for assessment of children with special needs:

- **Screening:** to identify students with severe learning problems
- **Eligibility:** to determine whether the student qualifies for special education
- **IEP planning:** to create annual goal and objectives, which are based on results of assessment

TABLE 10.1 Advantages and Limitations of Assessment Techniques

Formal		Informal	
Advantages	Limitations	Advantages	Limitations
Allows comparisons between individuals	May not be related to curriculum	Directly related to curriculum	Requires much preparation
Standard format	May not be appropriate for child	Can be designed for individual child	Difficult to compare children
Already prepared	May be misinterpreted		

- **Monitoring progress:** to gather information about the outcomes of instruction
- **Program evaluation:** to review the effectiveness of the educational program

Types of Assessment Procedures

There are many ways to gather the information necessary for the various purposes of assessment. In order to better understand the available options, it may be useful to examine the types of assessment procedures that are available. For example, there are *formal* and *informal* measures. Formal assessment procedures may be thought of as anything that has been published for use in assessment. This can include tests, observation forms, rating scales, and the like. Informal measures are developed by teachers and other practitioners to directly evaluate the skills of children with whom they are working.

In the field of assessment there is a great debate about the use of formal and informal assessment. Salvia and Ysseldyke (1995) note three frequently expressed areas of concern with formal testing. These include:

- **Overreliance on norm-referenced tests:** Norm-referenced tests have often been used to make placement and instructional decisions that go beyond what the tests can meaningfully assess.
- **Confusing what can and should be assessed:** To some extent, tests have dictated both what should be taught and how instruction is delivered.
- **Overreliance on objective and quantifiable measures:** Some skills (e.g., writing) are not easily measured with objective criteria.

Practitioners will have to make decisions about which kind of assessment procedures to use. In doing so, they might consider the advantages and shortcomings of each approach (see Table 10.1).

Most formal measures are *standardized*. According to Myers (1987) standardized assessment measures should have three criteria: set administration procedures, objective scoring criteria (including specific objective criteria for determining correct answers and reporting results), and a specified frame of reference (i.e., population to which the scores can be applied). The key feature of standardized

TABLE 10.2   Types of Assessment Procedures

Type of Assessment	Norm Referenced	Criterion Referenced
Formal	Commercially produced test that allows comparisons between subjects	Commercially produced test of specific skills
Informal	User-made test that uses local norms (e.g., all third grade classes in a school)	User-made test of specific skills (e.g., weekly spelling test)

assessment procedures is that they *must* be administered as the directions state. Otherwise, standardization is lost and it is not possible to compare across individuals.

Tests can be *norm referenced* or *criterion referenced.* Norm-referenced tests compare an individuals's performance to that of a comparison population, while criterion-referenced tests allow one to assess the individual's mastery of specific skills. Both norm-referenced and criterion-referenced tests can be formal or informal in format (see Table 10.2). Tests can evaluate broad areas of skill development (achievement tests) or focus on specific skill areas (diagnostic). In addition, tests can be administered either to groups or to individuals.

Assessment of Language

Language is one of the most difficult domains of human behavior to assess. There are many reasons why this is so. As we have seen throughout this book, understanding of language and language acquisition is incomplete. It is hard to assess something that cannot be clearly defined. As Sharon James (1993) points out, language is not a unitary phenomenon—it is "multidimensional, complex, and dynamic; it involves many interrelated processes and abilities; and it changes from situation to situation" (p. 186). In addition, language development and language disorders can vary widely. Both the sequence and the timing of normal language development can vary. Language disorders can range from mild to severe, receptive to expressive, from speech production to conversational competence.

Knowing that language is difficult to assess does not, of course, absolve us from doing so. It simply makes it all the more important to be clear about the purposes, the goals, and the means of language assessment. We also should keep in mind the limitations of language assessment and the need to relate assessment in other domains (e.g., intelligence testing and testing of academic skills) to assessment of language.

James (1993) has identified three purposes for assessment of language: **identifying** children with language disorders, **designing** appropriate language intervention programs, and **monitoring** changes resulting from intervention. The identification of children with language disorders includes two steps: screening, and determining the nature of the disability. Screening involves the testing of a large number of children, to identify those most in need of services. The instruments that are used must be relatively brief and easy to administer and interpret. Children who are identified as possibly having a language disorder can then be assessed more intensively. During the second step, the evaluator tries to determine whether the child does, in fact, have a language disorder and, if so, the type and severity of the problem.

In order to design appropriate language intervention programs, teachers and other educational professionals need to have specific information about the child's language abilities and difficulties. What aspects of language are involved? How delayed is the child? Does the child have difficulty understanding, as well as producing, language? Having information about how the child learns best and what instructional methods have been most successful are helpful to those planning language intervention programs.

It is essential that program outcomes be evaluated. How else can we know whether a particular instructional method is working and whether instructional objectives need to be changed? James (1993) points out the importance of assessing the child in a variety of settings, since generalization is such an important part of success in language.

What to Assess

What should be included in a comprehensive assessment of language? Although the answer to this question is affected by factors such as the characteristics of the child and the purposes for testing, there are some broad areas that should be included in most assessments of language. At the core of any assessment of language are the five basic elements of language discussed previously: phonology, morphology, syntax, semantics, and pragmatics. Both the child's understanding and production of each of these elements should be considered.

Phonology

In examining the child's production of speech sounds, professionals listen for intelligibility of speech and accuracy of sound production. Specific areas examined might include phonological errors such as those mentioned in Chapter 4 including: reduction of consonant clusters (*green* becomes *geen*), deletion of unstressed syllables (*banana* becomes *nana*), devoicing of the final consonant (*bed* becomes *bet*), and substitutions (*bus* becomes *but*). Phonological processing can also be assessed. Methods for the assessment of phonological awareness, including the detection of rhyme, division of words into sounds, and detection of beginning and ending sounds, were discussed in Chapter 5.

Morphology

We know from research discussed in Chapter 4 that there is a developmental sequence of morphology. We know, for example, that the use of the *-ing* ending usually precedes the use of prepositions such as *in* and *on*. We know that the use of the plural *s* generally emerges before the use of the regular past tense *ed*. In assessing a child's morphological development, we should know which word endings and prefixes the child is using. It is also important to test the child's use of morphemes in both real and nonsense words. Children may correctly use such constructions as the past tense because they have heard them previously. By asking them to use the correct morpheme with a nonsense word, we are assessing whether the child has acquired the morphological *rule*.

Syntax

There are two general areas that could be included in an assessment of syntactic development: use of phrase-structure rules and use of transformational rules. Phrase-structure rules are the basic building blocks of grammar. They include the basic syntactic elements (e.g., noun, verb, adjective) and the rules that govern word order (e.g., noun before verb). Assessment of syntax can include examining both the syntactic elements used by the child and the frequency of their usage, in addition to the types of sentences used by the child and the accuracy and frequency of their usage. For example, does the child use both simple and compound sentences? How frequently are compound sentences used? Are they used appropriately? One could also examine whether the child correctly produces and can interpret a variety of types of sentences, including complex sentences and sentences that contain negation. Assessment of syntax might also include the use of transformational rules, such as in the understanding and use of questions, imperative sentences, and the passive voice.

Semantics

The child's knowledge of meaning is typically assessed through examining vocabulary to see how many words and what types of words (e.g., objects, actions, social greetings) are in the child's vocabulary, as well as how quickly the child can access words. Speed of processing is a critical factor in language usage. In addition, evaluations of the child's understanding of word meanings and understanding and use of nonliteral language are used for some children. Can they understand and use figures of speech such as metaphor? Do they understand proverbs and humor?

Pragmatics

Assessment in pragmatics would help determine the child's understanding and use of a variety of speech acts and conversational rules. As children develop, they use an increasing variety of speech acts. Evaluating the child's use of speech acts, such as requesting, protesting, greeting, and answering, and the ability to understand both direct and indirect speech acts provides information on language development. Conversational rules include a number of aspects such as turn taking, conversational repairs, topic setting and maintenance, and awareness of the need to vary one's language in different conversational situations. All of these elements and many more could be included in an assessment of pragmatic competence (see Table 10.3).

TABLE 10.3   Language Elements Used in Assessment

Element	Expressive	Receptive

Phonology	Articulation of speech sounds
	Phonological errors:
	    reduction
	    deletion
	    devoicing
	    sounds
	    substitution
		Phonological awareness:
		    rhyme
		    division of words into sounds
		    adding/deleting beginning and ending

Morphology	Use of grammatical morphemes in real and nonsense words	Identification of grammatical morphemes

Syntax	Use of basic sentence elements
	    (e.g., noun, verb)
	Use of sentence types
	    (simple, complex)
	Use of transformational rules
	    (question, passive)
		Understanding and interpretation of sentence types and transformational rules

Semantics	Vocabulary use: amount types Speed of word retrieval Use of nonliteral language	Identification of words Comprehension of humor/proverbs, and the like

Pragmatics	Use of speech acts:
	    requesting
	    greeting
	    answering
	Use of conversational rules:
	    turn taking
	    repairs
	    topic setting
		Understanding of direct and indirect speech acts

Prerequisites of Language

A comprehensive assessment of language might also include the evaluation of social, cognitive, and physiological prerequisites of language. We know, for example, that normally developing children engage in a number of prelinguistic communicative routines with their parents. These include turn-taking exchanges, gaze behavior, and the like. Observation of these routines could be included in the assessment of a nonspeaking child. An evaluation of the child's level of cognitive development may provide helpful information on whether the child engages in symbolic play or whether the concept of object permanence seems to be established. Certainly one would need to know whether the child's speech-processing abilities are intact. An examination of the child's mouth and teeth to determine whether they are healthy and intact may be necessary. In addition, a neurological evaluation may be necessary to determine whether the child is physically capable of using and understanding language.

Making Assessment Decisions

With so many possible elements to use in a comprehensive assessment of language, how is one to decide what to include? The choices can be determined by several factors. The first consideration is the purpose of the assessment. Clearly, there will be different assessment goals for a language screening than for an assessment for the purposes of instructional planning. A screening evaluation will likely include just a few of the major aspects of language, while assessment for classification or instructional decision making should be both more comprehensive and more in-depth. The nature of the child is another important factor in determining what will be assessed. It should be obvious that it would not be appropriate to assess all elements of language in all children. Younger children and children with lower functional levels may need more comprehensive testing of phonological and morphological development, as well as language prerequisites. On the other hand, for older children and children at more advanced stages of development, assessment is likely to focus on the use of nonliteral language, complex sentences, and pragmatic skills.

It may also be useful to consider the child's language history and the results of observations of the child's use of language at home, in school, and/or in the community in making language-assessment decisions for any particular child. Parents' reports of the child's language development, though often inaccurate, may give general information of the course and timing of language development in the child. The goal, of course, is to include just the right elements in the assessment—not so many that the child will become bored and noncompliant but enough to develop a comprehensive picture of the child's language abilities.

Assessment Methods

As noted earlier in this chapter, there are two basic types of assessment procedures—formal and informal. We will first examine formal procedures for evaluating language, including tests, checklists, and observation systems and will then consider the many informal methods available.

Formal Procedures

Formal language assessment procedures consist primarily of standardized tests, that is, tests that have a standard set of directions and format. While standardized tests clearly have some advantages over informal techniques (e.g., objectivity and ease of use), Owens (1991) points out that standardized tests of language do not provide a complete picture of the richness and complexity of a child's language. He asserts, furthermore, that standardized tests of language fail to consider cultural diversity and can be misinterpreted.

Despite concerns such as those raised by Owens, use of formal, standardized tests of language continues. Therefore, it is important for practitioners to be aware of the great variety of language tests available, to keep in mind the limitations of these tests, and to learn about alternative assessment procedures—such as those discussed later in this chapter.

Formal tests of language can be divided into two main types: comprehensive measures and tests of specific language skills. The comprehensive tests of language are designed to test a broad range of language skills across a wide range of ages. For example, the Test of Language Development—Primary (2nd ed.) (Newcomer & Hammill, 1988) is designed to assess both expressive and receptive language in children from age 4 to 9 and comprises seven subtests that cover the areas of phonology, syntax, and semantics. The seven subtests include:

> *Picture vocabulary:* Choosing from a group of four pictures, the child points to the one that shows the stimulus word.
>
> *Oral vocabulary:* The tester reads a word. The child describes what the word means.
>
> *Grammatic understanding:* The child selects from a group of three pictures the one that best represents a sentence read by the tester.
>
> *Sentence imitation:* The child must repeat sentences that vary in length and grammatic complexity.
>
> *Grammatic completion:* The child must complete a stimulus sentence by supplying the appropriate word (e.g., use of possessive, plural, tense).
>
> *Word discrimination:* The child listens to pairs of words read by the tester and must say whether the words are the same or different from each other.
>
> *Word articulation:* The child describes a picture. The examiner makes a phonetic transcription of the child's speech.

Using scores for each subtest, practitioners can derive an overall language age, as well as gain composite scores for phonology, syntax, semantics, speaking, and listening. The test is relatively easy to administer and interpret. It requires no special training, other than requiring a very careful reading of the manual. Examples of other comprehensive tests of language skills include the Test of Language Development—Intermediate (2nd ed.) (Hammill & Newcomer, 1988) and the Clinical Evaluation of Language Fundamentals—Revised (Semel, Wiig, & Secord, 1987) (see Table 10.4 for these and other examples of comprehensive tests of language).

Comprehensive tests of language skills have several advantages, the most important being that they give a reasonably complete picture of the child's language functioning. They provide information about the child's skills in syntax and semantics, and some (but not all) evaluate skills in phonology (e.g., the Test of Language Development—Primary (2nd ed.)) and pragmatics (the Bankson Language Test). Most of these tests evaluate both receptive and expressive language skills. Because these tests evaluate a wide range of skills, the results reflect the child's skills in various domains of language. For example, look at the results below. What do they tell us about this child?

TABLE 10.4   Comprehensive Tests of Language

Test Name (authors)	Age Range (year, month)	Areas Assessed	
		Receptive	Expressive
Bankson Language Test—2 (Bankson, 1990)	3–0 to 6–11		syn, sem, prag
Clinical Evaluation of Language Fundamentals–R (Semel, Wiig, & Secord, 1987)	5–0 to 16–11	syn, sem	syn, sem
Test of Early Language Development (2nd ed.) (Hresko, Reid, & Hammill, 1991)	2–0 to 7–11	syn, sem	syn, sem
Test of Language Development—Primary (2nd ed.) (Newcomer & Hammill, 1988)	4–0 to 8–11	pho, syn, sem	pho, syn, sem
Test of Language Development—Intermediate (2nd ed.) (Hammill & Newcomer,1988)	8–6 to 12–11	syn, sem	syn, sem
Test of Adolescent Language—2 (Hammill, Brown, Larsen, & Wiederholt, 1987)	12–0 to 18–5	syn, sem	syn, sem

Note: syn = syntax   prag = pragmatics
         sem = semantics   pho = phonology

Test of Language Development—Primary (2nd ed.)

Name: Juanita M.
Chronological Age = 7 years, 4 months
Language Age = 6 years, 2 months
Subtests (standard scores: mean = 10, standard deviation = 3)

Receptive	*Expressive*
Picture Vocabulary = 10	Oral Vocabulary = 8
Grammatic Understanding = 9	Sentence Imitation = 6
	Grammatic completion = 5
Word Discrimination = 8	Word Articulation = 7

First, the child's overall language abilities are significantly below those of other children her age. And, her scores are much lower for expressive than for receptive language. Vocabulary appears to be a relative area of strength, while syntax appears to be a special problem area.

TABLE 10.5   Tests of Specific Language Skills

	Age Range (years)
Phonology	
Goldman-Fristoe Test of Articulation (Goldman & Fristoe, 1986)	2–16+
Wepman Auditory Discrimination Test (Wepman, 1973)	5–8
Goldman-Fristoe-Woodcock Test of Auditory Discrimination (Goldman, Fristoe, & Woodcock, 1970)	4–70+

	Age Range (years + months)
Syntax	
Northwestern Syntax Screening Test (Lee, 1971)	3–11 to 7–1
Carrow Elicited Language Inventory (Carrow-Woolfolk, 1974)	3 to 7–11
Test of Auditory Comprehension of Language (Carrow-Woolfolk, 1985)	3 to 9–11
Semantics	
Boehm Test of Basic Concepts—R (Boehm, 1986)	K to Grade 2
Peabody Picture Vocabulary Test—R (Dunn & Dunn, 1981)	2–6 to 40
Pragmatics	
Let's Talk Inventory for Children (Bray & Wiig, 1987)	4 to 8
Test of Pragmatic Skills—R (Shulman, 1986)	3–0 to 8–11

While these comprehensive tests of language can give us valuable information to use in making classification decisions, by their very nature they are limited in depth. Because they are designed to test a wide range of skills, they do not have a sufficient number of items for in-depth exploration of a specific language domain. Often such in-depth analysis is important for making instructional decisions, because teachers need to know whether *specific* language structures are present or absent.

Tests of specific domains of language can provide more specific level of information. These tests evaluate phonological, syntactic, semantic, or pragmatic skills in greater depth than most general tests of language can. Examples of these tests can be found in Table 10.5.

Formal, standardized tests can provide us with important information for making classification and instructional decisions. However, as noted earlier, there are significant limitations to the use of standardized tests. Salvia and Ysseldyke (1995) note three particularly troubling issues regarding language assessment. First, standardized tests may not accurately reflect the child's spontaneous language abilities. Since standardized tests must be administered in a very particular way, they do not allow for spontaneous language expression. The child may talk incessantly before and after the testing session, but this cannot be counted as part of the test. A good tester will, however, be sure to note everything about the testing session. A second issue raised by Salvia and Ysseldyke involves problems associated with the use of test results to plan intervention. They note that many language tests do not easily translate into therapeutic goals. They also caution, as an aside here, that clinicians may be tempted to teach in ways that will improve test scores rather than their focusing on the skills the child needs for success in the classroom and the community. Third, there is a danger that tests may not adequately assess children from diverse social and cultural backgrounds. This is an especially important concern with language testing, since language is so closely intertwined with social and cultural norms.

Informal Measures

Because of these and similar concerns, many researchers and clinicians have suggested that informal, nonstandardized assessment of language be included in a comprehensive assessment of language (Lahey, 1988; Owens, 1991). Informal assessment procedures range from relatively low-structured, spontaneous language samples to highly structured, elicited imitation tasks. Informal measures, even the more highly structured tasks, provide the clinician with greater opportunities to exercise judgment in the selection of assessment objectives and methods.

Language sampling.   One very useful way for obtaining information about a child's language abilities is through collecting and analyzing a sample of the child's language. Although language samples can be a rich source of information, they may also be seen as intimidating and too difficult for teachers to collect and analyze. Because language samples are such an important language assessment tool, it is important to know there are readily applicable methods for collecting and analyzing language samples within school settings.

Owens (1991) noted that "good language samples do not just occur. They are the result of careful planning and execution" (p. 61). This is important to keep in mind. Since the goal of any language sampling is to get a representative sample of the child's language, one cannot just put a child at a table, turn on a tape recorder, and hope for a good sample of language. Accomplishing this goal requires careful planning of the *context, materials,* and *techniques* that will be used.

The best context in which to obtain a language sample is a realistic setting. In other words, the child's classroom, home, or lunchroom are ideal places to record the sample. If possible, the child should be engaged in real activities, for example, recording a language sample from a group of three students with learning disabilities while they work together on a group science project. Recording the language sample in natural settings increases the likelihood that a representative sample of language will be obtained. This is especially true for young children. Research has found that younger children produce longer utterances when the speech sample is collected at home rather than in the clinic (Kramer, James, & Saxman, 1979).

Of course, each of these settings has some built-in limitations. There are usually background noises and many other distractions in the classroom and the lunchroom; however, obtaining samples of language used at home is not realistic for teachers and speech-language specialists. Therefore, the ideal of assessment in a natural setting must be balanced by the realities of the limitations. Sometimes it may be necessary to adapt the setting to make it more possible to record a language sample, for example, by bringing mom into a clinic room that is furnished in a homelike way or by sectioning off a portion of the classroom for language sampling.

The selection of materials used during the collection of the language sample is critical to the results. For young children, toys are often the most effective materials to use to elicit representative language samples. James (1993) suggests that toys with multiple pieces, such as the Fisher-Price school, are best. Owens (1991) suggests that blocks, dishes, and dolls work well for 2-year-olds, while 3-year-olds prefer books, clothes, and puppets. Wanska, Bedrosian, and Pohlman (1986) examined the effects of different types of play materials on pragmatic aspects of language. They found that the children in their study produced more conversation centered on the here and now when they played with a toy hospital set than when they assembled Legos. When the children were playing with Legos, they were more likely to talk about things other than what they were presently doing. Whatever materials are used, it is essential that the items be interesting, age-appropriate, and effective in eliciting language.

Sometimes pictures are used as the stimulus for a language sample. These, too, must be carefully selected. A single, static picture (for example, a mountain and stream) is likely to elicit a brief, descriptive response (e.g., *there is a mountain* or *there is a stream*). Using a series of pictures showing action (such as a cartoon strip), for example, is the best way to elicit a variety of language. Recently, video narration has also been used as a way to obtain a language sample (Dollaghan, Campbell, & Tomlin, 1990). The child watches the video and responds either during the video or afterward. One of the advantages of video elicitation is that, if carefully selected, video may do a better job than other methods of language elicitation holding the child's attention.

The choice of actual technique of language elicitation is also critical—in addition to the choice of context and the materials used. For example, children may be recorded during either spontaneous language situations, during structured activities, or during an interview. Each of these techniques has some advantages and weaknesses.

The spontaneous language sample is undoubtedly the ideal way to elicit the most representative sample of language, but it is also the most difficult. If you have ever tried to obtain a spontaneous sample, you know how difficult this can be. Most children (and most adults) freeze up or get silly when they know they are being taped or observed and then may fail to produce the kind of language practitioners are looking for. Unplanned interruptions—from doorbells to fire drills to fights—tend to interfere with the session. Although spontaneous language samples are an ideal, it is probably impossible to obtain a totally spontaneous sample. We should think about what we can do to approximate this ideal.

Structured samples use an activity or a material to elicit a sample. The science project example discussed earlier is an example of a structured, language-sample activity. Wren (1985) used three types of formats to elicit language samples: spontaneous interaction, elicited interaction, and specific tasks. She used a variety of tasks to elicit language, including free play with puppets, explanation of a game, and storytelling. However, she found that a mock birthday party activity in which the children were prompted to respond yielded the most language responses. She used a prompt, such as *Today is _____'s birthday. Let's have a party. What are some of the things that we'll need?* Structured activities have the advantage of increasing the likelihood of getting the desired language response. On the other hand, they tend to constrain the language sample by using a contrived procedure. As a result, certain vocabulary and language structures may be prompted by the task itself.

Coggins, Olswang, and Guthrie (1987) compared the results of using a low-structured observation to that of using an elicitation task in assessing the pragmatic skills of young children. In the elicitation condition, the children were presented with objects that they could not use by themselves (e.g., a plastic jar with a screw-on lid, a remote-control toy car). The examiner then waited for the child to make a request. In the low-structured condition, the examiner simply watched the child and mother as they played together. Coggins et al. found that the two methods were complementary. For example, they found that the children produced very few spontaneous requests in the low-structured situation but produced numerous requests with the more structured task. The results of this study, as well as more recent research (Wetherby & Rodriguez, 1992) suggest that it is best to use a variety of techniques to elicit a representative sample of language.

Recently, Evans and Craig (1992) reported on their use of a structured interview procedure to elicit a language sample. Using open-ended questions, such as *What can you tell me about your family?* and *What do you like to do after school?*, the authors found that their interview procedure could be as good as—or better than—a spontaneous language sample is in eliciting representative language samples from 8- and 9-year-old children with speech and language impairments. Specifically, they found that the children in their study produced more utterances and were more responsive during the interview session. One of the reasons for the success of this technique is the type of questions the authors asked. It is important that questions are asked in such a way that the children have a good deal of latitude in their responses. Questions such as *What is your name?* and *How many people live in your house?* will get nothing more than one-word answers.

Language samples can be videotaped, audiotaped, or transcribed as they happen. As James (1993) points out, videotaping is especially useful—even essential—for recording multiperson conversations and interactions in which the context is important. On the other hand, it can also be disrupting. She suggests that audiotape recording, supplemented by good notes about nonverbal behavior and context, can be almost as useful as videotaping. Keeping running notes of nonverbal behaviors, even when videotaping, is important. Sometimes the tape fails to capture the raised eyebrow or facial expression that is an important part of conversation.

How long should the language sample be? There is no simple answer to this question. It depends, in part, on how talkative children are, the length of their utterances, and the number of conversational exchanges. Experts have suggested that 50 to 100 utterances is an optimal length (Lahey, 1988; Lee, 1974; Owens, 1991). Others have suggested that 30 minutes is a good length (Miller, 1981). While there are no hard and fast guidelines, research by Cole, Mills, and Dale (1989) found that it is important to get more than one sample of language and that several shorter samples over varying days and times give the most representative picture of the child's language.

After the language sample has been collected, it must be transcribed. This is a tedious task that must be performed with great accuracy. However, it is essential for the transcriber to record the language as accurately as possible. Utterances should never be interpreted or improved. Natural spoken language is a bit messy. There are frequent stops and starts. Speakers frequently interrupt and overlap each other and speakers sometimes stray from the topic. All of these idiosyncrasies of language must be preserved in the language sample. There is often a great temptation on the part of the transcriber to edit or interpret the speech, thinking, "The child *must* have meant to say this, I'll just 'clean it up." The recorder must constantly listen for what was *actually* said rather than what *should* or *might* have been said. This is sometimes not as easy as it sounds. Look at the sample below, taken from a 7-year-old child with a severe expressive-language disorder:

Nick: Umm, army crows.
Teacher: Tell me again?
N: Army crows.
T: An army crawl?
N: Yeah.
T: I don't know what an army crawl is. Tell me about that?
N: Du dut craw on da mat.

When this exchange began, we did not know what Nicholas meant by an *army crow*. Later, it became more clear that he was talking about a way of crawling on your belly. It would have been easy to go back and "clean up" the transcript. But this sample shows just how difficult it is to understand Nick.

When transcribing a language sample, practitioners must develop some method for labeling the utterances. In the sample above, each utterance is numbered, thus allowing the clinician to refer to the appropriate sentence to illustrate a point.

One of the more difficult tasks in transcribing language samples is making decisions about when one utterance stops and the next begins. Look at this example from Owens (1991):

"We went in a bus and we saw monkeys and we had a picnic and we petted the sheeps and one sheep sneezed on me and we had sodas and we came home" (p. 81).

Is this *really* one sentence? Owens suggests that there are really four utterances contained in this sentence. He suggests that utterances should be interpreted as containing no more than one *and*. Intonation provides another clue to determine where utterance breaks occur. Careful listeners can often hear the pitch drops that signal the end of an utterance. Probably the most useful advice for anyone attempting to analyze language samples is to be consistent. Whatever conventions you adopt, if you use them consistently, you are more likely to get a representative sample of language.

The next step in the language-sample assessment is to analyze the results. In doing so, we will look at the basic elements of language as our guide, beginning with syntax, the most accessible element in the transcript.

Syntactic analysis of language samples usually begins with calculation of *mean length of utterance (MLU)*. MLU is a rough measure of the complexity of a child's language. It is derived by adding all of the morphemes produced in a sample of language and dividing by the number of utterances. For example, if a child produced 125 morphemes in 50 utterances, the MLU would be 2.5 (125/50). The rules for counting morphemes can become rather complex (see Owens, 1991). One rule states that only the first instance of a repeated word should be counted. Therefore, if a child says *I go, go, go to school,* only the first *go* is counted. The best advice for anyone trying to calculate MLU is to be consistent in whatever decisions you make about counting morphemes.

MLU is a reasonably accurate measure of syntactic complexity until the child reaches an MLU of 4.0. After this point the child's use of complex sentence structures can actually reduce rather than increase MLU. For example, look at the following sentences:

1. The boy is playing and the girl is playing.
2. The boy and girl are playing.

Sentence 1 consists of 11 morphemes, while there are only 7 morphemes in sentence 2. Yet sentence 2 illustrates a more sophisticated use of conjunction. Therefore, MLU becomes a less accurate measure of language complexity. Although the use of MLU has sometimes been criticized (e.g., Johnston & Kamhi, 1984; Lund & Duchan, 1988), MLU is a widely used measure of syntactic complexity. But MLU can give only a very general indication of the child's syntactic development. In addition to MLU, some of the following could be included in an analysis of the child's syntactic development:

- word endings used *(-s, -ed, -ing)*
- sentence types (declarative, question, imperative)
- sentence complexity (simple, compound, embedded)
- verb tenses (present, past, future)
- advanced structures (gerunds, passive voice)

Like MLU, *type-token ratio (TTR)* is a rough measure of semantic development. Type-token ratio is calculated by counting the number of *different* words used in a language sample and dividing by the total number of words in the sample. For example, look at the sentence *The dog chased the cat around the house.* There are eight words in the sentence, but only six different words *(the, dog, chased, cat, around, house).* If the next sentence were, *The dog caught the cat*, there would be only one new word *(caught).* In a language sample of 100 words with 50 different words, the type-token ratio would be .50. A language sample of 100 words with 80 different words would yield a TTR of .80. Thus, a higher type-token ratio indicates that a greater variety of words is being used in the language sample. This is an indicator of a larger vocabulary,

Other analyses of semantic skills are also possible, such as in looking for overextensions and underextensions. For example, does the child use some words to stand for larger classes of things (e.g., *dog* for all domestic animals), or does the child use some words in a very narrow way (e.g., *cup* used only for a particular cup)? In addition, the child's use of figurative language (e.g., metaphor and humor) and the use of a variety of semantic functions (action, actor, state of being) could be examined. Of course, it is essential that words are used accurately—with correct meaning and in the appropriate context—and that notations are made of the speaker's violations of any of the rules of semantic relationships (for example, *the married bachelor is here*).

Language samples may also be analyzed for pragmatic, as well as syntactic and semantic, usage. Johnson, Johnston, and Weinrich (1984) reported a number of pragmatic-functioning problems that could be identified from samples of children's language. These included:

- Problems with topicalization

  - Problems establishing the topic and making comments
  - Problems in maintaining a topic

- Problems with conversation

  - Difficulty in initiating and closing a conversation
  - Inability to respond
  - Not knowing how to take a conversational turn

- Problems with register

  - Giving insufficient information to the listener
  - Inability to adjust language to the listener

Each of these pragmatic trouble spots could be included in a language-sample analysis. In addition, one could look for the use of a variety of pragmatic functions. Halliday (1975) identified several ways in which language is used in young children (see Table 10.6). Language samples can reveal which pragmatic functions are being used by the child.

TABLE 10.6   Pragmatic Functions in Child Language

1. Instrumental—language used to satisfy needs and desires ("I want more milk")
2. Regulatory—language used to control or regulate the actions of others ("Open the door")
3. Interactional—language used to establish interactions ("Hi"; "goodbye")
4. Personal—language used to express personal feelings, attitudes, and interest ("I love you")
5. Heuristic—language used to explore and organize the environment ("That's a kitty")
6. Imaginative—language used to create an imaginary environment

Source: Adapted from M. Halliday. (1975). *Explorations in the function of language.* London: Edward Arnold.

In order to analyze language samples for pragmatic usage, one must be careful to note what is going on during the language sampling. Other participants, the context, and objects in the environment may all affect the child's language usage.

Sometimes phonological development is examined via a language sample. A phonological analysis examining the child's use of speech sounds can reveal speech errors such as substitutions (*go* becomes *do*) and deletion of sounds *(banana* becomes *nana),* as well as whether errors usually appear in the initial, final, or middle position within words.

For a thorough analysis of phonological development, it is necessary to do a phonetic transcription of the language sample—rewriting each utterance using a standard simple of speech-sound coding. This is a laborious process that requires great expertise. Usually only a trained speech-language specialist can do a phonetic transcription.

It is possible to use a computer program to assist with language-sample analysis. The SALT program (Systematic Analysis of Language Transcripts) can calculate MLU and TTR, as well as many other measures of syntax, semantics, morphology, and pragmatics (Miller & Chapman, 1985). Although the computer can be very helpful, other judgments are required about the language sample itself—such as where utterances begin and end. Computer analysis of language samples can assist, but not replace, clinical judgment.

Language samples are a very good way of finding out more about the language of a particular child. They can give a more realistic picture of the child's use of language in realistic conversational contexts. Careful analysis of the samples can yield information that can be used for instructional planning. One should be careful, however, in using language samples as a way of comparing children. Research has found that although language samples are reasonably consistent for any particular child, they are not a reliable way to compare the language performance of children (Cole et al., 1989).

Language elicitation tasks.   Sometimes it is necessary to structure a language elicitation activity in a way that will prompt a certain kind of response. Let's say, for example, that you wanted to find out whether a child had developed the use of the past tense *(-ed)* ending. Although children just might use a few *-ed* endings in a spontaneous language sample, they would be unlikely to produce more than a few. Alternatively, you might want to use a task that prompts the use of *-ed* endings, for example, by showing a brief video of a cartoon character fishing and then asking questions about what the child saw. The responses should be mostly in the past tense.

There are many ways to elicit specific language responses. One widely used method is imitation. Using this technique, the examiner says a sentence and asks the child to repeat it. To prompt the use of the present progressive ending, the examiner might say, *The girl is riding a bike.* The theory behind the use of imitation tasks is that children will only be able to repeat those language structures that they have already mastered (Menyuk, 1968). Research on the use of imitation tasks has yielded mixed results. Some studies have found imitation to be a poor way of measuring language performance (Connell & Myles-Zizter, 1982); others have found that the usefulness of these activities varied from child to child (Fujiki & Brinton, 1987). While imitation tasks can be useful, they should be used in combination with other measures of language use, such as those that follow.

Morphology. Berko (1958) developed a classic task that required that children complete a sentence that described a picture. For this task, the examiner prompts a response by saying, *This is a wug. Now there are two of them. There are two _____.* The child has to fill in the blank. By using nonsense words, this task is able to assess the child's knowledge of morphological rules.

Syntax. Owens (1991) gives two suggestions for eliciting negatives. The first he calls "The emperor's new clothes." The examiner makes an untrue statement *(Oh Shirley, what beautiful yellow boots),* which should prompt the subject to respond with a negative *(I'm not wearing boots).* He calls the second technique "Screw up." The examiner makes a statement that does not match the action *(Here's your snack*—said as the examiner hands the subject a pencil). The subject should respond by saying, *That's not a snack.* These examples show the creativity that teachers and others can apply to elicit specific syntactic structures. For example, to elicit the use of possessives, one could say, *Who does that book belong to?* as a way to prompt the response, *It's John's book.*

Semantics. Howell, Fox, and Morehead (1993) present several ways to elicit vocabulary knowledge (p. 281). One suggestion goes as follows:

Target word: *drill*
Directions: "Select the words which make sentence 2 most like sentence 1."
Sentence 1: We need *drill* on our skills.
Sentence 2: If we want to get better at our skills we should
    . . . study them.
    . . . put a hole in them.
    . . . do them a lot.

Wiig and Semel (1984) suggest the use of an "identification and selection" task to assess word knowledge. With this task, the child chooses a word or picture that corresponds to a target word. For example, the child might be asked to point to *the big one* in an array of objects of different sizes.

Pragmatics.   There are many ways to elicit aspects of pragmatics. For example, Owens (1991) suggested some of the following activities:

Target	Technique	Example
Requests for information	Pass it on	*Clinician:* John do you know where Linda's project is? *Client:* No. *Clinician:* Oh, see if she does. *Client:* Linda, where's your project?
Contingent query	Mumble	*Clinician:* (finishing a story) And, so, just as the giant got to the door, (mumble). *Client:* What? (If the child makes no response, prompt with a question)
Initiating conversation	Request for assistance	*Clinician:* John, can you ask Keith to help me? *Client:* Keith, can you help us?

Other methods for examining pragmatic language include asking a child to teach a task to another, asking the child to request a cookie from different people (e.g., a friend, a teacher), and asking two children to act as host and guest on a talk show (see Activity 2, Chapter 5).

The development of elicited language tasks is limited only by one's creativity and knowledge of language. These tasks can be fun for the child while also providing important information about the child's language development.

Summary

In this chapter we have considered the many ways that language can be assessed. We examined formal, standardized language; language samples; and elicited language tasks. Development of a comprehensive plan of language assessment should include the following elements:

- Testing of hearing
- Examination of the child's mouth, teeth, and tongue to determine whether malformations may be affecting language production
- Assessment of cognitive functioning
- Observation of language use in school
- A language sample
- Formal tests of language
- Elicted language tasks

The case study following (adapted from Wiig & Semel, 1984) illustrates how a variety of assessment procedures can be used to produce a comprehensive picture of an individual's language skills.

Case Study: Bob

When Bob was referred for an in-depth language evaluation, he was 14 years old and attended the eighth grade in a suburban public school. His parents were concerned about his failing academic achievement. At the time of referral, Bob's performance on a test of academic achievement placed him three grades below his actual grade level in reading and spelling.

Bob's early developmental milestones in motor, speech, language, and social development were reported to have occurred within the expected age ranges. The results of an assessment of intelligence, using the WISC-R, placed Bob's verbal scale IQ in the average range and his performance scale IQ in the high-average–bright range. More important, however, is that the school psychologist reported a discrepancy of 18 IQ points between the verbal and performance scale IQs, observing areas of relative weakness on verbal tasks probing the recall of general information, stored knowledge, and word knowledge.

Bob was then given several formal tests of language ability, including the *Peabody Picture Vocabulary Test (PPVT)* and selected subtests of the *Illinois Test of Psycholinguistic Abilities* and the *Detroit Tests of Learning Aptitude (DTLA)*. These tests were complemented by informal testing of specific language functions and tasks.

On tests of word knowledge, Bob's ability to perform depended upon the task requirements. When he was asked to match words to pictures (PPVT), his performance was only 6 months below age level, within normal limits. When he was asked to tell how two words were alike and how they were different (DTLA), his performance level fell about 2 years below age expectations. When Bob was asked to define words (DTLA), his performance level fell about 3½ years below age level.

Several subtests were administered to probe Bob's ability to recall spoken words, sentences, and oral directions. His performances on all tests fell well below age-level expectations. The error patterns on all the tests of recall of spoken words, sentences, and directions proved revealing. In all instances, associative, antonym, or synonym word substitutions appeared to present a barrier. As examples, Bob substituted *east* for *south*, and *nice* for *good* when repeating words and sentences. When Bob performed actions in response to oral directions, he consistently substituted spatial and directional words. Bob's error patterns indicated significant word-substitution problems on listening tasks, which may have interfered with his performance in school.

Review Questions

   1. What is the difference between *assessment* and *testing?*

   2. What makes language especially difficult to assess?

   3. Discuss the advantages and limitations of formal and informal methods of language assessment.

4. Calculate the mean length of utterance (MLU) for the language-sample information given below:

Number of morphemes	Number of utterances	MLU
250	75	
327	90	
340	85	

5. What is type-token ratio? How is it calculated? What does it indicate about language development?

6. Compare the advantages and the limitations of two methods for eliciting language samples.

7. Describe an informal elicitation technique that could be used to prompt a child to ask questions.

Suggested Activities

1. Informal language-elicitation tasks are designed to prompt the child to produce a specific language structure. Your task is to develop elicitation activities for the following language elements:

possessives *(his, yours, mine)*

multiple meaning words *(table, swing, left)*

use of politeness terms *(please, thank you)*

You must select materials and formats that will cause the individual to produce the desired responses. Include in your report:

– a description of the materials and format you selected
– the age and disability (if any) of the individual being tested
– the results of your assessment
– your interpretation of the results

2. Compare using two of the techniques for eliciting language samples (pictures, interviews, structured-task, spontaneous) discussed in the chapter. You will need to collect two language samples of approximately 50 utterances each (a total of 100 utterances) from one individual using each of the techniques. Analyze the resulting samples for the MLU, TTR, and language-complexity topics discussed.

In your report, include the following:

– a description of the procedures used
– a description of the subject (e.g., age, disability, if any)
– a report of the results
– your conclusion about what the results indicate about the two methods you used for eliciting language samples

References

Bankson, N. (1990) *Bankson language test* (2nd ed.). Austin TX: Pro-Ed.

Berko, J. (1958). The child's learning of English morphology. *Word, 14*, 150–177.

Boehm, A. (1986). *Boehm test of basic concepts—Revised*. San Antonio, TX: Psychological Corporation.

Bray, C., & Wiig, E. (1987). *Let's talk inventory for children*. San Antonio, TX: Psychological Corporation.

Carrow-Woolfolk, E. (1974). *Carrow elicited language inventory*. Chicago: Riverside.

Carrow-Woolfolk, E. (1985). *Test for auditory comprehension of language—Revised*. Chicago: Riverside.

Coggins, T., Olswang, L., & Guthrie, J. (1987). Assessing communicative intent in young children: Low structured observation or elicitation tasks? *Journal of Speech and Hearing Disorders, 52*, 44–49.

Cohen, R., Swerdlik, M., & Smith, D. (1992). *Psychological testing and measurement* (2nd ed). Mountain View, CA: Mayfield.

Cole, K., Mills, P., & Dale, P. (1989). Examination of test-retest and split-half reliability for measures derived from language samples of young handicapped children. *Language, Speech, and Hearing Services in Schools, 20*, 259–268.

Connell, P., & Myles-Zitzer, C. (1982). An analysis of elicited imitation as a language evaluation procedure. *Journal of Speech and Hearing Disorders, 47*, 390–396.

Dollaghan, C., Campbell, T., & Tomlin, R. (1990). Video narration as a language sampling context. *Journal of Speech and Hearing Disorders, 55*, 582–590.

Dunn, L., & Dunn, L. (1981). *Peabody picture vocabulary test—Revised*. Circle Pines, MN: American Guidance Service.

Evans, J., & Craig, H. (1992). Language sample collection and analysis: Interview compared to freeplay assessment contexts. *Journal of Speech and Hearing Research, 35*, 343–353.

Fujiki, M., & Brinton, B. (1987). Elicited imitation revisited: A comparison with spontaneous language production. *Language,*

Speech, and Hearing Services in Schools, 18, 301–311.

Goldman, R., & Fristoe, M. (1986). *Goldman-Fristoe test of articulation*. Circle Pines, MN: American Guidance.

Goldman, R., Fristoe, M., & Woodcock (1970). *Goldman-Fristoe-Woodcock test of auditory discrimination*. Circle Pines, MN: American Guidance.

Halliday, M. (1975). *Explorations in the function of language*. London: Edward Arnold.

Hammill, D., Brown, V., Larsen, S., & Wiederholt, J. (1987). *Test of adolescent language–2*. Austin, TX: Pro-Ed.

Hammill, D., & Newcomer, P. (1988). *Test of Language Development—Intermediate* (2nd ed.). Austin, TX: Pro-Ed.

Howell, K., Fox, S., & Morehead, M. (1993). *Curriculum-Based Evaluation: Teaching and Decision Making* (2nd ed.). Pacific Grove, CA: Brooks/Cole.

Hresko, W., Reid, D., & Hammill, D. (1991). *Test of early language development* (2nd ed.). Austin, TX: Pro-Ed.

James, S. (1993). Assessing children with language disorders. In D. Bernstein & E. Tiegerman (Eds.), *Language and communication disorders in children* (3rd ed.) (pp. 185–228). New York: Merrill.

Johnson, A., Johnston, E., & Weinrich, B. (1984). Assessing pragmatic skills in children's language. *Language, Speech, and Hearing Services in Schools, 15*, 2–9.

Johnston, J., & Kamhi, A. (1984). Syntactic and semantic aspects of the utterances of language-impaired children: The same can be less. *Merrill-Palmer Quarterly, 30*, 65–86.

Kramer, C., James, S., & Saxman, J. (1979). A comparison of language samples elicited at home and in the clinic. *Journal of Speech and Hearing Disorders, 44*, 321–330.

Lahey, M. (1988). *Language disorders and language development*. New York: Macmillan.

Lee, L. (1971). *Northwestern syntax screening test*. Evanston, IL: Northwestern University Press.

Lee, L. (1974). *Developmental sentence analysis.* Evanston, IL: Northwestern University Press.

Lund, N., & Duchan, J. (1988). *Assessing children's language in naturalistic contexts.* Englewood Cliffs, NJ: Prentice-Hall.

McLoughlin, J., & Lewis, R. (1994). *Assessing special students* (4th ed.). New York: Merrill.

Menyuk, P. (1968). Children's learning and reproduction of grammatical and nongrammatical phonological sequences. *Child Development, 39,* 849–859.

Miller, J. (1981). *Assessing language production in children.* Baltimore: University Park Press.

Miller, J., & Chapman, R. (1985). *Systematic analysis of language transcripts.* Madison, WI: Weisman Center on Mental Retardation and Human Development.

Myers, P. (1987). Assessing oral language. In D. Hammill (Ed.), *Assessing the abilities and instructional needs of students* (pp. 38–158). Austin, TX: Pro-Ed.

Newcomer, P., & Hammill, D. (1988). *Test of language development—Primary* (2nd ed.). Austin, TX: Pro-Ed.

Owens, R. (1991). *Language disorders: A functional approach to assessment and intervention.* New York: Merrill.

Salvia, J., & Ysseldyke, J. (1995). *Assessment* (6th ed.). Boston: Houghton-Mifflin.

Semel, E., Wiig, E., & Secord, W. (1987). *Clinical evaluation of language fundamentals—revised.* San Antonio, TX: Psychological Corporation.

Shulman, B. (1986). Test of pragmatic skills-revised. Tucson, AZ: Communication Skill Builders.

Wanska, S., Bedrosian, J., & Pohlman, J. (1986). Effects of play materials on the topic performance of preschool children. *Language, Speech, and Hearing Services in Schools, 17,* 152–159.

Wepman, J. (1973). *Auditory discrimination test.* Palm Springs, CA: Research Associates.

Wetherby, A., & Rodriguez, G. (1992). Measurement of communicative intentions in normally developing children during structured and unstructured contexts. *Journal of Speech and Hearing Research, 35,* 130–138.

Wiig, E., Semel, E. (1984). *Language assessment and intervention for the learning disabled* (2nd ed.). Columbus, OH: Merrill.

Wren, C. (1985). Collecting language samples from children with syntax problems. *Language, Speech, and Hearing Services in Schools, 16,* 83–102.

Chapter *11*

Intervention Models and Procedures

As we know from the preceding chapters, there are children who, despite exposure to language, fail to develop language skills at the same rate or to the same extent as other children. Difficulty with the development and use of effective speech, language, and communication skills affects the ability of students to understand classroom instruction, socialize with their peers, and become full members of society. What are we to do about children with language disorders?

We could wait for them to catch up. Some may do so, but most children with language disorders not only do not catch up, they fall further and further behind. Since we cannot usually count on spontaneous recovery to take care of the problem, it is often necessary to develop intervention strategies to help students with language disorders enhance their speech, language, and communication skills.

In this chapter and the next one we will examine effective language intervention practices. Chapter 11 presents the major models of language intervention. Principles and guidelines for intervention are suggested. There are also descriptions of effective programs and examples of intervention strategies for specific elements of language.

After completion of this chapter, you should be able to:

1. Discuss the rationale for language intervention.
2. Describe decisions that need to be made prior to language intervention.
3. Describe a functional approach to language intervention.
4. Discuss how information about language development can be used in the design of effective language-intervention strategies.
5. Describe naturalistic approaches to language intervention and explain how these differ from structured approaches.
6. Discuss what type of language intervention works best.
7. Describe how language acquisition models can be applied to the development of language intervention procedures.

Rationale for Language Intervention

Cole and Dale (1986) pose three questions to address in evaluating language intervention for children with disabilities. First, is intervention necessary? They answer this question by pointing out that a large number of studies have found that young children with language disorders are much more likely to have academic, social, and language difficulties later in life than are children with normally developing language (Aram & Nation, 1980; Aram, Ekelman, & Nation, 1984; King, Jones, & Laskey, 1982). So it appears that intervention is, indeed, necessary if we hope to improve the chances of success in school and in life for children with early language disorders.

The second question posed by Cole and Dale is whether effective interventions exist. Again, there are numerous studies that support the effectiveness of language intervention for improving language skills. This is true for young children with mild to moderate language disorders (Goldstein & Hockenberger, 1991), as well as for individuals with significant disabilities (Bryen & Joyce, 1985). In addition to their enhancing language and communication skills, language intervention programs can also have positive effects on other areas of functioning. For example, a number of studies have found that when students with significant behavior problems are taught to improve their communication skills, their behavior problems decrease (Doss & Reichle, 1989; Durand, 1993).

The third question raised by Cole and Dale is, however, the most critical one. What type of intervention is the most effective? Despite a great deal of research on this subject, there is no simple answer to this question. We can show that certain kinds of intervention work for particular children, under specific conditions, and to achieve particular goals. In this chapter we will examine some of the research on language intervention as we try to answer the question, what language intervention methods are most effective?

Preparing for Language Intervention

Language intervention, in the words of Olswang and Bain (1991), "is viewed as focused, intensive stimulation designed to alter specific behaviors" (p. 255). As they note, intervention involves more than monitoring, or providing general suggestions to encourage communication. Intervention is targeted at specific language skills and is intensive enough to cause an improvement in these skills. Although clinicians may disagree about the particular methods for intervention, most would agree that the goal of language intervention is to make intervention itself unnecessary.

Developing a plan for language intervention requires addressing four questions. The first question is *when* to intervene. In order to answer this question, we need to know if there is a need for intervention. Answering this question might seem like a relatively simple task. By using the assessment procedures outlined in the previous chapter, we can establish that the child does, in fact, have a significant language disorder. Yet, this is really not sufficient. As Olswang and Bain

(1991) point out, a child's being eligible for intervention does not necessarily mean that the child is a good candidate for intervention. They suggest that speech-language specialists consider the child's cognitive abilities and potential for change before intervening. Olswang and Bain contend that children whose language scores are similar to their scores on cognitive tests may not be good candidates for specific language intervention, since their development is uniformly delayed. They also note that some research has suggested that children will benefit most from intervention when it is delivered just at that point when they are ready to learn, and they suggest methods of assessment that can be used to determine when a child is most likely to benefit from intervention.

Teachers and parents are most interested in knowing if and when to refer a child for intervention. Again, knowing that the child has difficulty with some aspect of language may not be enough. Concerned parents may want to know whether their child will benefit from speech therapy when there is no question that the child exhibits some speech impairment. They wonder, is it serious enough to justify intervention and will the problem go away without intervention? In order to answer these questions, we have to ask some more questions:

1. **Is the child having difficulty with academic tasks?** For example, does the child have difficulty with reading, spelling, or writing?
2. **Does the child have difficulty participating in classroom interactions?** Does the child have difficulty understanding directions, following discussions, or contributing to classroom interactions?
3. **Does the child have difficulty getting along with others?** Are language difficulties causing the child to be teased by others, be misunderstood, or be left out of social activities?
4. **Is the language problem getting worse, getting better, or staying about the same?** If the child is making steady progress, intervention may not be needed. Instead, the child may need to be carefully monitored for a while.

If the answer to at least one of the first three questions is yes, and the problem appears to be getting worse or not improving, the child should probably receive intervention for the speech or language difficulty.

Once a decision is made that the child needs intervention, the next question is *where* such intervention should take place. The answer to this question used to be easy. As Miller (1989) notes in her retrospective review of language intervention, until the 1970s most language intervention was carried out in a speech clinic. The child was pulled out of the classroom for specialized—usually one-on-one—instruction. Miller points out that two developments changed this approach. First, theories of language began to put more emphasis on pragmatics—the use of language in natural contexts. Second was the realization that language is an integral part of classroom success. In addition, many researchers and practitioners were concerned about the stigma of removing children from their peers. As a result of these trends, the classroom-based, service-delivery model has become more widespread. With classroom-based intervention, the speech-language specialist becomes a partner with the classroom teacher in service delivery.

TABLE 11.1   Advantages/Limitations of Speech-Language Service-Delivery Models

Model	Advantages	Limitations
Pull out	Specific skills can be focused on Distraction reduced for student	Student may be stigmatized No opportunity for realistic practice
In-class therapy	Opportunities for immediate application Availability of curricular materials	Distractions in classroom Stigma may still be attached
Consultation	Opportunity to share/discuss language goals for student Teacher involved as communicator	Relies on teacher's knowledge of language Need for planning time
Collaboration	Speech-language specialist can support instruction Language instruction embedded in classroom activities	Less focus, possibly, on language goals Need for planning time
Team teaching	Complete integration of language and academic goals No stigma for child	Less direct focus on language goals Need for planning time

Even if the speech-language specialist is working one-on-one with the child in a corner of the room, there is an increased opportunity to observe the child in the natural setting of the classroom, for the child to immediately practice a new skill, and for the clinician to use actual curriculum materials from the classroom. So the preferred location for service delivery today is in the child's classroom. Occasionally it may be necessary to remove the child from the classroom. For example, when a new skill is being presented, the quiet and concentration available in a speech therapy room may be helpful. But these times should be limited in number and duration.

Answering the question about *where* intervention should take place suggests an answer to the third question—*who* should deliver intervention. With classroom-based intervention there is a greater role for the classroom teacher in the child's intervention. This is as it should be. After all, it is the classroom teacher— regular or special—who knows the child the best and will see that child for most of the school day. This is the professional who has the greatest opportunity to help the child improve his or her language skills. In classroom-based intervention models, the teacher becomes a significant partner in the intervention program. The speech-language specialist's role may be to act as a consulting or collaborating professional with the classroom teacher. As a consultant, the specialist can advise the teacher on the best methods and materials to help the child learn and practice the targeted language skill. In collaborative service-delivery models, the teacher and speech-language specialist divide their classroom responsibilities (Montgomery, 1992). As the teacher presents the lesson the speech-language specialist may check for understanding or coach the child in how to respond. These roles may be difficult for teachers and speech-language specialists to accept at first, but the goal is to present a more natural setting for language intervention (see Table 11.1).

The fourth question is undoubtedly the most difficult one and, indeed, the one that will be the focus for the remainder of this chapter—*how* to intervene. As we noted in the chapter introduction, research on language intervention has failed to find one method that works under all circumstances. Rather, factors such as the child's level of cognitive and language functioning (Yoder, Kaiser, & Alpert, 1991) and the element of language targeted for intervention have to be considered.

Although clinicians and researchers cannot always agree on what constitutes the most effective methods for language intervention, there are some practices that most would agree are preferable. Owens (1995) has called these practices *functional* intervention. Functional-intervention approaches recognize that language skills need to be *integrated* and *applied* to natural settings. Functional intervention emphasizes use of *conversational* skills rather than isolated syntactic or semantic rules and is usually delivered in *natural* settings, where there is an opportunity for immediate application and *generalization*.

Owens (1995) suggests eight principles for implementing a *functional* approach to language intervention. These are

1. The language facilitator serves as reinforcer: By demonstrating attentiveness, responsiveness, and respect for the child, the language facilitator will encourage language interaction.

2. Closely approximate natural learning: As much as possible, language intervention procedures should follow the natural process of language acquisition. Using natural environments with parents and teachers as models are ways to implement this principle.

3. Follow developmental guidelines: The language development of nondisabled children is used as a guide for the selection of intervention targets. Easier, less complex structures are taught first.

4. Follow the child's lead: The language facilitator should be prepared to follow the child's lead in selecting topics for conversation and means of expression. The facilitator should be sensitive to the child's communicative intent rather than focus solely on structure. Rather than correcting children the language facilitator should be responsive to the child's attempt to communicate.

5. Actively involve the child: Language learning is not a passive process. The interests of the child should be considered in planning language intervention activities.

6. Language is heavily influenced by context: Language intervention should occur in the natural context. The language facilitator can manipulate the context to focus on desired intervention goals.

7. Familiar events provide scripts: Scripts are sequences of events that provide structure. Familiar activities, such as making popcorn, can be used as context for language learning.

8. Design a generalization plan first: Language intervention is of little use if the child does not use the newly acquired skills. Therefore, it is essential that intervention be designed in such a way that generalization to new environments will be likely.

Despite widespread agreement about the effectiveness of functional approaches to language intervention, debates continue about the best way to implement procedures such as those suggested by Owens. In the next section, we will focus on two major areas of debate about language intervention: developmental versus remedial approaches and structural versus naturalistic approaches. In addition, we will see how theories of language acquisition can help guide intervention decisions.

Methods for Language Intervention

Developmental versus Remedial Approaches

One of the major questions in language intervention is how information about language acquisition can and should be used in planning therapy for children with language disorders. It is important for professionals to understand normal language development. After all, how are we to recognize developmental problems if we do not have a fair idea of what constitutes the norm? Knowledge of the usual steps and timing of normal language development provides a benchmark against which the language development of any individual child can be compared. In addition, with knowledge of normal language development, the teacher or speech-language specialist can better develop instructional goals for a child. Knowing what *should* come next can help in determining what should be taught next.

Since we know that children with disabilities often acquire language in the same sequence (although more slowly) as nondisabled children, it makes sense to follow developmental guidelines in planning language goals. This was the hypothesis tested by Dyer, Santarcangelo, and Luce (1987). In a series of studies, they taught phonetic sounds and syntactic structures to children with severe language disabilities. They found that earlier-emerging forms (e.g., *b* sounds) were learned in fewer trials than were later-emerging forms (e.g., *z* sounds). Moreover, later-emerging forms were never acquired unless the earlier forms had been learned. Here, using normal language development as a guideline turned out to be a useful way of planning instructional goals for these students with severe language disorders.

Although knowledge of normal language development can be helpful in planning language intervention, Owens (1995) cautions against using this knowledge too strictly. He points out, for example, that it would be a mistake to teach children with language delays to go through all of the steps that normally developing children use to get to the final form of a language structure. It is not necessary for a child to say *goded* before learning the correct irregular past tense form, *went*. Owens suggests that developmental hierarchies can best be used as broad guidelines for intervention—for help in determining which structures are less complex and, thus, should be taught prior to more complex structures. Having knowledge of language development can also help the instructor avoid leaps that are too great for the child to master.

Some still argue that using normal language development as a guideline for language intervention is a mistake even if it is used with the above cautions in mind. They argue that considerable research on children with disabilities (some of which has been reviewed in previous chapters) shows that these children sometimes do not develop language in the same way as nondisabled children. For example, we know that there may be limits to the development of syntactic skills in children with mental retardation (Kamhi & Johnston, 1982) and idiosyncrasies in the spoken language of children with autism (Volden & Lord, 1991). Children with disabilities may skip developmental steps, develop splinter skills, and fail altogether to develop some steps. For these reasons, normal development may not always be a good guideline to planning intervention for children with disabilities. There is a real danger that too strict an adherence to developmental guidelines may result in denying a child services. It may be determined that a particular child is not ready to learn a skill—even though the child has demonstrated the skill on several occasions—because he or she has failed to acquire the prerequisite skills. Similarly, there is a danger that intervention may focus inappropriately on a skill the child does not need, causing frustration for the child and delays in teaching needed skills.

Another argument against using normal language development as a guide for language intervention is that sometimes techniques that work for normally developing children may not work for children with disabilities. For example, Connell (1987) and Connell and Stone (1992) found that modeling correct language was sufficient to improve the language skills of normally developing children but did not have the same effect on the language of children with specific language impairments. In the first study, Connell (1987) compared the use of imitation (a highly structured approach) and modeling (a less structured approach) in teaching an invented language rule to children with specific language impairments and to normally developing children. Those children who received *imitation* instruction were told to repeat the target word after the teacher. If they did so correctly, they were praised. The *modeling* group simply listened as the teacher showed a picture and said the corresponding word. The children were to make no response at all. Connell found that normally developing children learned more from the modeling procedure than from the imitation procedure. However, the imitation procedure was the best one for the children with language delays. More recent research by Connell and Stone (1992) has continued to find that structured training using imitation works well for children with significant language impairments.

As a result of concerns about the role of normal development in planning language intervention, some have suggested that intervention should focus on teaching specific skills that the children will need in their immediate environment. Sometimes called *remedial* or *functional* approaches, these intervention programs seek to identify skills that the children need to be successful in their present environment or in one which they will soon be entering.

TABLE 11.2 Examples of Functional (Integrated) and Nonfunctional (Nonintegrated) Objectives

Integrated (functional)	Nonintegrated (nonfunctional)
Given that John is seated at a table in the cafeteria and is missing an eating utensil that he needs, on 3 consecutive days he will request the utensil by pointing to the corresponding photograph on his communication board.	When seated at a table in the cafeteria, upon which is a spoon, a knife, and a fork, John will correctly place photographs of each of these three utensils on the corresponding object, with 80 percent or greater accuracy in three out of four consecutive sessions.
Given that John is dressing himself for school and requires assistance, on 5 consecutive days he will request his mother's attention and then point to the article of clothing with which he needs help.	While getting dressed following gym class, upon his aide's request John will correctly point to his shoes, socks, shirt, and pants 80 percent or more of the time on 2 out of 3 consecutive days.
Given that John is not feeling well, he will issue unambiguous yes/no responses 80 percent or more of the time to an adult who is attempting to identify what is wrong with him.	John will accurately indicate *yes* and *no* in his communication book 80 percent or more of the time, on 2 out of 3 consecutive days, in response to his mother's asking him a series of questions soliciting personal information.

Source: Adapted from S. N. Calculator & C. M. Jorgensen. (1991). Integrating AAC instruction into regular education settings: Expounding on best practices. *Augmentative and Alternative Communication, 7,* 204–213.

To better understand how functional communication differs from nonfunctional, consider the situations that appear in Table 11.2, described by Calculator and Jorgensen (1991). Calculator and Jorgensen use these situations as examples of what they call *integrated* and *nonintegrated* objectives. In the first example, the functional goal stipulates that John request an object (utensil) that he actually needs. The nonfunctional goal simply requires that John match pictures with objects. Similarly, in the other examples the emphasis is on the utilization of skills that John actually needs to use rather then on performing a task simply to accomplish an instructional objective. These examples demonstrate that it is possible to change a nonintegrated (or nonfunctional) objective to one that is integrated (or functional).

Similarly, Mire and Chisholm (1990) provide examples of functional goals for adolescent or adult students with moderate to severe mental retardation. They studied students who had received many years of language training focusing on isolated semantic and syntactic skills. Despite their having many years of intervention, these students had failed to acquire functional communication abilities. Now, rather than focusing on developmental language goals, their students are learning language that will lead to specific functional outcomes (see Table 11.3). The examples in Table 11.3 utilize real community-based situations that require that the individual use communication skills.

How, then, should teachers and other professionals use developmental information in planning language intervention? Normal language development

TABLE 11.3 Functional Goal Formats

Goal: Independently place an order at a fast food restaurant
   A. Begin order with phrase "I want _____."
   B. Use appropriate eye contact when ordering
   C. Specify size of items.
   D. Use appropriate semantic referents when ordering (including names of specific items, such as Big Mac, Whopper).
   E. Deny request for order when cashier suggests items not desired by student.
   F. Cancel order or part of order.
   G. Terminate interaction.

Goal: Independently complete shopping routine
   A. Request assistance.
   B. Request change.

Goal: Independently communicate needs/comments during leisure-time activities
   A. Purchase ticket.
   B. Request information, if necessary.
   C. Participate appropriately in leisure-time conversation.

Goal: Independently communicate needs while traveling
   A. Request amount of fare and/or where to deposit.
   B. Phone for taxi.
   C. Respond to request for destination.
   D. Request directions.

Source: From S. Mire & R. Chisholm, "Functional Communication Goals for Adolescents and Adults Who Are Severely and Moderately Mentally Handicapped," *Language, Speech, and Hearing Services in Schools,* 21(1990), 57–58. © American Speech-Language-Hearing Association. Reprinted by permission of the American Speech-Language-Hearing Association and the author.

should be seen as a framework within which there can be considerable variation. This is true for normally developing children and even more true for children with disabilities. Information about normal language development should be used as a way to identify children at risk for language disorders and as a way to develop an overall sequence of skills. The child's age and status should most importantly determine how developmental guidelines are used. In general, developmental hierarchies are less valid for older children and children with more severe disabilities. These children are more likely to benefit from programs that focus on skills needed in their current environment, skills of functional communication and general literacy.

Structured versus Naturalistic Approaches

As language acquisition theories have focused more on pragmatics and the role of social interaction, traditional language-intervention approaches have been modified or abandoned altogether. The result, as Yoder et al. (1991) point out, is that contemporary language intervention procedures exist along a continuum, from highly structured, didactic teaching to more naturalistic, child-oriented approaches. Among the more highly structured procedures are behavior-based methods

TABLE 11.4   Structured Intervention Contrasted with Naturalistic

Structured	Naturalistic
Uses clinical setting	Uses natural environment contexts
Uses drill and practice activities	Uses conversational activities
Uses massed trials	Uses dispersed trials
Follows rigid hierarchy of goals	Follows child's lead
Uses reinforcers determined by instructor	Uses reinforcers based on child's interest
Reinforces correct responding	Reinforces attempts at communication

Source: Adapted from: K. N. Cole & P. Dale. (1986). Direct language instruction and interactive language instruction with language-delayed preschool children: A comparison study. *Journal of Speech and Hearing Research, 29,* 206–217.
Warren, S. F., & Kaiser, A. P. (1986). Incidental language teaching: A critical review. *Journal of Speech and Hearing Disorders, 51,* 291–299.

that use imitation, modeling, and/or reinforcement (such as the DISTAR language program) and highly structured programs that teach syntactic rules (e.g., Fokes Sentence Builder). Typically these programs come with a standardized set of instructions and materials. They take the child through a highly structured sequence of steps toward a goal that is set prior to instruction. Although highly structured programs *can* work, they have been criticized for being unnatural (Goetz, Schuler, and Sailor, 1981); that is, the instructional procedures are unlike what the child is likely to encounter in the real world, and as a result, children may master *splinter* skills—skills that are relatively useless.

Naturalistic approaches emphasize the delivery of language instruction in natural settings, utilizing dispersed trials which follow the child's lead and use reinforcers indicated by the child's preferences (Warren & Kaiser, 1986). Although language-instruction goals may be set prior to instruction, the language facilitator is encouraged to be responsive to the child. The language facilitator may structure the environment in ways that will lead toward a language goal but should follow the child's lead and be responsive to the child rather than to a set of instructions (see Table 11.4). Therefore, if the child uses structures that were not anticipated or wants to talk about topics that were not part of the plan, the facilitator should follow the child's lead.

A number of different instructional approaches can be grouped under the general heading of naturalistic instruction. One example is the **milieu** model. This approach to language instruction emphasizes the use of ongoing activities as its basis (Warren, 1991). Several specific instructional procedures can be grouped under this general model. For example, the **mand-model** method (see Chapter 6) is an example of a milieu procedure that uses the child's activity as the basis for language teaching. Another example of a milieu teaching procedure is **time delay.** When using this procedure, the language facilitator moves close to the child and looks at the child for 5 to 15 seconds, while waiting for the child to talk. If the child does not initiate an interaction, the adult can provide a verbal prompt or model an initiation. **Incidental teaching** is still another milieu approach. Warren and Kaiser (1986) describe incidental teaching as including the following elements:

1. Arranging the environment to increase the likelihood that the child will initiate to the adult.
2. Selecting language targets appropriate for the child's skill level, interests, and the environment.
3. Responding to the child's initiations with requests for elaborated language.
4. Reinforcing the child's communicative attempts with attention and access to the objects and activities with which the child has expressed interest.

Warren and Kaiser give the following example to illustrate the use of incidental teaching in practice:

Child (points to box of crayons, looks toward adult and says): Colors.

Adult (focusing attention on child): What do you want?

Child: Want color.

Adult (modeling): Say, I want colors.

Child: I want colors.

Adult (giving child the crayons): Good, here are the colors.

As Table 11.4 shows, there are many differences between structured and functional approaches to language instruction. Yet there is research to support each approach. For example, the studies by Connell (1987) and by Connell and Stone (1992) that were described earlier in this chapter have found that children with more severe language disorders learn best in more highly structured language instruction programs. Other researchers (e.g., Courtright & Courthright, 1979; Friedman & Friedman, 1980) have found similar results.

However, research reported by Yoder et al. (1991) called into question the long-held assumption that direct, structured methods of language teaching are more effective for students with significant language disorders. In their study, Yoder et al. compared a less structured (milieu) approach to a more structured (Communication Training Program) language-instruction program for teaching language skills to 40 preschool children with significant delays in both language and cognitive development. The milieu program was designed to follow the child's lead in determining the goals and pace of the program. Milieu training sessions were described as conversational in nature. The Communication Training Program used a drill and practice procedure to teach previously specified language goals. Unlike the research by Connell and others, cited above, Yoder et al. found that the milieu approach worked best for the children with the most serious language impairments. The more structured program worked best for the higher functioning children. The authors speculated that one reason for their findings may have been that the lower functioning children benefited more from a program that emphasized the generalization of language skills (the milieu approach).

Still other research has failed to find any difference at all between structured and naturalistic language-instruction programs. Cole and Dale (1986) compared the use of the DISTAR language program to an interactive language program. The DISTAR program uses predetermined teacher-initiated instructional formats to teach a carefully sequenced hierarchy of language skills. Imitation and reinforcement are important components of the program. The interactive program used natural training opportunities (e.g., snack time) to teach goals that were individualized for each child. Materials were carefully selected to elicit interaction, and facilitators were encouraged to engage in communication with the child rather than to directly reinforce a response. Unlike the studies reviewed previously, Cole and Dale found little difference between the two instructional models in teaching language skills to the preschool children with language delays who served as the subjects of their study. The authors note that one reason there may have been no difference could be that both methods were implemented effectively. In other words, when there are adequate staffing, clear goals, and continual monitoring of progress, children may learn no matter what the theoretical basis of the instructional program.

The results of the Cole and Dale study suggest that some combination of structured and naturalistic language teaching methods might work best. The authors themselves suggest presenting a concept initially using direct instruction, then practicing using a more naturalistic approach. An alternative could be to introduce a language concept through naturalistic communication, then to practice using more highly structured, drill and practice procedures.

One example of a procedure that combines structured and naturalistic procedures is the **interrupted-behavior-chain** strategy (previously described in Chapter 6). In this approach, a targeted language skill is inserted in the middle of an already established sequence of behaviors. Caro and Snell (1989) give an example of the application of this strategy in grocery shopping. Having taught an individual to read a grocery list, locate items on the shelf, and pay the cashier, the teacher could interrupt the behavior sequence to ask the student to say which items had already been placed in the grocery cart, and then praise a correct response. If the student produced an incorrect response, the instructor would model the correct response and prompt the student to produce it. This is an example of the combination of a natural environment (grocery shopping) with a structured instructional technique (prompting, modeling, reinforcement).

Intervention Based on Language Acquisition Models

The major theories of language acquisition were discussed in Chapter 3. These theories are useful for what they can tell us about the process of learning language and about language itself. But they can also be used as guidelines for language intervention. Each of the theoretical models we reviewed—behavioral, psycholinguistic, semantic-cognitive, and pragmatic-interactionist—has implications for the selection of language teaching goals and for instructional methods (see Table 11.5).

TABLE 11.5   Intervention Procedures Based on Language-Acquisition Models

Model	Goals	Procedures	Example
Behavioral	Specific, discrete language behaviors Assessment of prerequisite skills	Prompting Reinforcement	DISTAR Language Program
Psycholinguistic	Developmental guidelines Rule learning	Discovery of underlying rules	Fokes Sentence Builders
Semantic-cognitive	Cognitive prerequisites Semantic concepts	Stimulation activities	Peabody Language Kits
Pragmatic-interactionist	Communication	Extension of conversation (expansion)	Let's Talk kits

The **behavioral** theory of language acquisition suggests that language is learned just like any other behavior; that is, the processes of imitation, modeling, and reinforcement are critical components in the child's acquisition of language. In the behavioral model, teachers choose specific, discrete language behaviors as the focus of instruction and, through assessment, determine that the child has acquired the prerequisite skills. The child is *prompted* to make a response (say, *I want a cookie*) and is *reinforced* for making a correct response *(Good talking!)*. Instruction continues until mastery of the skill is achieved. The *DISTAR Language Program* (SRA) is an example of a commercial program that is based on a behavioral theory of language acquisition. DISTAR uses a highly structured sequence of lessons to teach discrete language skills through the use of modeling, imitation, and reinforcement.

The **psycholinguistic** theory of language acquisition places most of its emphasis on biological development, on the idea that language emerges as the individual develops. Although there is little that teachers can do to directly influence biological maturation, they may still apply the psycholinguistic model to language instruction. First, this theory suggests using *developmental guidelines* for instructional goals, and second, that instruction should focus on *rule learning*. According to the psycholinguistic theory, the most important developments in early language learning involve the acquisition of the underlying rules of language. Instruction that helps children become aware of language rules, discover underlying rules, and apply these rules in new situations is most useful. The *Fokes Sentence Builder* (DLM) is an example of a commercial program based on the psycholinguistic model of language acquisition. Students learn to build sentences of increasing length by combining sentence elements.

Using the **semantic-cognitive** model of language learning as a guide to teaching language involves focusing on the acquisition of cognitive prerequisites to language and on the development of semantic concepts. As discussed earlier in this book, some theorists (e.g., Piaget) claim that certain cognitive prerequisites (e.g., object permanence) must precede the emergence of spoken language. If children lack these prerequisites, it may be necessary to help them acquire the necessary skills. Although there has been a great debate as to whether it is possible to teach cognitive skills, many researchers believe it is possible to help children who are ready to take the next step do so just a bit more quickly. The formal name for this idea is the *zone of proximal development.* As proposed by Vygotsky (1962), the notion is that when children are just at the edge of developing a new skill, experiences and instruction can help them take this step. In addition to its helping children develop cognitive prerequisites, the semantic-cognitive model suggests that language learning can be facilitated by the development of new semantic concepts. When children have something to talk about, the theory suggests, they will find a way to express their new ideas. The *Peabody Language Development Kits* (American Guidance Service) emphasize the development of cognitive concepts and thinking.

The **pragmatic-interactionist** model implies that the goal of language intervention should be to enhance communication. Children should be encouraged to interact with parents, peers, and teachers. Language facilitators should be responsive to the child, letting the child take the lead in language interaction by setting the conversational topic. Reed (1994) gives several examples of techniques that can be used to extend conversation (see Chapter 12 for a more detailed discussion). One example is *expansion.* Using this technique, the adult takes a child's utterance and repeats it using a higher-level language model. Reed gives the following example:

Target: Attributive *big* + noun

Situation: Adult and child are putting toys away.

Adult: Now, what do you have?

Child: Big car.

Adult: Big car. That's right. That is a big car (expansion). I want the big car (expansion).

Another example is the *Let's Talk* programs (Psychological Corporation), which use picture cards and structured training activities to teach social-interaction skills to students ages preschool to adult.

What Works

In this section we have reviewed several different language-intervention approaches, noting that for students with disabilities, some research supports the use of developmental guidelines in selecting language instruction goals, while other research suggests this is not the best approach. In addition, some research has found that highly structured intervention techniques work best with students with severe language disabilities, while other studies have found that less structured, more naturalistic methods work best. Language-acquisition theories suggest still other ways that language instruction can be delivered. How is one to decide which approach to use?

Part of the answer to this question comes, as it should, from research on language intervention programs. Bryen and Joyce (1985) reviewed 43 published studies from the 1970s on the type and effectiveness of language-intervention programs for students with severe disabilities. They concluded that there were some methods that worked and that successful intervention programs:

- Took into account the cognitive, social, motor, and language abilities of students prior to intervention.
- Conducted intervention in an environment-based context.
- Established goals that stressed the importance of spontaneous communication for a variety of purposes.
- Used interactional methods of intervention (e.g., ongoing modeling, play, commenting, waiting, responsiveness to communicative intent).
- Viewed and measured the interdependence of the various communicative, cognitive, social, and environmental systems.

Nye, Foster, and Seaman (1987) examined the effects of language intervention techniques used with children with language/learning disabilities. Using a meta-analysis technique that allowed them to examine the relative effectiveness of 61 studies, they found that the modeling technique was the most powerful. This was followed by the elicitation technique (where the child completes a statement). The least effective technique was general stimulation. They found that syntactic skills were most amenable to change, while pragmatic skills were the most difficult to alter.

The results of research on language intervention suggest that factors such as the child's age and degree of disability, as well as the aspect of language being taught, should be considered when making decisions about the goals and methods of intervention. Developmental guidelines seem to be most appropriate for younger children. Goals developed from the demands of the environment (functional goals) are also useful—especially for older students and students with more severe disabilities. Structured intervention procedures work best for teaching syntactic skills. Instruction that takes place in natural settings can be effective if there are clear goals.

The ultimate goal of language intervention should always be to make the child a more effective communicator. Therefore, no matter what intervention method teachers choose to use, they should always consider that the skills taught should be generalized to new environments. There are many ways to increase generalization of language instruction, including:

- **Use instructional methods that enhance generalization:** These include more naturalistic approaches (like milieu teaching) and those that integrate discrete-skill instruction into the natural environment (like the interrupted-behavior-chain strategy).

- **Use instructional materials that enhance generalization:** Use both a variety of materials, and materials that are familiar to the child, that is, are likely to be found in the child's environment.
- **Give the child many opportunities for interaction:** Structure training so the child has an opportunity to interact frequently with a variety of people (teachers, peers, therapists, parents).
- **Use natural contexts whenever possible:** It will be much easier for the child to use a language skill if it is taught in the environment where it will be practiced.

Teaching for generalization is especially important today as children with disabilities are more completely included into the regular education classroom.

It is sometimes instructive to examine what does not work, in addition to looking at what works. Damico (1988) presented a case study of a therapy plan that failed. Debbie was referred to the speech-language pathologist at the age of 6 because of her "lack of pronouns and omission of words during conversation" (p. 52). After extensive testing, she received about 7 months of group and individual therapy, at the end of which she was judged to have made sufficient progress to no longer need speech and language intervention. Six years later Debbie was referred once again to the speech-language pathologist. Her problems were now worse than ever. She was shy and quiet, with poor social skills, and was reading four grade levels below the norm for her age. Language testing indicated that she had a severe language disorder. What went wrong?

Damico suggests five things that may have caused the failure of language intervention for Debbie:

1. The fragmentation fallacy: Speech and language therapy tends to focus on discrete aspects of language rather than on language as a whole. As a result there was no focus on Debbie's ability to understand and use language in natural settings.

2. Therapist bias: In this case, the therapist was biased to perceive Debbie as successful. After all, she was a pretty, outgoing, and cooperative child from an upper-middle-class family. Test results were interpreted in the most positive light. Had the therapist been biased against Debbie, of course, Debbie might never have completed therapy.

3. Acquiescence: Parents and teachers acquiesced in response to the "expert"—the speech-language pathologist.

4. Lack of follow-up: Had there been a follow-up examination, Debbie's continuing problems might have been identified. But none was required and none was given.

5. Bureaucratic policies and procedures: Regulations required the use of tests that focused on discrete language skills. A large case load contributed to the fact that Debbie was released from therapy so quickly and was not followed.

The factors cited by Damico for the failure of language intervention in Debbie's case are not uncommon in school environments. We would do well to be aware of these potential problems and do our best to avoid them.

Specific Intervention Techniques

So far we have considered research-based principles that can be applied to the development of language intervention programs. This section provides specific examples of intervention techniques for each of the five aspects of language, describing, for each element of language, two informal and one formal (commercial) intervention procedures. These suggestions are a small sample of the many methods that can be used to enhance language. The best ways are often those that the classroom teacher develops with the materials and situations that are natural to the classroom.

Phonology

Mercer and Mercer (1993) suggest an activity called *phonetic bingo*. Each player receives a bingo card containing letters. The caller calls out a column number and a phoneme (4, t). The player having that phoneme in the correct column places a marker over the letter. The winner is the first player to cover five letters in a row.

Owens (1995) describes a backward-chaining technique to help the child become aware of unstressed syllables. Children often have difficulty perceiving unstressed syllables and may make errors in production.The teacher begins by teaching the last sound first. For example, in words like *monkey* and *turkey,* the last syllable is *key.* In order to enhance learning, a picture of a *key* can be paired with the sound. The actual teaching procedure goes like this:

1. The teacher presents and names the picture for the child *(key).*
2. The child repeats the sound *(key).*
3. Using the picture, the teacher produces the target word *(monkey)* with equal stress on both syllables.
4. Using the picture, the teacher says the target word with natural stress, while the child repeats the word.
5. Without using the picture, the teacher says the target word with natural stress, while the child repeats the word.
6. The child produces the target word independently.
7. The child uses the target word in a sentence and in conversation.

Pro-Ed distributes a program entitled *Remediation of Common Phonological Processes,* developed by Dana Broudy. With this program, 426 illustrated word-pair cards are provided to help teach children from preschool through grade 4 to hear minimal sound differences between words.

Morphology

Following are two of Wiig and Semel's (1984) many suggestions for improving morphological skills. They suggest the following activity for practicing the use of the present progressive *(ing)* ending:

The boy is _____.	(walking/walks)
The boy _____ every day.	(walking/walks)
The boy is _____.	(sleeping/sleeps)
During the night the boy _____.	(walks/sleeps)

Another technique to practice morphological skills is to reformulate sentences. For example:

Usually the boy eats cereal.
Yesterday _____.
Tomorrow _____.
Right now _____.

Teaching Morphology Developmentally (Communication Skill Builders) is an example of a commercially produced material that is designed to enhance skills in morphology. Color stimulus cards are provided to teach features such as the present progressive, past tense, and plurals to children between 2½ and 10 years of age.

Syntax

Hammill and Bartel (1995) suggest using a version of the children's game "I Spy" to teach the effective use of noun and verb phrases. One player must identify an object in the room by describing it *(I see two large red books and one large blue book)*. The other player must guess what object the first player has in mind. The teacher can help by encouraging the students to use precise language (not just, *I see a book)*.

Mercer and Mercer (1993) describe a self-correcting activity they call "Make It Say a Sentence" that can be used to practice sentence order. The student receives a card with a scrambled sentence *(ran school she was she since to late)*. The student must unscramble the sentence, write down the correct word order, and then check for the correct answer from a list of the answers in an accompanying envelope.

There are many commercially available materials to teach syntax skills. One example is *Syntax One; Syntax Two* (Communication Skill Builders). *Syntax One*, designed to help students develop awareness of word order and word endings, uses a syntax wheel that rotates to reveal stimulus pictures designed to elicit specific syntactic forms. In *Syntax Two*, students are presented with problem-solving situations in which they must ask questions.

Semantics

Atkinson and Longman (1985) suggest the use of sniglets to teach vocabulary development to adolescents and adults. *Sniglets* are words that do not appear in a dictionary but should. For example *bathquake* means the loud sound you sometimes hear when the water faucet is turned on. By experimenting with *new* words and trying to define sniglets, students learn about word meaning.

Wiig and Semel (1984) also provide many suggestions for enhancing students' skills in semantics. For example, they suggest using verbal analogies *[Trees have leaves and birds have _____ (feathers)]*, riddles *(You can ride on it. It rides on tracks. It has an engine. It has a caboose. It is a _____.)*, and twenty-question games to help children practice semantic skills.

The *Peabody Language Development Kits* (American Guidance Service) are probably the best known and most widely used materials for developing language skills. Although the kits focus on several aspects of language, they are especially useful for teaching semantic concepts. Three levels of kits span the age range from preschool to 7 years old and use a multimedia approach that includes picture cards, puppets, and posters. Children are taught to use receptive and expressive language, as well as to develop thinking skills.

Pragmatics

Hammill and Bartel (1995) suggest several role-playing activities designed to help students practice their communication skills. They suggest that students be assigned the role of speaker or responder in situations such as the following:

- Speaker (customer) is returning a defective appliance to the store. Speaker wants the responder (store representative) to refund the purchase price. Responder must try to implement the store policy,which is to make exchanges only.
- Speaker believes his/her examination has not been scored correctly. Speaker must try to convince responder (teacher) to give him/her some extra points on an essay question.

Mercer and Mercer (1993) suggest providing the student with a tape of sentences such as the following, to help them practice identifying indirect requests:

- What time is it?
- Can you shut the door?
- Can't you finish your work?
- Is the water running?
- Can't you sit still?

The student's job is to decide if each sentence is an indirect request or a question. An answer key could be provided so students can check their work.

Let's Talk for Children (Psychological Corporation) is designed to help students from 4 to 9 years old acquire, maintain, and generalize communicative functions. Communication activity cards prompt children to use a variety of speech acts. A home activities manual provides suggestions for the generalization of skills to the home environment.

Summary

In this chapter we have sampled the great variety of intervention models and procedures that are available for enhancing language skills in children with language disorders. Research on language intervention has suggested that the procedures that usually work best combine clearly stated outcomes with practice in natural settings. It is important that those planning intervention activities consider the strengths and limitations of the individual child, as well as the various environments in which the child will have to apply the skills. If research has done nothing else, it has made us aware that teaching isolated skills outside natural environments does not work.

Review Questions

1. Why is language intervention needed?

2. In addition to knowing that a child has a language disorder, what other criteria should be considered before making a decision to intervene?

3. Describe three ways that speech-language specialists could work with regular or special education teachers to deliver services.

4. What does Owens mean by *functional* intervention?

5. List three arguments in support of, and three arguments against, the use of developmental guidelines for planning language intervention in children with language disabilities.

6. Contrast the behavioral model to the psycholinguistic model on goals and methods of language intervention.

7. Mr. Clark is teaching Maria to use *-ing* endings. Give three suggestions that Mr. Clark can use to increase the probability that Maria will generalize this skill to new situations.

Suggested Activities

1. Teachers often have to develop informal intervention activities using materials and methods readily available in the classroom. Develop informal intervention suggestions for the following language skills:

- Understanding idioms: *foot in your mouth; two left feet*
- Using conjunctions: because; but
- Developing turn-taking skills

2. Mercer and Mercer (1993) describe a technique that they call *Does it mean the same thing?* This instructional method is designed to help students recognize the underlying (deep) structure of sentences.

The student receives a card that contains two sentences. One is a simple sentence *(The boy hit the ball)*; one is a sentence with a more complex structure *(The ball was hit by the boy).*

The student must indicate whether the two sentences have the *same* or *different* underlying meanings (deep structure).

Your task is to make up additional sentences that include questions, embedded sentences, and passive constructions. Try to design this task so it is self-correcting.

3. If you have the opportunity to work with a student with more severe language difficulties, try the *interrupted behavior-chain* strategy.

First, identify a task that the student can perform with success. Then try interrupting the activity at some point by asking the student to say what he/she is doing now or what they want.

Report on: (1) The task selected; (2) Your intervention strategy; and (3) The student's response (if any).

References

Aram, D. M., Ekelman, B. L., & Nation, J. E. (1984). Preschoolers with language disorders: 10 years later. *Journal of Speech and Hearing Research, 27,* 232–244.

Aram, D. M, & Nation, J. E. (1980). Preschool language disorders and subsequent language and academic difficulties. *Journal of Communication Disorders, 13,* 159–170.

Atkinson, R. H., & Longman, D. G. (1985). Sniglets: Give a twist to teenage and adult vocabulary instruction. *Journal of Reading, 29,* 103–105.

Bryen, D., & Joyce, D. (1985). Language intervention with the severely handicapped: A decade of research. *Journal of Special Education, 19,* 7–39.

Calculator, S. N., & Jorgensen, C. M. (1991). Integrating AAC instruction into regular education settings: Expounding on best practices. *Augmentative and Alternative Communication, 7,* 204–213.

Caro, P., & Snell, M. (1989). Characteristics of teaching communication to people with moderate and severe disabilities. *Education and Training in Mental Retardation, 29,* 63–77.

Cole, K. N., & Dale, P. (1986). Direct language instruction and interactive language instruction with language-delayed preschool children: A comparison study. *Journal of Speech and Hearing Research, 29,* 206–217.

Connell, P. J. (1987). A comparison of modeling and imitation teaching procedures on language-disordered children. *Journal of Speech and Hearing Research, 30,* 105–113.

Connell, P. J., & Stone, C. (1992). Morpheme learning of children with specific language impairments under controlled conditions. *Journal of Speech and Hearing Research, 35,* 844–852.

Courtright, J., & Courtright, I. (1979). Imitative modeling as a language intervention strategy: The effects of two mediating variables. *Journal of Speech and Hearing Research, 22,* 389–402.

Damico, J. S. (1988). The lack of efficacy in language therapy: A case study. *Language, Speech, and Hearing Services in Schools, 19,* 51–66.

Doss, S., & Reichle, J. (1989). Establishing communicative alternatives to the emission of socially motivated excess behavior: A review. *Journal of the Association for Persons with Severe Handicaps, 14,* 101–112.

Durand, V. M. (1993). Functional communication training using assistive devices: effects on challenging behavior and affect. *Augmentative and Alternative Communication, 9,* 168–176.

Dyer, K., Santarcangelo, S., & Luce, S. (1987). Developmental influences in teaching language forms to individuals with developmental disabilities. *Journal of Speech and Hearing Disorders, 52,* 335–347.

Friedman, P., & Friedman, K. (1980). Accounting for individual differences when comparing the effectiveness of remedial language teaching methods. *Applied Psycholinguistics, 1,* 151–171.

Goetz, L., Schuler, A., & Sailor, W. (1981). Functional competence as a factor in communication instruction. *Exceptional Education Quarterly, 2*, 51–60.

Goldstein, H., & Hockenberger, E. H. (1991). Significant progress in child language intervention: an 11-year retrospective. *Research and Developmental Disabilities, 12*, 401–424.

Hammill, D. D., & Bartel, N. R. (1995). *Teaching students with learning and behavior problems.* Austin, TX: Pro-Ed.

Kamhi, A. G., & Johnston, J. R. (1982). Towards an understanding of retarded children's linguistic deficiencies. *Journal of Speech and Hearing Research, 25*, 435–445.

King, R., Jones, D., & Lasky, E. (1982). In retrospect: A fifteen year follow-up of speech-language-disordered children. *Language, Speech, and Hearing Services in Schools, 13*, 24–32.

Mercer, C. D., & Mercer, A. R. (1993). *Teaching students with learning problems.* New York: Merrill.

Miller, L. (1989). Classroom-based language intervention. *Language, Speech, and Hearing Services in Schools, 20*, 153–169.

Mire, S., & Chisholm, R. (1990). Functional communication goals for adolescents and adults who are severely and moderately mentally handicapped. *Language, Speech, and Hearing Services in Schools, 21*, 57–58.

Montgomery, J. K. (1992). Perspectives from the field: Language, speech, and hearing services in schools. *Language, Speech, and Hearing Services in Schools, 23*, 363–364.

Nye, C., Foster, S. H. & Seaman, D. (1987). Effectiveness of language intervention with the language/learning disabled. *Journal of Speech and Hearing Disorders, 52*, 348–357.

Olswang, L. & Bain, B. (1991). When to recommend intervention. *Language, Speech, and Hearing Services in Schools, 22*, 255–263.

Owens, R. E. (1995). *Language disorders: A functional approach to assessment and intervention.* Boston: Allyn and Bacon.

Reed, V. A. (1994). *An introduction to children with language disorders.* New York: Merrill.

Volden, J., & Lord, C. (1991). Neologisms and idiosyncratic language in autistic speakers. *Journal of Autism and Developmental Disorders, 21*, 109–130.

Vygotsky, L. (1962). *Thought and language.* Cambridge, MA: MIT Press.

Warren, S. F. (1991). Enhancing communication and language development with milieu teaching procedures. In E. Cipani (Ed.), *A guide for developing language competence in preschool children with severe and moderate handicaps* (pp. 68–93). Springfield, IL: Charles Thomas.

Warren, S. F., & Kaiser, A. P. (1986). Incidental language teaching: A critical review. *Journal of Speech and Hearing Disorders, 51*, 291–299.

Wiig, E. H., & Semel, E. (1984). *Language assessment and intervention for the learning disabled.* Columbus, OH: Merrill.

Yoder, P. J., Kaiser, A. P., & Alpert, C. L. (1991). An exploratory study of the interaction between language teaching methods and child characteristics. *Journal of Speech and Hearing Research, 34*, 155–167.

Chapter **12**

Classroom-Based Intervention

Skill in the understanding and use of language is essential for school success. Just think for a moment about the many ways that language is used in the classroom. Language is used to give directions, ask and answer questions, and provide feedback. Language is embedded in reading and writing and in all of the academic subject areas that rely on reading and writing. Language is used for social interaction—in the classroom, in the lunchroom, and on the playground.

Despite the importance of language in the classroom and the many opportunities for using language that classroom environments present, until recently most speech and language intervention was done outside the classroom. Today, however, there is a trend toward integrating speech and language instruction in the classroom and including teachers—regular and special education—in the language-intervention process.

This chapter examines the changing service-delivery system for speech and language intervention and provides the rationale for these changes. The chapter also examines the many ways that language is used in the classroom, detailing how to recognize children with speech and language problems and providing specific suggestions for enhancing the language and communication skills of preschool through secondary-level children. Also included here are models of collaboration between teachers and speech-language professionals and, finally, some of the research on the outcomes of classroom-based language intervention.

After completion of this chapter, you should be able to:

1. Explain the ways in which language is used in schools.
2. Provide a rationale for the delivery of language intervention in the classroom.
3. Identify children with language difficulties.
4. Develop specific suggestions for enhancing language and communication skills of students at the preschool, elementary, and secondary levels.
5. Describe the skills needed for an effective collaboration with other professionals.
6. Explain the effectiveness of classroom-based interventions.

Language in the Classroom

The classroom—regular or special education—can be a rich source of language experience. Throughout the school day, teachers and children are engaged in communicative interaction. Whenever teachers give directions, ask a question, or provide verbal feedback to students, language is likely to be the mode of interaction. When students are asked to respond to questions, to work in groups, or to give reports, language is the means of expression. Many academic subject areas are directly dependent on language (e.g., reading and writing), while others rely on language in less obvious, but no less important, ways. For example, good language skills are necessary to understand the vocabulary and perform the complex problem-solving required for success in math.

Bashir and Scavuzzo (1992) identified seven language functions to facilitate learning that they found reported in the research literature on classroom interaction. These functions include structuring a lesson, delivering a lecture, organizing information, constructing knowledge, managing and clarifying information, developing and directing inquiry, and conversing with teachers and peers.

Although the classroom can be a wonderful source for language stimulation and practice, it can be a minefield for children with language difficulties. Consider this vignette from an actual classroom of young (5- to 7-year-old) children with communication disabilities:

Teacher (directed to three children in the first row): Can you get your books and come here?

Students: (No response, puzzled looks on their faces)

Teacher (raising her voice): Can you come here?

Students: (More puzzled looks, still no response)

Teacher (exasperated): Get your books and come here!

Students: (Picked up their books and walked to the teacher's desk)

What was going on here? It seems rather clear that the children were unable to understand the teacher's language. Because the teacher used an indirect request and gave multiple directions, the children were confused. They were not sure how to respond. When the teacher gave a direct command, the children responded appropriately. The teacher might have concluded that the children had hearing impairments or auditory perception problems, or even had emotional disturbances (resistance to authority).

This example is intended to show just how important it is for teachers to be aware of the language they direct toward students. At first this teacher seemed to be unaware of the effect that her language was having on the students. Had she not modified her language, the students could have been left confused and may have missed an opportunity for learning. This teacher had the advantage of teaching in a classroom with a small number of children whom she had reason to believe had difficulties with language. In a regular education classroom with 25 or 30 children, the teacher may have been too busy helping other children to notice that some did not understand the directions.

Identifying Children with Language Difficulties

Since language is so important for school success, it is important that teachers be aware of children who may be having language difficulties. Research has shown that many children with early language disorders continue to have problems throughout the school years (Bashir & Scavuzzo, 1992). A substantial percentage (40–75%, according to Aram, Ekelman, & Nation, 1984) have problems in reading. Since classroom teachers are able to observe students for most of the school day, they are in the best position to identify children with language and communication difficulties. Owens (1995) suggests that teachers look for the following signs of a child with language difficulty:

- Seems to fail to understand and follow directions
- Is unable to use language to meet daily living needs
- Violates rules of social interaction, including politeness
- Lacks ability to read signs or other symbols and to perform written tasks
- Has problems using speech to communicate effectively
- Demonstrates a lack of appropriate organization and sequence in verbal and written efforts
- Does not remember significant information presented orally and/or in written form
- May not recognize humor or indirect comments
- Seems unable to interpret the emotions or predict the intentions of others
- Responds inappropriately for the situation

Children who have difficulty answering questions, following directions, and using language to communicate with their peers may be having language problems. To get additional information about language abilities teachers can use a checklist such as the one in Table 12.1.

Another classroom-based method for gathering information about language functioning is *curriculum-based assessment.* Nelson (1989) defines curriculum-based assessment as "the use of curriculum contexts and content for measuring a student's language intervention needs and progress" (p. 171). In other words, when using curriculum-based assessment to assess language skills, teachers can compare the child's language skills to those required by the curriculum in that classroom. Nelson suggests that teachers observe the child's ability to use the various language rule systems (phonological, morphological, and so on) in all modalities demanded by the curriculum (listening, speaking, reading, writing, and thinking). She also suggests that teachers pay attention to the child's ability to think about and use language (metalinguistic skills) (see Table 12.2).

TABLE 12.1 Checklist for Identification of Language Impairment

The following behaviors may indicate that a child in your classroom has a language impairment that is in need of clinical intervention. Please check the appropriate items.

_____ Child mispronounces sounds and words.

_____ Child omits word endings, such as plural -s and past tense -ed.

_____ Child omits small unemphasized words, such as auxiliary verbs or prepositions.

_____ Child uses an immature vocabulary, overuses empty words, such as one and thing, or seems to have difficulty recalling or finding the right word.

_____ Child has difficulty comprehending new words and concepts.

_____ Child's sentence structure seems immature or overreliant on forms, such as subject-verb-object. It's unoriginal, dull.

_____ Child's question and/or negative sentence style is immature.

_____ Child has difficulty with one of the following:

_____ Verb tensing	_____ Articles	_____ Auxiliary verbs
_____ Pronouns	_____ Irreg. verbs	_____ Prepositions
_____ Word order	_____ Irreg. plurals	_____ Conjunctions

_____ Child has difficulty relating sequential events.

_____ Child has difficulty following directions.

_____ Child's questions often inaccurate or vague.

_____ Child's questions often poorly formed.

_____ Child has difficulty answering questions.

_____ Child's comments often off topic or inappropriate for the conversation.

_____ There are long pauses between a remark and the child's reply or between successive remarks by the child. It's as if the child is searching for a response or is confused.

_____ Child appears to be attending to communication but remembers little of what is said.

_____ Child has difficulty using language socially for the following purposes:

_____ Request needs	_____ Pretend/imagine	_____ Protest
_____ Greet	_____ Request information	_____ Gain attention
_____ Respond/reply	_____ Share ideas, feelings	_____ Clarify
_____ Relate events	_____ Entertain	_____ Reason

_____ Child has difficulty interpreting the following:

_____ Figurative language	_____ Humor	_____ Gestures
	_____ Emotions	_____ Body language

_____ Child does not alter production for different audiences and locations.

_____ Child does not seem to consider the effect of language on the listener.

_____ Child often has verbal misunderstandings with others.

_____ Child has difficulty with reading and writing.

_____ Child's language skills seem to be much lower than other areas, such as mechanical, artistic, or social skills.

TABLE 12.2 Areas of Consideration for Curriculum-Based Language Assessment

Rule Systems	Modalities	Linguistic Levels	Contexts
Phonological	Listening	Sound	Formal tests
Morphological	Speaking	Syllable	Spontaneous samples
Syntactic	Reading	Word	Academic materials:
Semantic	Writing	Sentence	• Workbook pages
Pragmatic	Thinking	Text	• Reading text
			Grade level
			Reading level
			• Science text
			• Math activities

Source: From N. W. Nelson, "Curriculum-Based Language Assessment and Intervention," *Language, Speech, and Hearing Services in Schools, 20(1989),* 170–184. © American Speech-Language-Hearing Association. Reprinted by permission of the American Speech-Language-Hearing Association and the author.

In addition to simply observing children in their classrooms, teachers can gather informal, curriculum-based information about language use in many other ways, for instance, by participating with the child in answering questions at the end of a chapter. In this way teachers can evaluate the ability of the child to understand text, to paraphrase, and to formulate a response. Other possibilities are to ask the student to retell a story or explain the steps to solving a math problem (Nelson, 1989). Each of these activities can yield important information about the child's ability to understand and use language in the classroom.

Classroom teachers play a critical role in the identification of children with speech and language problems. It is important for teachers to be aware of the signs of language difficulty and methods of structuring activities to create opportunities to observe language. When coupled with information from other types of assessment (such as formal and informal testing), teachers' observations can help identify those children who are most in need of intervention.

Delivering Language Intervention in the Classroom

In the last ten years or so there have been great changes in the way that services are delivered to children with disabilities. These changes have occurred in special education and speech-language services as well as in many other professions that serve children with disabilities. The result of these changes has been that more children with disabilities are being served within the regular education classroom. There are both theoretical and political reasons why these changes have occurred. We will look at some of these factors and how they have affected the delivery of language intervention.

Changes in Special Education

Anyone who works with children with special needs is aware that there has been a major shift in thinking about the best way to serve these children. Prior to the

1970s, most students with special needs were taught in self-contained special education classrooms. As early as 1968, Dunn (1968) questioned the effectiveness of special education classrooms. When Public Law 94-142 was written (1975), the principle of the *least restrictive environment* was included. Public Law 94-142 required that students with disabilities be educated with their nondisabled peers as much as possible. *Mainstreaming* (the practice of returning students with special needs to the regular education classroom for part of the day) developed as a procedure for implementing the mandate of the least restrictive environment principle. Even as mainstreaming was developing, some questioned the effectiveness of this delivery system (Wang & Birch, 1984; Reynolds, Wang, & Walberg, 1987). By the 1980s, concerns about mainstreaming had coalesced into the *Regular Education Initiative (REI)*. Advocates of REI argued that there should be no distinction between regular and special education—that all children should be educated in the same classroom (Will, 1986). *Inclusion* is the term currently used to describe a service delivery model where children with disabilities receive most or all of their education in a regular education classroom in their neighborhood school.

Today, children with special needs are placed in self-contained special education classrooms, in resource rooms, or in regular education classrooms, but there is an increasing trend toward less restrictive settings. This trend presents both opportunities and challenges for the delivery of language intervention. When children with disabilities are placed in regular education classrooms, there is the opportunity for interaction with nondisabled peers and the chance to see appropriate models of language (Stainback & Stainback, 1984). At the same time, there is the danger that the children with special needs may not receive the services that they need (Kauffman, 1989).

Speech-Language Services

Paralleling the changes in service delivery for special education are changes in the way that speech and language services are being delivered. In describing the evolution of models of speech and language service delivery, Cirrin and Penner (1995) noted that the profession of speech-language pathology has moved from reliance on pull-out services to delivery of speech and language intervention in the classroom. Cirrin and Penner discuss four reasons for this change:

1. **Growing evidence and concern regarding the efficacy of providing language intervention in pullout settings** because of concerns about students' lack of generalization, and the possible negative effects of removing children with disabilities from the classroom.

2. **Holistic views of language and literacy** that emphasize the role that language plays in learning and classroom success.

3. **The emphasis on—and impact of—collaboration in business and industry.**

4. **Recent policy changes** that have taken place in special education.

As Cirrin and Penner note, one of the reasons for the move to classroom delivery of speech and language intervention is changes in our views about language and literacy. Miller (1989) describes how intervention procedures for speech-language problems have changed from emphasizing voice and articulation goals to a greater emphasis on the use of language for communication. At the same time, both speech-language professionals and educators have come to recognize the interrelatedness of language skills. The *whole language* view of learning recognizes that language is an integrated system that involves cognition and social development, as well as language skills (Norris & Hoffman, 1990). With this recognition has come the development of instructional procedures—such as incidental teaching—that emphasize teaching language skills in natural settings. The key elements of a naturalistic approach to language intervention, according to McCormick (1986), are that (1) children learn and have ample opportunities to use words for preferred and interesting objects, events, and relations; and (2) that they have numerous opportunities to practice newly acquired communication skills in naturally occurring activities.

As the field of speech-language pathology has shifted from an emphasis on speech therapy in pull-out settings to naturalistic, classroom-based intervention, a number of models have been developed to implement this change. Miller (1989) describes five ways that speech and language professionals can deliver services to the classroom:

1. The language specialist teaches in a self-contained classroom: The language specialist teaches children with significant language difficulties in a special classroom. The teacher focuses on language skills that will help the children make the transition to literacy.

2. The language specialist team teaches: Team teaching may take place in a regular classroom with a regular education teacher, in a self-contained classroom with a special education or reading teacher, or in a resource setting with a special education teacher. Whatever the setting, the teachers should jointly plan, instruct, and evaluate.

3. The language specialist provides one-to-one classroom-based intervention: The language specialist can use actual classroom materials to help the child with significant difficulties improve his/her vocabulary, study skills, writing, and test-taking strategies. The language specialist must collaborate closely with the classroom teacher.

4. The language specialist consults: The language specialist provides information and support to the classroom teacher. The teacher is responsible for carrying out the mutually agreed-upon instructional strategies.

5. The language specialist provides staff, curriculum, or program development: Language specialist may provide in-service training, participate in curriculum development activities, and develop parent education programs.

We began this section by noting the increasing trend to educate children with disabilities in regular education settings. This trend is found both in special education and in the speech-language field. A crucial question is whether this new delivery system *works*. There has been a great deal of debate on this question (e.g., Reynolds et al., 1987; Fuchs & Fuchs, 1988). Most actual studies on the effectiveness of inclusive education have found that, at the least, children with disabilities did no worse in regular education classrooms than they did in special class placements (Bear & Proctor, 1990; Zigmond & Baker, 1990). One study that compared the effectiveness of a pull-out program to a classroom-based language-intervention program for preschool children found little difference between the two approaches (Wilcox, Kouri, & Caswell, 1991). In other words, the classroom-based approach was as effective as the pull-out program. Therefore, even if classroom-based intervention programs are no more effective than pull-out programs, they are the preferred model, in most cases, because of their inherent advantages (socialization opportunities, reduced stigma, generalization).

Enhancing Language Skills in the Classroom

So far our focus has been on *where* language intervention should take place. Although this is certainly an important issue, an equally important question is *what* teachers and speech-language specialists should do to help children enhance their language skills. Having already reviewed a number of intervention models and suggestions in Chapter 11, we will now focus on techniques that may be especially effective in classroom settings.

Enhancing Classroom Interaction

One of the most important things teachers can do is to teach in ways that will enhance the language and communication of children in their classroom. Sociolinguists who have carefully observed classroom interactions have found that teachers dominate the conversation, ask a lot of questions that require minimal responses (one-word answers), and initiate most of the interactions (Cazden, 1986). As a result, in the typical classroom, children are rather passive recipients of communication rather than active partners in such interaction. Even worse, many teachers actively discourage interaction between students and even between the student and the teacher. Of course, there is a limit to how much interaction can be tolerated, but if language learning is an important goal, some interaction should not only be tolerated but encouraged. Without the chance to interact, children with language-learning difficulties will have little opportunity to develop crucial language skills.

Fortunately, it is possible to enhance classroom communication. Dudley-Marling and Searle (1988) have provided four suggestions that teachers can use to enhance the language-learning environment. They suggest that (1) the physical setting must promote talk; (2) the teacher must provide opportunities for children to interact and use language as they learn; (3) the teacher needs to provide opportunities for children to use language for a variety of purposes, for a variety of audiences; and (4) the teacher needs to respond to student talk in ways that encourage continued talk. Let's look at each of these suggestions in more detail.

The physical setting must promote talk: Dudley-Marling and Searle note that many classrooms are organized to discourage interaction. Individual work stations, carrels, and widely spaced rows are all designed to help students concentrate, but they also have the effect of reducing interaction. While there is certainly a need for concentration, many students also need opportunities to interact with their peers. Providing large tables where groups can work, learning centers, and interactive classroom displays can give students opportunities to interact in the classroom.

The teacher must provide opportunities for children to interact and use language as they learn: Teachers can structure classroom conversation around academic tasks. For example, children reading a story about fishing can be encouraged to share their previous fishing experiences with the group. Teachers are sometimes reluctant to let students engage in these kinds of conversations because students may stray from the topic. If this happens, students can be redirected back to the topic. Remember, communication is a goal for many students and conversation is not an off-task behavior. Other examples of using instructional activities for language interaction are encouraging the students to say aloud their strategies for solving a math problem or having them read a story to the class.

The teacher needs to provide opportunities for children to use language for a variety of purposes, for a variety of audiences: Teachers can encourage class decision-making and problem-solving and provide opportunities for discussion and sharing. Look at the following example (taken from Lindfors, 1987):

S_1: Did even Martin Luther King have to sit in the back of the bus?

T: All black people did.

S_2: That was really no fair.

S_3: That reminds me. Why do we always have to sit at the same lunch table?

T: What would you rather do?

S_3: Sit anywhere we want.

T: That might become confusing. Most people would rather know exactly where they sit.

S_2: I don't would rather know.

T: How does everyone else feel about this?

In this example, the class went from discussing the life of Martin Luther King to talking about lunchroom seating. By pursuing the discussion the students had the opportunity to really understand the concepts of freedom and responsibility. Teachers can provide opportunities for students to talk to each other, to younger children (through cross-age tutoring), and to adults (parents and visitors).

The teacher needs to respond to student talk in ways that encourage continued talk: Teachers often ask questions in ways that give the student little opportunity to respond. When students do respond, the teacher may not respond in ways that encourage further interaction. Dudley-Marling and Searle give an example of a teacher discouraging interaction:

S: Boy, you should have seen the neat stuff at the circus.

T: Really, Johnny, you shouldn't say "neat stuff."

The authors suggest that this interaction could have been turned into a longer communicative interaction if the teacher had said something like, *Oh, you had a good time at the circus.* Consider another example of classroom interaction adapted from Lindfors (1987):

T: What does the earth revolve around?

S: The sun.

T: The sun. Right. But as it moves around the sun, it also keeps turning like this (turns ball) on its own . . .

S: Center.

T: Well, its kind of . . .

S: Axis.

T: Its own axis, right.

Was this an effective instructional interaction? If we look just at the content of the lesson, it appears that the child knows the appropriate science facts. But, if communication is our concern, the interaction is not satisfactory. There was little opportunity for the child to participate in a prolonged interaction. The teacher asked questions that required only one-word answers. No discussion was required or expected.

Teachers should be careful not to dominate the conversation, and they should follow the child's lead in setting the conversational topic. One simple but effective strategy for increasing interaction is to pause several seconds for a response to a question. Research has found that teachers wait less than one second for a response (Rowe, 1974). Longer wait-time increases the likelihood that students will respond (Rowe, 1986).

Throughout the school day there are numerous opportunities for teachers to prompt interaction and respond to students in ways that encourage interaction. Two effective ways of increasing interaction are through use of *self-talk* and *parallel talk.* When using self-talk, teachers or speech-language specialists talk about what they are doing as they do it. For example, an adult playing with a set of farm animals might say, *Look, now I'm moving the horse. There goes the pig. Now, why did the chickens go over there?* With parallel talk, the adult describes the action for the child as the child performs the action. The adult might use language similar to the above as the child plays with the animals.

Norris and Hoffman (1990) give other examples of strategies that teachers and speech-language specialists can use to assist children. One example is *restating and rewording*. When using this technique, the adult acknowledges what the child has said and provides alternative models for communicating the same information. Norris and Hoffman give the following example:

Child: I want brush.

Adult: Right, give me the brush.
It's my turn.
I want the brush now.

Other examples include *expansion* and *extension*. When using expansion, the adult repeats the child's utterance using a more advanced language model. (Child: *Brush hair.* Adult: *That's right. You need to brush your dolly's hair.*) Extensions add new ideas to what the child has said. (Child: *Brush hair.* Adult: *Right, we need to brush it and then put on her hat.*)

All of these techniques are designed to take naturally occurring classroom situations and turn them into opportunities for language teaching. As McCormick (1986) stated, the focus of instruction "should be on increasing the quantity and quality of child-initiated communications (verbal and nonverbal) to obtain desired objects and regulate the actions of others" (p. 124). McCormick gives five suggestions that teachers can use to enhance classroom communication:

1. Seek participation of as many persons as possible in language training (aides, volunteers, parents, related services personnel, peers).
2. Arrange opportunities for language training and practice in a range and variety of contexts.
3. Assure opportunities for language training and practice throughout the school day.
4. Accumulate an appealing assortment of materials.
5. Use natural, response-specific reinforcers.

Enhancing Communication in Specific Classroom Environments

The techniques considered so far for enhancing language and communication skills are useful in nearly any classroom. But there are some strategies that are more effective in particular classroom environments or with children at certain ages or developmental levels.

Preschool Classrooms

Language and communication development is often a major goal in preschool classrooms. Teachers of preschool children usually include many activities to involve their students in such interaction. For example, Watson, Layton, Pierce, and Abraham (1994) describe a preschool program for children with language disorders that incorporates instruction in emerging literacy skills into activities that most teachers of preschool children will recognize. These activities include

Circle time: When the bell rings, children get their mats and bring them to the circle. Children must recognize their names in order to get their mats. After an opening song, children discuss the job chart that has jobs listed in print, supplemented by pictures. When there is a song, the words are written out on a poster board and the teacher points to the words as they are sung.

Storytime: Books that follow a classroom theme (animals, communities, and so on) are selected. As the teacher reads the story, each child is asked for some kind of response. In addition, there are opportunities for choral responding. Because repeated readings help children improve their comprehension skills, the story is reread at least three times in a week.

Story-related group activity: The teacher uses follow-up activities to reinforce concepts from the story. Children may role-play parts from the story or make puppets to represent characters from the story.

Literacy-rich centers: Watson et al. describe three literacy centers that are used in their classroom. At the *art and writing center,* children draw pictures related to the *story of the week* and tell about their picture. The *role-playing center* contains dress-up clothes, dolls, and toys that the children can use to act out action from the story or from their own *scripts.* During free time the children can go to the *book and library center* to look at books and listen to tapes.

Snack time: Often snack time is integrated with the weekly theme. Snack packaging is used as reading material for the child, rather than being thrown away.

Gross motor play/outdoor activities: Even during gross motor activities there are opportunities to practice literacy skills. When teaching exercises, the teacher also introduces the written word (e.g., *arm, body*).

Closing circle: This provides a final opportunity during the day for children to recall and talk about their experiences. When children are given printed materials to take home, the child is told about the purpose of the message, reinforcing the idea that print has a purpose.

Elementary Classrooms

As children enter the elementary school years, language becomes important not only as a means of communication but as a part of the curriculum. Students are asked to analyze sentences and apply their language skills to reading and writing. In the past decade there has been a major shift in the elementary curriculum to the concept of *whole-language* instruction. While there are many variations on the basic whole-language theme, Lerner (1993) identifies the basic tenets of the whole-language approach as follows:

- **Reading is viewed as part of the integrated language system, closely linked to other forms of language—oral and written.** Underlying language skills are thought to be critical, but developments in any area (writing, reading, or language) support the development of skills in related areas.
- **Both oral and written language are acquired through natural usage.** Since children learn to talk without special exercises and drills (at least, most do) whole language advocates such as Goodman (1990) propose that children can learn to read by being immersed in books.
- **The whole-language curriculum capitalizes on the use of authentic literature, and it provides abundant opportunities for expressive literacy—or writing.** Whole-language instruction is based on children's literature rather than on basal texts.
- **The whole-language philosophy avoids the teaching of separate nonmeaningful parts of language or the use of isolated exercises and drills.** There is much less emphasis on sound-symbol relationships and greater emphasis on extracting meaning from text. Decoding skills can be learned in context.

Rather than presenting reading, writing, and language as separate units, teachers using whole-language instruction acknowledge the interrelationships between these domains. Reading becomes the basis for writing and language activities, discussions precede and follow reading, and writers talk before they write. The whole-language approach assumes that the child has a firm grasp on spoken-language skills. Clearly, children who are having difficulty with spoken language are at risk for learning problems when a whole-language approach is used.

The whole-language approach creates many opportunities for teachers to integrate language skills with other academic tasks. Norris (1989) gives an example of a procedure for integrating language-skills instruction with reading. She calls this approach *communicative reading strategies*. The teacher or clinician selects a text passage at the child's reading level. The passage selected should reflect a language problem the child is experiencing. The child reads the passage aloud while the adult listens for miscues, hesitations, or other problems. Then the adult asks the child for an explanation of what was read, a clarification of the text, or an extension of the ideas. Any errors occurring in the initial reading become targets for feedback from the adult. Norris points out that this technique can be used in the child's classroom, with available materials.

Many other instructional techniques utilize whole-language principles to teach language-arts skills. For example, in the directed reading-thinking activity (DRTA) (Stauffer, 1975) students are encouraged to predict what will happen in a reading passage. They are encouraged to think and work in groups to arrive at predictions. Using the K-W-L (know-want-learn) technique (Ogle, 1986), teachers help their students identify (1) **what I know** about the topic of the reading, (2) **what I want to find out** about the subjects, and (3) **what I learned** after reading the selection.

Secondary Classrooms

Secondary-age students do not necessarily outgrow speech and language problems (Aram, et al., 1984). Instead, as they respond to the demands of the secondary setting, their problems may surface in new ways. Lecturing, note-taking, and independent research projects pose difficult challenges to the student with language difficulties.

Buttrill, Niizawa, Biemer, Takahashi, and Hearn (1989) described a program they developed to support secondary-age students with language disorders. In the program, students attend a *language/study skills* class for one period a day; the remainder of the day they attend regular, general-education classes. Seven major elements are included in the *language/study skills* curriculum:

> **Academic organization:** Students are helped to organize their assignments, organize their time, and monitor their own performance.
>
> **Study skills:** Students learn *how* to study, also receiving instruction in note taking, text reading, and test taking.
>
> **Critical thinking:** Students are helped to enhance their ability to observe and describe, solve problems, and use inductive and deductive reasoning.
>
> **Listening:** Students are given strategies for focusing their attention. They are taught to recognize lecture cues that will help them to identify important information.
>
> **Oral language:** Students are taught word retrieval skills, helped with their use of figurative language, and given practice in being a good listener and an effective speaker.
>
> **Written language:** Students are given numerous opportunities to write. Writing includes note taking, use of computers, and research papers.
>
> **Pragmatics:** Students learn about conversational roles. They role-play various conversational situations.

The special language problems of secondary-age students may sometimes be overlooked because of the emphasis put on content in secondary skills. The program described by Buttrill et al. reminds us that learning language does not stop at the preschool or elementary years but continues through adolescence and beyond.

Classrooms for Students with Severe Disabilities

There are some new and promising ideas about teaching language skills to children with more severe disabilities. These new strategies emphasize the integration of students with disabilities into school and the community. These newer procedures include an emphasis on functional skills, exposure to literacy activities, and the use of computers to enhance language skills.

Owens (1995) describes an *integrated, functional* model of language intervention for students with severe disabilities. This approach uses natural environments such as the school, home, and community to teach functional skills—skills demanded by these environments. Owens describes three instructional procedures that are compatible with integrated, functional intervention:

Incidental teaching: The adult enhances the child's skills in communication within naturally occurring communicative interactions. Ongoing activities and routines are the context for training.

Stimulation: Adults can stimulate language by providing a slightly more complex model than language the child is presently using. Owens suggests that care givers respond to all attempts at communication, while providing feedback and an appropriate model.

Formal training: Owens suggests that formal training may also be necessary, in addition to use of the very naturalistic approaches. He suggests that this occur a few times each day, for brief periods.

Individuals with disabilities often have significant difficulty developing literacy skills. Until recently these difficulties had been attributed largely to disabilities within the individual. But Koppenhaver, Pierce, Steelman, and Yoder (1995) suggest that literacy-learning difficulties may also be due to the way parents and professionals respond to individuals with disabilities and to learning contexts. For example, their research has shown that parents of children who use augmentative communication devices had relatively low expectations for their child's ability to acquire reading and writing skills (Light, Koppenhaver, Lee, & Riffle, 1994). Other research has discovered that children with severe disabilities are rarely exposed to text-length material. Most of their instruction is with isolated words and sentences.

Koppenhaver et al. (1995) also reported on a project developed by Pierce and Steelman (1994) that was designed to enhance the literacy skills of young (2- to 8-year-old) students with severe disabilities. The program has five elements:

1. Developmentally appropriate activities and strategies are used to enhance listening, speaking, reading, and writing skills.
2. Generalization is emphasized by teaching concepts across contexts rather than focusing on drill-and-practice sessions.
3. Many purposeful, print-related experiences are provided to help children understand the function of print.
4. A thematic approach is used to integrate classroom experiences.
5. Collaboration between teachers, therapists, and parents is stressed so that classroom literacy activities are integrated into home and clinical environments.

The work of Koppenhaver and his colleagues at the Center for Literacy Studies at the University of North Carolina has helped us to rethink the role of literacy education for students with severe disabilities. Their research suggests that *all* students can benefit from exposure to—and participation in—literacy-based activities. We should be careful not to limit the development of students with severe disabilities because of our preconceived notions about what they cannot do.

The development of powerful, portable, and relatively inexpensive computers and peripherals has the potential for significantly enhancing the learning of students with severe disabilities. Schery and O'Connor (1992) compared the outcomes of a computer-based language instruction program (Programs for Early Acquisition of Language) to regular classroom language instruction for 52 students with severe disabilities. The results indicated that the group that used the computer program outperformed the comparison group on a vocabulary posttest. In addition, the computer group also made significant gains in social/interpersonal behaviors. The authors caution that although computers are certainly not a panacea, they do represent an important instructional tool for students with severe disabilities, as evidenced by research results.

Specific Intervention Suggestions

In the preceding two sections we have reviewed useful methods for enhancing classroom interaction in a variety of environments, as well as strategies found effective in specific types of classrooms. Here are some activities that you may find helpful for enhancing language in the classroom:

1. **Group decision making:** Give a group of students an assignment to complete a project (such as making a poster to illustrate a science concept). Give the group some pictures from which they must select four to use on their poster. Encourage group discussion and decision making.

2. **Missing materials:** For younger children, set up a group project so that each member of the group has something that the other group members need. For example, one student has markers, one has crayons, one has scissors, and so on. Encourage the students to ask others when they need something. If necessary, provide a model for requesting.

3. **Rewriting:** One way to practice using different registers of communication is to rewrite a story for three different audiences. For example, one version could be for the students' peers, one for parents, and one for younger children.

4. **Classroom routines:** Teachers can use routine classroom tasks as the vehicle for classroom interaction. If your class has a snack time, for example, use this as a communication time. Even students with little or no spoken language can benefit from this. Students can be required to indicate either verbally or nonverbally which of two items they prefer. They get their snack only after making a response.

5. **Computers for socialization:** We don't usually think of computers as a forum for social interaction, but they can be. Computer programs that emphasize problem solving (e.g., Oregon Trail) are a great way to get a group talking to each other. You might group three students together and encourage them to come up with a group solution to the dilemmas posed by the software.

Summary

In this chapter we have examined language in the classroom, considering the important roles that language plays as an instructional tool and as the primary means of communication between teacher and students. We have also examined methods for identifying children who may be experiencing difficulty understanding and/or using language in the classroom. Research studies have provided general suggestions for enhancing language interaction, as well as ideas for specific types of classrooms. Such research has also demonstrated that teachers can provide a more enriching language environment for *all* students if they are aware of the role that language plays in the classroom and if they plan to enhance language and communication in the classroom.

Review Questions

1. List and briefly discuss three ways that language is used in the classroom.

2. List five signs of language difficulties that could be observed by teachers within the classroom.

3. How have changes in service-delivery models affected the delivery of speech-language intervention?

4. Describe how a classroom could be restructured to enhance language interaction.

5. Describe the following and give an example of each: self-talk; expansion.

6. Describe some of the challenges that face secondary-level students with language difficulties.

7. Give three suggestions for enhancing the literacy of students with moderate to severe mental retardation.

Suggested Activities

1. Observe language interaction between a teacher and a group of students. As you observe, note who initiates the interaction, what response (if any) is made, and who responds. Also note the type of interaction that takes place. If the teacher asks questions, are they open ended or do they require little response? Does the teacher use a lot of directives (e.g., *Sit down, Open your book*).

After completing your observation, analyze your results and answer the following questions:

   a. Who initiates most of the interaction?
   b. Do the students respond? If so, describe the types of responses (e.g., verbal/non-verbal, short/long).
   c. What could the teacher have done to increase interaction and responsiveness in the classroom?

2. Observe a child who may have language difficulties. Look for the following:

a. How often the teacher and peers initiate interaction with the child
b. How frequently the child initiates interaction
c. The child's ability to follow directions
d. Any other evidence of possible difficulties with language understanding or expression

3. If you have the opportunity to work with a young child (5 or younger) or a child with disabilities who is functioning at approximately this level, try to use *expansion*. You will need to set up a play activity that will give the child the opportunity to interact. As the child plays, ask questions to prompt a response. When the opportunity arises, use expansion to model a more adult form of language for the child.

Try to video- or audiotape your play session.

References

Aram, D. M., Ekelman, B. L., & Nation, J. E. (1984). Preschoolers with language disorders: 10 years later. *Journal of Speech and Hearing Research, 27,* 232–244.

Bashir, A. S., & Scavuzzo, A. (1992). Children with language disorders: Natural history and academic success. *Journal of Learning Disabilities, 25,* 53–65.

Bear, G. G., & Proctor, W. A. (1990). Impact of a full-time integrated program on the achievement of nonhandicapped and mildly handicapped children. *Exceptionality, 1,* 227–238.

Buttrill, J., Niizawa, J., Biemer, C., Takahashi, C., & Hearn, S. (1989). Serving the language learning disabled adolescent: A strategies-based model. *Language, Speech, and Hearing Services in Schools, 20,* 185– 204.

Cazden, C. B. (1986). Classroom discourse. In M. C. Wittrock (Ed.), *Handbook of research on teaching* (pp. 432–464). New York: Macmillan.

Cirrin, F. M., & Penner, S. G. (1995). Classroom-based and consultative service delivery models for language intervention. In M. E. Fey, J. Windsor, & S. F. Warren (Eds.), *Language intervention: Preschool through the elementary years* (pp. 333–362). Baltimore: Paul H. Brooks.

Dudley-Marling, C., & Searle, D. (1988). Enriching language learning environments for students with learning disabilities. *Journal of Learning Disabilities, 21,* 140–143.

Dunn, L. (1968). Special education for the mildly retarded: Is much of it justifiable? *Exceptional Children, 35,* 5–22.

Fuchs, D., & Fuchs, L. S. (1988). Evaluation of the adaptive learning environments model. *Exceptional Children, 55,* 115–127.

Goodman, K. S. (1990). The past, present, and future of literacy education: Comments from the pens of distinguished educators, Part I. *The Reading Teacher, 43,* 302–311.

Kauffman, J. M. (1989). The regular education initiative as Reagan-Bush education policy: A trickle-down theory of education of the hard-to-teach. *The Journal of Special Education, 23,* 256–278.

Koppenhaver, D. A., Pierce, P. L., Steelman, J. D., & Yoder, D. E. (1995). Contexts of early literacy intervention for children with developmental disabilities. In M. E. Fey, J. Windsor, & S. F. Warren (Eds.), *Language intervention: Preschool through the elementary years* (pp. 241–274). Baltimore: Paul H. Brooks.

Lerner, J. W. (1993). *Learning disabilities: Theories, diagnosis, and teaching strategies.* Boston: Houghton-Mifflin.

Light, J., Koppenhaver, D., Lee, E., & Riffle, L. (1994). *The home and school literacy experiences of students who use AAC systems.* Unpublished manuscript.

Lindfors, J. W. (1987). *Children's language and learning.* Englewood Cliffs, NJ: Prentice-Hall.

McCormick, L. (1986). Keeping up with language intervention trends. *Teaching Exceptional Children, 18* (winter), 123–129.

Miller, L. (1989). Classroom-based language intervention. *Language, Speech, and Hearing Services in Schools, 20,* 153–169.

Nelson, N. W. (1989). Curriculum-based language assessment and intervention. *Language, Speech, and Hearing Services in Schools, 20,* 170–184.

Norris, J. (1989). Providing language remediation in the classroom: An integrated language-to-reading intervention model. *Language, Speech, and Hearing Services in Schools, 20,* 205–218.

Norris, J. A., & Hoffman, P. R. (1990). Language intervention within naturalistic environments. *Language, Speech, and Hearing Services in Schools, 21,* 72–84.

Ogle, D. (1986). K-W-L: A teaching model that develops active reading of expository text. *The Reading Teacher, 39,* 564–570.

Owens, R. E. (1995). *Language disorders: A functional approach to assessment and intervention.* Boston: Allyn and Bacon.

Pierce, P. L., & Steelman, J. D. (1993). *The O.W.L. (oral and written language) curriculum for young children with disabilities.* Chapel Hill: Center for Literacy and Disability Studies, University of North Carolina.

Reynolds, M. C., Wang, M. C., & Walberg, H. J. (1987). The necessary restructuring of special and regular education. *Exceptional Children, 53,* 391–398.

Rowe, M. (1974). Wait-time and rewards as instructional variables, their influence in language, logic, and fate control: Part I—Wait time. *Journal of Research in Science Teaching, 11,* 81–94.

Rowe, M. (1986). Wait time: Slowing down may be a way of speeding up! *Journal of Teacher Education, 37,* 43–50.

Schery, T. K., & O'Connor, L. C. (1992). The effectiveness of school-based computer language intervention with severely handicapped children. *Language, Speech, and Hearing Services in Schools, 23,* 43–47.

Stainback, W., & Stainback, S. (1984). A rationale for the merger of special and regular education. *Exceptional Children, 51,* 102–111.

Stauffer, R. G. (1975). *Directing the reading-thinking process.* New York: Harper and Row.

Wang, M. C., & Birch, J. W. (1984). Comparison of a full-time mainstreaming program and a resource room approach. *Exceptional Children, 51,* 33–40.

Watson, L. R., Layton, T. L., Pierce, P. L., & Abraham, L. M. (1994). Enhancing emerging literacy in a language preschool. *Language, Speech, and Hearing Services in Schools, 25,* 136–145.

Wilcox, M. J., Kouri, T., & Caswell, S. (1990). Early language intervention: A comparison of classroom and individual treatment. *American Journal of Speech-Language Pathology, 1(3),* 49–62.

Will, M. (1986). Educating children with learning problems: A shared responsibility. *Exceptional Children, 52,* 411–415.

Zigmond, N., & Baker, J. (1990). Mainstream experiences for learning disabled students (Project MELD): Preliminary report. *Exceptional Children, 57,* 176–185.

Chapter 13

Augmentative and Alternative Communication

Despite our best efforts to provide appropriate intervention for speech, language, and communication difficulties, many school-age children fail to develop spoken language. Until recently there was little that could be done for these children. They were often relegated to the back wards of institutions or employed in nonproductive sheltered workshop activities. But today new technologies offer hope for these individuals who previously lacked access to that most important human characteristic—communication. These new approaches are called augmentative and alternative communication (AAC).

This chapter examines the rapidly developing field of augmentative and alternative communication, describing a variety of approaches—from sign systems to sophisticated electronic devices. Most important, instructional methods that are designed to develop the functional use of AAC systems are discussed. The goal of this chapter is to help you become aware of the many options that are available for persons who do not speak and how to best utilize these procedures in classroom settings.

Specifically, after reading this chapter you should be able to:

1. Define *augmentative and alternative communication.*
2. Describe the options that are available to enhance the communication of non-speaking persons.
3. Understand the criteria for selecting AAC systems.
4. Know the outcomes that can be expected from the use of AAC procedures.
5. Describe methods found effective for enhancing the communicative interaction of AAC users.

Howard, a student with mental retardation, has severe articulation problems that make his speech very difficult to understand. He carries a communication wallet with pictures he shows others so they can understand what he is talking about. When he goes to McDonald's, he uses pictures from the wallet to help him order his meal. Melissa, a 16-year-old girl with autism, rarely talks. She has learned to communicate with a Touch Talker. Now, she can respond to questions from her teacher by touching a symbol on her display, activating a voice output device that serves as her voice. Tony, a 9-year-old student with cerebral palsy, attends a regular education classroom. Because of his limited motor abilities, he uses a head pointer to touch an electronic keyboard to formulate written messages and produce a voice output. Tamika, a student with moderate mental retardation, has learned a repertoire of eight signs that she uses to supplement her limited spoken output.

What all of these individuals have in common is that they are using some type of AAC procedure. For many, if not most, children with severe disorders of language and communication, AAC represents their best hope for the development of communication skills (Romski & Sevcik, 1988).

It is estimated that there are approximately 900,000 individuals in the United States who are nonspeaking because of disabilities such as cerebral palsy, mental retardation, and autism (Blackstone & Painter, 1985). Zangari, Lloyd, and Vicker (1994) cite evidence from several studies that suggests that from .3 to 1 percent of the school-age population may be in need of AAC services. This means that from 150,00 to 500,000 children could require AAC services. Although there is no accurate count of the number of school-age children who actually use augmentative and alternative communication, there are undoubtedly many children who could benefit from the use of AAC procedures but who do not yet have the opportunity to do so.

Components of Augmentative and Alternative Communication

The term *augmentative communication* refers to methods and devices that supplement existing verbal communication skills (Mustonen, Locke, Reichle, Solbrack, & Lindgren, 1991). In other words, the objective is to enhance the communication skills that the individual already exhibits. *Alternative communication* refers to techniques that substitute for spoken communication for those individuals who appear unable or unlikely to develop spoken-language skills (McCormick & Shane, 1990). In practice, the distinction between augmentative and alternative communication is sometimes not clear. There are times when use of an alternative communication procedure represents the best way to enhance speech output for the individual. In other instances, an approach designed to augment spoken language production could become the primary communicative mode for that person. Since both achieve the same end, for the purposes of this text, the approaches are grouped under the term *augmentative and alternative communication*.

Augmentative and alternative communication systems consist of three components: *communication devices, symbol systems, and communication skills* (McCormick & Shane, 1990). Each of these components must be considered when an AAC procedure is being developed. Sometimes most attention is lavished on the communication device—especially if it is a particularly high-tech system. Teachers and speech language specialists must be careful not to become so caught up in the technical sophistication of the device that they ignore the other components of AAC systems. After all, the device is of little use if the user cannot understand it or does not use it.

Devices

There are two basic kinds of AAC devices (or systems)—*aided* and *unaided* (Vanderheiden & Lloyd, 1986). **Unaided techniques** do not require external support devices or procedures in order to operate. They include techniques such as speech, sign language, and facial expressions. Unaided techniques have the obvious advantages of portability and ease of use. With the exception of during an occasional bout of laryngitis, the voice, hands, and facial expressions cannot be lost or broken. There are no concerns about electrical outlets or battery packs. The "device" is always ready for use. With spoken language or facial expressions, although the users may have difficulty expressing themselves, listeners are usually familiar with the means of communication (spoken or nonverbal language) being used. Of course, when a sign language is used as the mode of communication (e.g., American Sign Language [ASL] or Signed English), there will be a more limited number of potential communication partners.

Aided devices employ communication means that may be as simple as a communication board (see Box 13.1) or as complex as a computer with a synthetic speech output device. They may be *electronic or nonelectronic,* and they employ a *selection procedure* and use some type of *symbol system.* Mustonen et al. (1991) note several advantages of electronic communication devices. For example, use of electronic devices can enable users to produce more complex messages than their own language skills allow. As an example, Mustonen et al. describe how by pressing a symbol for a soft drink, an electronic aid could produce the expression, *Gee, I'm thirsty. I'd like a medium Diet Cherry Coke.* If the device has voice output capabilities, there is the further advantage of communication from a distance. Another advantage of electronic devices is the capability to store messages for future use.

Rounsefell, Zucker, and Roberts (1993) discuss four features that are common to all communication aids, electronic or not: output, selection technique, vocabulary capability, and portability.

Output refers to the appearance of the display and how it enhances communication with a listener. Communication boards typically consist of a flat surface on which drawn or written symbols are displayed. They can be placed on a wheelchair lap tray, bound in a book, or folded into a wallet-sized container. The output is a visual display, which the user accesses by pointing.

Electronic devices may use a visual display, a printed output, or a voice output. Visual displays allow listeners to check their understanding of the message and to even offer corrections or suggestions for extension of the communication. Printed output (such as that produced by a Canon Communicator) has the advan-

---

BOX 13.1 Developing Communication Boards

Communication boards are one option for enhancing the communication of nonspeaking students. Before designing the board itself, you will need to

1. List the communicative functions (requesting, greeting, informing) and/or topics (actions, people, events) that compose the student's communicative repertoire.
2. Describe the objects, pictures, signs and/or symbols that will be on the board, including the:

   – number
   – size
   – distance
   – arrangement

3. Describe the pictures/signs/symbols that will permit the user to indicate:

   – that needed concepts/messages cannot be conveyed because the needed picture/sign/symbol is not available
   – instructions for communication partners

4. Delineate such construction-relevant factors as:

   – what size the board should be
   – how many pages it will have
   – where it will be used
   – how portable it must be
   – how it is to be mounted or carried
   – whether it should have a washable surface

Source: Adapted from L. McCormick and H. Shane. (1990). Communication system options for students who are nonspeaking. In L. McCormick & R. Schiefelbusch (Eds.), *Early language interventions: An introduction.* Columbus, OH: Merrill.

tage of producing a written record of interaction. This record can be used for assessment purposes or as a basis for further instruction in communication. Voice-output devices (VOCAS) have the advantage of being the closest approximation to natural speech.

According to Scherz and Beer (1995) the use of voice output systems has increased dramatically in the last decade. There are two types of voice output devices currently in use: *synthesized speech* and *digitized speech*. Devices that use synthesized speech are more widely used at this time because they have been in use longer and are generally less expensive. Examples include the Touch Talker (Prentke-Romich) and the WOLF (AdamLab). They can be used in text-to-speech applications where typed text is converted to vocal output. The intelligibility of synthesized-speech output devices can vary widely (Mirenda & Beukelman, 1990). In addition, factors such as the age and gender of the voice output can affect the acceptance of a voice-output device (Crabtree, Mirenda, & Beukelman, 1990). For example, a young girl may be reluctant to use a device that has an adult male voice as its output. These factors should be considered when selecting a synthesized-speech voice-output device. Digitized voice-output systems are nearly as intelligible as human speech (Mustonen et al., 1991) but, because of their high computer memory requirements, are not very useful for text-to-speech applications. Examples of devices that use digitized speech include the MaCaw (Zygo) and the Introtalker (Prentke-Romich).

A second common feature of communication aids is the **selection technique** employed. Users of a communication aid must indicate to their communication partner which letter or symbol they wish to select. Individuals with intact motor skills may use *direct selection*. In this case, the "speaker" simply points to a selected item. For those who have little or no voluntary control of their arms, adaptations can be used to allow them to make direct selections. These might be a head pointer (a rod attached to a headband) or an eyegaze system that identifies the selected item when the user looks at it for a period of time.

Direct selection is usually the fastest type of selection technique, however some individuals with significant motor impairments need another type of selection method. *Scanning* is an alternative. Scanning involves making a selection from the presented choices. Rather than directly selecting the desired word or symbol, with scanning, choices are displayed for the individual. Typically, scanning is associated with electronic displays that present a blinking light (cursor) which moves from item to item on the display panel. The user selects an item by merely pressing a button (or a switch or pad), or making some other motor movement that stops the scanning. The cursor may move across the display in a linear motion, in up-and-down columns, or in any other preprogrammed way. Scanning devices can be coupled with various types of switches so that the individual who has any voluntary muscle control at all can operate a communication device.

Vocabulary capability is defined by Rounsefell et al. (1993) as "the capability of an aid to allow the individual to have the vocabulary that he or she wants displayed or stored in the aid" (p. 298). Communication boards can be designed with overlays that can be changed for various settings and activities. Most electronic devices can be reprogrammed and the overlay changed to meet changing communicative needs. The ease with which such changes can be made and the number and usefulness of the items on the display are factors that should be considered in the design and/or selection of a communication aid.

Portability is the final feature of communication aids discussed by Rounsefell et al. (1993). Portability is an important concern in an era when emphasis is on the integration of persons with disabilities into their schools and communities. As technology advances, the devices are becoming smaller and more powerful. Clearly, a communication device is of little help if it cannot be used in the settings where it is really needed. Therefore, it is essential that portability be considered when decisions about communication devices are being made.

There are advantages and limitations to the use of either aided or unaided procedures (see Table 13.1). Ideally, unaided communication techniques would be the choice for everyone. But there are many individuals who are unable to develop spoken language or understand and use nonverbal communication or sign language. For these persons, aided communication methods are the best alternative. When appropriately designed or selected, aided communication devices permit people with severe impairments in motor and/or cognitive abilities to communicate with others.

TABLE 13.1 Advantages and Disadvantages of Aided and Unaided AAC Systems

	Advantages	Disadvantages
Unaided Systems	No external support devices needed Portable No cost (other than training)	Potential communication partners limited Relies on user's memory ability Signs may be difficult to learn
Aided Systems	Can produce message that is more complex than user's own language Can communicate at a distance (with VOCAS)	Electronic device may break or lose power Portability may be limited May be expensive

Symbol Systems

Unaided AAC systems typically use some type of sign system (e.g., American Sign Language, Signed English). These approaches have been used with various populations of individuals with disabilities, including those with mental retardation and autism (Bryen & Joyce, 1986). Studies examining the acquisition of sign systems by individuals with disabilities have generally found that such persons can acquire at least a basic sign vocabulary (Kiernan, 1983). Although a sign language system may be a useful form of communication for some students, for many students with disabilities, sign language is not an effective approach to the development of communication skills. Results of a survey reported by Bryen, Goldman, and Quinlisk-Gill (1988) indicated that despite years of training, few students with significant disabilities used signs in spontaneous conversation. In addition, with signing there is the obvious problem of the limited number of potential communication partners available. If the goal for persons with disabilities is community inclusion, sign language may not be the most effective approach. Therefore, many of these students require some sort of alternative approach that might include an aided AAC system.

Any AAC device must have some sort of symbol system as the mode of communication. For individuals with severe motor disorders but good literacy skills, letters and words can be the symbolic mode. But many users of AAC systems either have not had the opportunity to acquire literacy skills or have cognitive disabilities that impair their acquisition of written language. A variety of symbol systems, ranging from real objects to photographs to abstract-symbol systems, have been developed to aid these persons in communicating with an AAC system.

Photographs have the advantage of clearly representing an item. Of course, the quality of the photograph will affect its usefulness. The context in which an item appears also affects its recognizability (Mustonen et al., 1991). Photos that include a contextual background (a spoon that appears next to a plate) are more recognizable. Additionally, in general, color photographs are more easily recognized than black-and-white photos (Mirenda & Locke, 1989). An alternative to photos is line drawings. These usually are composed of black lines drawn on a white background.

A number of abstract symbol-systems are available, including *Picture Communication Symbols* (PCS) (Johnson, 1981), *Picsyms* (Carlson, 1984), *Sigsymbols* (Creagan, 1982), and *Blissymbols* (Bliss, 1965). As illustrated in Figure 13.1, all of these graphic symbol systems include pictorial representations of the items they name. In addition, Sigsymbols include ideographs (ideas represented through graphic symbols) and Blissymbols include both ideographs and arbitrary symbols (ideas assigned arbitrary configurations of lines). *Rebus* symbols are another form of line drawing used with AAC systems. Rebuses use pictures of objects to replace the word in a sentence. A number of rebus systems are commercially available (e.g., Clark, Davies, & Woodcock, 1974).

Several types of arbitrary symbols have also been used for alternative and augmentative communication purposes. Non-SLIP (Non-Speech Language Initiation Program), a symbol system developed by Carrier (1974), is based on the symbol system developed by David Premack in his research on teaching language to chimpanzees. The Non-SLIP program uses plastic, geometric shapes to represent words. The items are color-coded by part of speech, and the shapes can be put together to form sentences. Romski and her colleagues (Romski, Sevcik, & Pate, 1988; Romski, Sevcik, & Wilkinson, 1994; Romski, Sevcik, Robinson, & Bakeman, 1994) have reported that adults and school-age children with severe mental retardation can successfully use lexigrams for symbolic communication. The lexigrams are arbitrary visual-graphic symbols made up of combinations of geometric shapes, and are derived from those originally used to teach language skills to a chimpanzee (Rumbaugh, 1977) (see Figure 13.2).

Communication Skills

AAC procedures and devices present wonderful opportunities for nonspeaking persons to communicate with others. Yet, if the systems are not used—or not used effectively—the intervention is of no use, no matter how high-tech the device. As Janice Light (1988) put it, "One of the most critical issues for clinicians in the field of augmentative and alternative communication (AAC) is to determine how non-speaking individuals can best facilitate their daily interactions in educational, vocational, community, and home environments" (p. 66).

Research on the use of AAC systems has found that users tend to be relatively passive communicative partners. They rely on their speaking listeners to direct the conversation and rarely initiate interaction themselves (Calculator & Dollaghan, 1982; Light, Collier, & Parnes, 1985; Mirenda & Iacono, 1990). Calculator (1988) has described many AAC users as "underfunctioning." That is, they are not expected to communicate effectively and tend to live down to these expectations. Instead of asking for more food, for example, a student may simply throw the plate on the floor. The staff member's response may be to simply clean up the mess, rather than ask the student why he or she threw the plate. Con-

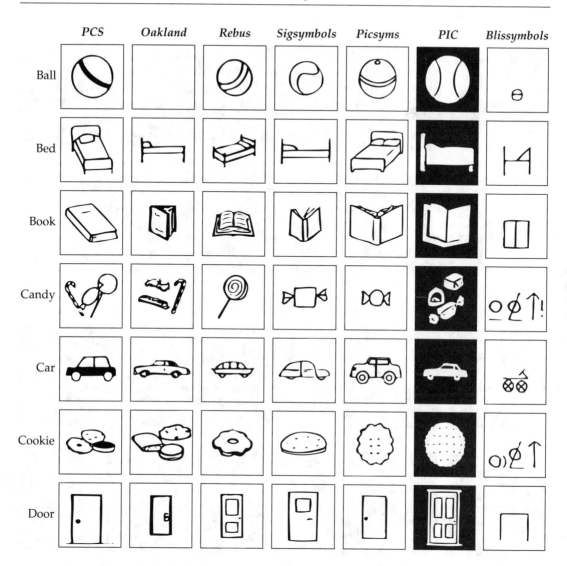

FIGURE 13.1   Examples of Line-Drawn Symbols

Source: Reprinted from *Augmentative Communication: An Introduction,* S. W. Blackstone, Editor, 1986, with permission from the American Speech-Language-Hearing Association.

versational partners tend to limit the interaction of AAC users in other ways. For example, they tend to ask questions that require only yes/no answers (Light et al., 1985) and initiate conversations that require no response (e.g., making a comment like "Nice work.") (Reichle, 1991).

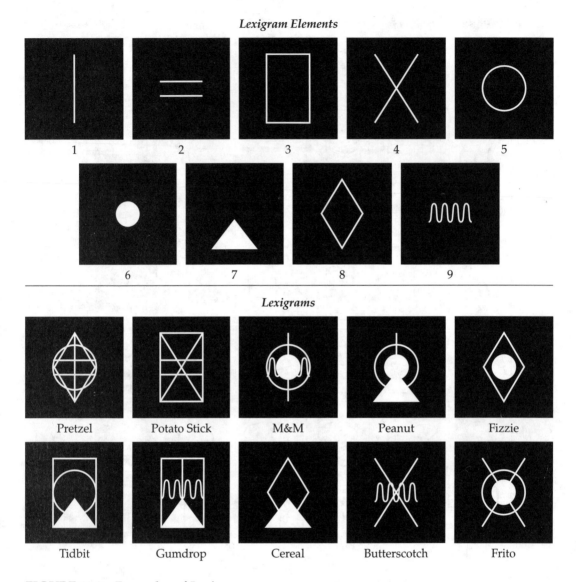

FIGURE 13.2   Examples of Lexigrams

Source: From M. A. Romski, R. A. Sevcik, and J. L. Pate, "Establishment of Symbolic Communication in Persons with Severe Retardation," *Journal of Speech and Hearing Disorders, 53*(1988), 94–107. © American Speech-Language-Hearing Association. Reprinted by permission of the American Speech-Language-Hearing Association and the author.

In addition to their rarely initiating conversation, AAC users have been found to have difficulty terminating conversations (Reichle, 1991). Some simply do not know how to do this. Others want to extend the conversation as long as possible, even if the interaction is no longer meaningful. Some AAC users have even been reported to make untrue statements, simply to keep a conversation going

(Reichle, 1991). While there is considerable variation in communicative abilities among AAC users (Light, 1988), the picture provided by most of the research suggests that most are not communicating effectively.

Implementing AAC Systems

Prerequisite Skills

One of the major issues in AAC involves prerequisites to its use. For many years it was claimed that in order to be successful, potential users of AAC systems had to have achieved certain cognitive and language prerequisites (Shane & Bashir, 1980). Sometimes called the *candidacy* model (Mirenda & Iacono, 1990), this approach suggested that the potential AAC user should be able to demonstrate development to at least stage V (means-end relations) on Piaget's description of cognitive development and show evidence of intentional communication before being introduced to an AAC system. The idea that AAC users needed these cognitive and language prerequisites was based on data from spoken language acquisition in normally developing children. These data indicated that specific cognitive and communicative behaviors preceded the emergence of spoken language. However, as Romski and Sevcik (1988) have noted, the exact relationship between cognition and communication development, and language acquisition has never been clearly defined. Moreover, there is a rapidly expanding body of research that indicates that persons with disabilities can benefit from AAC systems even if they lack these cognitive and communicative prerequisites. For example, Reichle and Yoder (1985) were able to teach preschoolers who functioned at stage IV on a Piagetian scale to label objects using graphic symbols. Although the preschoolers were unable to generalize this skill to functional communication, such as commenting and requesting, they were able to label. Romski, Sevcik, and Pate (1988) taught young adults with severe mental retardation to request foods and objects by using graphic symbols on a computer display panel, despite the subjects' lack of spoken language comprehension skills.

Because of research such as that described above and the realization that research from normal language development is not always easily translated to individuals with disabilities, most clinicians and researchers are today suggesting a try-and-see, rather than a wait-and-see, model for potential AAC users (McGregor, Young, Gerak, Thomas, & Vogelsberg, 1992). Use of this approach requires a careful analysis of the communicative environments in which the AAC user functions and of what would be required to make it possible for the individual to communicate (Mirenda & Iacono, 1990).

Preassessment

As with any kind of intervention, the development of an AAC system begins with assessment. The most useful kind of assessment is one that is ecological in nature, that is, one that surveys the communicative environments and communicative needs in which the individual will function. According to Sigafoos and York (1991), an ecological inventory for potential AAC users should include the following elements:

- **Priority instructional targets:** These include both the communication *demands* and *opportunities* presented by the environment. Demands might include asking for help in a classroom or vocational environment, whereas opportunities for communication may exist in many environments.
- **Specific communication content:** This domain includes specific *communicative intents* demanded by the environment (requesting, rejecting, and so on), specific *vocabulary* needed by the learner, and *modes of communication* that may be effective within particular environments. For example, sign language is only useful if others in the signer's environment know the sign system.
- **Instructional design information:** This area includes analysis of *when to teach communication*, of *specific cues and consequences* available in the environment (e.g., running out of materials is a natural cue for communication), and of information on *how to sequence trials*.

In addition to assessing the environment, practitioners must gather information about the potential AAC user. The purpose of this assessment is to *describe* the learner's present communication status rather than to make decisions about whether the individual should or should not use an AAC device. Mirenda and Iacono (1990) have suggested that the following learner characteristics be considered when developing AAC systems:

- **Mobility:** The student's positioning and ability to walk should be evaluated. These factors need to be considered in making decisions about AAC methods.
- **Manipulation:** The individual's fine motor skills should be evaluated to determine if the student can use a gestural communication system or what, if any, adaptations to a communication device will be necessary.
- **Communication:** The focus should be on *how* the student communicates. Does the student have any speech? Does the student use gestures or other sorts of nonspoken communication?
- **Cognitive/linguistic:** The purpose of this assessment is to determine which types of symbol systems are likely to be successful with this student.
- **Sensory/perceptual:** It is necessary to gather information about the learner's vision and hearing abilities.

Developing an AAC System

Training can be developed using information from the assessment of both the individual and of the environment, goals, and objectives for augmentative and alternative communication. McCormick and Shane (1990) suggest that AAC instructional programs should (1) enhance the child's ability to participate in aca-

TABLE 13.2 Examples of Goals for AAC Instruction

Overall Goals	Second-Level Specific Objectives	Objectives
To enhance the child's ability to participate in academic, functional, and social activities in normal environments	Increasing the frequency and variety of basic communicative behaviors, especially such functions as requesting and commenting Increasing the sophistication and complexity of language forms and structures and other communicative devices Increasing the student's opportunities for communication, communicative modes, and use of available sign and/or symbol systems	Jason will initiate a request for drink (milk, juice, Koolaid) and food (cookie, cracker, apple) at morning and afternoon snack times by pointing to the appropriate symbols on his communication board. Randy will demonstrate increased assertiveness and participation in science class by raising his hand and asking or answering (with his communication board and gestures) at least three questions each day.

Source: From L. McCormick and R. L. Schiefelbusch, *Early Language Interventions: An Introduction* (2nd ed.). Copyright © 1990 by Allyn and Bacon. Reprinted by permission.

demic, functional, and social activities in normal environments and (2) improve the quality and quantity of the child's language and communication skills.

With these general goals in mind, educators can then develop specific objectives and plans, such as those that appear in Table 13.2. As with any educational plan, it is important that instructional outcomes be clearly defined before teaching begins. Only then will educators know if their instruction has been successful.

The establishment of instructional objectives paves the way for decisions about the AAC system. These decisions relate to the *type* of system to be used (aided or unaided), the nature of the *symbol system* (e.g., gestural, pictorial, symbolic), and the communication instruction required.

Deciding the type of system to be used—aided or unaided— is the first decision needed in designing an AAC system. The provider must weigh the advantages and limitations of each type of system in combination with information about the learner and the communicative environment. Characteristics of the learner, such as sensory and motor skills, may determine what kind of system is possible. Similarly, environmental demands and opportunities will also have an impact on this decision. If potential communication partners are not familiar with American Sign Language, this might be a poor choice for an AAC system.

In many cases, the choice of a communication system is not as critical as it might seem. Frequently, a combination of communication systems, including both aided and unaided, are preferable. For example, Barrerra, Lobato-Barrera, and Sulzer-Azaroff (1980) found that a combined gestural and vocal mode intervention was more effective than either mode used alone. Keogh and Reichle (1985)

TABLE 13.3   Strategies for Selecting Signs

Strategy	Interpretation
Select contact signs over noncontact signs	Contact signs are those where there is contact between the hands or between the hand and another part of the body.
Select symmetric signs over asymmetric signs	Symmetric signs are those where each hand makes identical shapes or movements.
Select translucent signs over nontranslucent signs	Translucent (or iconic) signs are those that resemble the item being signed.
Select signs where there are maximal locational differences	Signs that are made in different locations relative to the signer's body are more easily learned (e.g., signs made at the side).
Select visible over invisible signs	Visible signs are those that signers can easily see as they produce them. Some signs are made out of the field of vision (e.g., from the top of one's head).
Select reduplicated over nonreduplicated signs	Reduplicated signs are those that are repeated two or more times.
Group signs to be taught in close proximity to each other into conceptually dissimilar sets	Signs that differ in meaning may be learned more easily.
Select single-handshape over multiple-handshape signs	
Select one-handed signs over two-handed signs	
Select single-movement over multiple-movement signs	

Source: Adapted from J. E. Doherty. (1985). The effects of sign characteristics on sign acquisition and retention: An integrative review of the literature. *Augmentative and Alternative Communication, 1,* 108–121.

suggested that a mixed mode, in which some vocabulary items are taught via one mode and others are taught in another, might be beneficial for some learners. Another alternative is to teach students to use two modes of communication. Depending on the situation, they can choose the method that works best. For example, signing may work well in school with a teacher who knows sign language but a communication wallet might be necessary when ordering at McDonald's (Reichle, Mirenda, Locke, Piche, & Johnston, 1992; Romski, Sevcik, Robinson, & Bakeman, 1994).

Once a method of communication (or combination of methods) has been selected, the next decision involves selection of an appropriate symbol system. For an unaided communication procedure, the choice will be among the variety of gestural languages in existence (see Chapter 8 for a review). Research has found that some signs are easier to learn than others. Doherty (1985) has suggested several specific strategies for selecting signs. They are presented in Table 13.3.

Regardless of which communication system is selected, a decision must be made as to which vocabulary items to include. Unfortunately, decisions about vocabulary are often based on what the teacher or clinician *thinks* the student needs to know rather than on what the environment demands (Reichle, et al., 1992). In fact, when Reichle (1983) asked interventionists how they made decisions about vocabulary selection, he got the following responses (in order of frequency): (1) selected vocabulary that the interventionist thought would be important, (2) selected vocabulary from the first 50 word developmental data, (3) selected vocabulary from word lists obtained from surveying service providers, (4) selected vocabulary from word lists derived from vocabulary used by learners with developmental disabilities. A better strategy would be to select vocabulary demanded by the learner's environment. This vocabulary could be derived from the results of the preassessment ecological inventory.

Three factors should be considered when selecting AAC symbol systems— guessability, learnability, and generalization. Symbols range in *guessability* from those that are *very transparent* (easily guessed) to those that are *translucent* (need additional information to decode) (Mustonen et al., 1991). The term *iconic* is also used to describe guessability. Iconic symbols are similar in appearance to the items that they represent. For example, the drawings of the ball in figure 13.1 are all reasonably transparent (or iconic); that is, naive viewers would likely call the drawing a ball. The Sigsymbol drawing of a cookie, however, may not be as readily guessable. In general, however, Picsyms and Rebus symbols have been found to be easier to guess than the meanings of Blissymbols (Musselwhite & Ruscello, 1984). Research by Mirenda and Locke (1989) on subjects with mild to severe mental retardation, found the following order of guessability: real objects, color photographs, black-and-white photographs, miniature objects, black-and-white line symbols (Picsyms, Picture Communication Symbols) (Mayer-Johnson Co., 1986), Rebuses, Self-Talk symbols (Johnson, 1986)), Blissymbols, and written words.

Learnability refers to the ease or difficulty of learning a particular symbol set. Generally, studies with nondisabled children have found that learnability is related to iconicity (guessability). Symbols that are more iconic (similar to the object being named) are more easily learned. Rebus symbols are easier to learn than Blissymbols which are, in turn, easier to learn than Non-SLIP chips or words (Clark, 1981; Carrier & Peak, 1975). Research on persons with disabilities has found that, for them, matching photographs with objects is easier than matching line drawings with objects (Sevcik & Romski, 1986) and that Rebus symbols are also more easily learned than Blissymbols (Hurlbut, Iwata, & Green, 1982).

According to Mustonen et al. (1991) iconic symbols facilitate the acquisition, generalization, and maintenance of graphic communication systems. The researchers acknowledge, on the other hand, that for students who can acquire higher-order symbolic information, iconic symbols may not be necessary. Another consideration is determining the ease with which symbols can be combined to make sentences. Lexigrams and Blissymbols are readily combined into sentences. Of course, printed words are easily generalized, but lexigrams have been shown to be easier to discriminate than printed words for persons with severe mental retardation (Romski, Sevcik, Pate & Rumbaugh, 1985).

When graphic symbols are selected for use with an AAC system, Reichle (1991) suggests that four questions should guide their selection:

- **What types of symbols should be used?** Choices include photographs, line drawings, abstract symbols, and the like. The selection should be made on the basis of what works for a particular learner.
- **How large will the symbols be?** Learners with poor visual acuity will require larger displays.
- **How will the learner select the symbols?** Direct selection, scanning, or a combination of these could be used.
- **How will the symbols be displayed?** A board (electronic or nonelectronic), wallet, or book could be used to display the symbols.

Again, as with most decisions involving augmentative and alternative communication, the decision about which symbol system to use must include considerations of the abilities and needs of the individual student: their literacy skills, cognitive abilities, and potential communicative partners. Romski and Sevcik (1988) have suggested, however, that the most important decisions may regard the instructional strategies for enhancing communicative competence rather than the mode of communication employed.

Earlier in this chapter, we reviewed some of the research on the communication difficulties encountered by users of AAC and found that AAC users often lack opportunities to communicate. When they do communicate, they have been reported to have a lot of difficulty communicating effectively with others and are, therefore, relatively passive communicators who rarely initiate interactions.

Recently, researchers and clinicians have focused more attention on the problem of how to enhance the communication skills of AAC users. A variety of techniques, from highly structured, direct-teaching procedures to more naturalistic methods have been used with some success (Mirenda & Iacono, 1990). In reviewing the research on teaching conversational skills to students who have severe disabilities and are using AAC systems, Calculator (1988) identified two major approaches that appear to work: *teaching in natural environments* and *teaching functional skills*.

As stated previously natural environments have proven to be the best place to teach conversation skills. When instruction is designed so that students have opportunities to talk about real situations with conversational partners who actually exist in those settings, not only does interaction increase but there is a greater chance for generalization of the skill as well (Calculator, 1988). In addition to being provided with opportunities for interaction in natural environments, AAC users should be taught to use their systems for functional purposes—that is, to accomplish some real task in the environment rather than one contrived for instructional purposes. Calculator (1988) gives the following example of how instruction for 8-year-old, nonspeaking Joshua was made more functional. For two years, Joshua's instructional program consisted of his teacher presenting two objects at a time and requesting that he indicate through eye gaze the one named by his teacher. Since, after two years of instruction Joshua still had not reached criterion levels, his program was redesigned to give him opportunities to use eye gaze during various activities in the school day. For example, at nap time Joshua was prompted to choose, using eye gaze, one of two locations for his nap. At snack time he selected between two snacks. Within six months he was able to accurately indicate his preferences in a number of different contexts.

Spiegel, Benjamin, and Spiegel (1993) give another example of the integration of functional communication within natural environments. They taught a 19-year-old male with cerebral palsy and moderate mental retardation to increase his use of an AAC device (Touch Talker) (Prentke-Romich). Although the student had learned to use the Touch Talker, he used it infrequently for interaction with others. He learned to respond to conversational prompts that utilized sentences he had previously learned. For example, the student learned to produce the sentence *I need to go to the bank.* After demonstrating that he could produce this sentence, he was given the following prompt: *You just received your S.S.I. check in the mail. You want to put it in your savings account, and Ruby can drive you to the bank. Now, here comes Ruby to talk to you.* The student was then expected to type his previously learned sentence. Using this procedure, the student not only learned to respond to the vignettes appropriately but increased his spontaneous use of his AAC device as well.

Apparently, merely teaching an individual to use an AAC device is not enough to ensure that the person will use it. The results of the Spiegel et al. (1993) study suggest this. So do the results of a training study conducted by Dattilo and Camarata (1991). They first taught two adults with severe motor impairments to use a Touch Talker. There was no significant increase in the initiation of interaction by either subject following this Touch Talker instruction. But when subjects were specifically taught to use their device to initiate conversations, the number of initiations increased rapidly.

McGregor et al. (1992) taught a 20-year-old student with cerebral palsy and mental retardation to initiate interaction in three school settings (classroom, speech therapy room, and vocational training area). After a short (5-minute) preinstruction phase, the student, Winston, was simply reminded to use his AAC device (Touch Talker) if he wanted something. The teacher made sure she responded and gave Winston reinforcement for his use of this device. Using this simple intervention procedure, Winston significantly increased use of his Touch Talker in all three school environments.

Not only the AAC user, but also the listener, requires training. Often, listeners have to be very patient as AAC users formulate their messages. But patience alone may not be enough. Researchers have found that instruction in understanding the speech produced by voice output communication devices can increase the responsiveness of listeners to AAC messages. (Rounsefell, Zucker, & Roberts, 1993). Communication between AAC users and their conversational partners can also benefit from instruction given to the listener on how to elicit communication from others (Hunt, Alwell, & Goetz, 1991).

Calculator (1988) suggests the following guidelines for planning communication goals for AAC users:

- **Increase the environments in which AAC is used:** Students should have the opportunity to practice their skills in many different types of settings.
- **Engage in age appropriate interactions:** Conversation should be consistent with that which would be expected with normally developing peers of the same age.
- **Increase opportunities for AAC use:** Students must be provided with both the vocabulary needed in the environments they are likely to encounter and the opportunities to use their conversational skills.
- **Focus conversation on topics valued by individual:** When students have the opportunity to request desired things and reject items they really dislike, they tend to value their communication skills.
- **Focus conversation on topics valued by parents and guardians:** Parents must recognize the need for AAC and the value of communication that meets real needs.
- **Consider ease of acquisition:** Systems should be designed to be readily used so that students have the maximum opportunity for communication.
- **Consider enhancement of status for the AAC user:** Intervention should target skills that will enhance the status of the AAC users in their own eyes as well as in society's view.

There is increasing evidence that users of augmentative and alternative communication can be helped to be effective communicators. It seems clear, however, that general instruction in the use of an AAC system is not sufficient. Rather, AAC users have to be taught specifically to use their system in effective communication interactions. Instruction in natural environments on functional skills appears to be effective, as does instruction that considers the special needs of the listener.

To summarize, the process of planning an AAC instructional program consists of five steps:

1. **Preassessment,** including an ecological inventory and assessment of the learner
2. **Development of goals** that should enhance the child's ability to participate in all environments.
3. **Selection of a mode of communication,** either aided, unaided, or a combination
4. **Selection of a symbol system,** gestural or graphic
5. **Selection of methods to enhance communication** for both the AAC user and communication partners

There is evidence from research that with careful planning and the use of effective instructional techniques, nonspeaking individuals can develop effective communication skills.

TABLE 13.4   Suggestions for Integrating AAC Users into Regular Education Settings

1. Educational priorities should be established collaboratively with parents, advocates, and other team members (as opposed to discipline-referenced priorities).
2. Observation, assessment, and intervention should occur in the natural settings in which individuals spend their time.
3. Functional skills should be taught systematically throughout the day, rather than at designated times.
4. Anyone coming in contact with the augmented communicator is a potential instructor of communication skills.
5. The effectiveness of intervention procedures should be evaluated relative to individuals' performances in their natural settings.
6. Educational plans should specify desired communication behaviors relative to clusters of skills associated with the effective performance of a broader skill or activity.

Source: From Calculator SN, Jorgensen CM. "Integrating AAC Instruction into Regular Education Settings: Expounding on Best Practices," *Augmentative and Alternative Communication* 1991; 7: 204–212. Reprinted with permission.

Integrating AAC Use into Regular Education Settings

As more and more students with severe disabilities, including students with severe communication disabilities, are included in regular education settings, it becomes increasingly important for teachers—both regular and special education—to be aware of methods that will help these students become more fully integrated. For those students who use AAC systems, there are many challenges. Not only may teachers and students be unfamiliar with AAC devices, but many AAC users require a significant amount of help with their own communication skills.

Calculator and Jorgensen (1991) have provided some suggestions for integrating AAC users into regular education settings (see Table 13.4). They emphasize collaboration in planning for and teaching students with severe disabilities who use AAC systems. Since communication is a necessary skill in all the environments in which the student is expected to function, it is important that all staff be familiar with the AAC system used by the student. Both staff and student peers can benefit from instruction in the special listening skills required for augmentative and alternative communication.

As team members responsible for working with students using AAC systems, special educators may be called on to perform a variety of functions. A survey conducted by Locke and Mirenda (1992) found that many of these functions are traditional teacher-related responsibilities: adapting the curriculum, preparing and maintaining documentation, and writing goals and objectives for AAC users. However, some of the responsibilities are less traditional: identifying vocabulary, determining students' motivation and attitudes toward AAC techniques, and determining the communication needs of students. Two of the major concerns expressed by the teachers in this survey were the need for more training in AAC and the need for more time to work as a team.

It seems clear that as more children using AAC systems enter the public schools, staff will need to become better educated about augmentative and alternative communication—not only in understanding of how the systems work, but in their awareness of the necessity for creating meaningful communication opportunities within the natural school environments.

Outcomes of AAC System Usage

One of the questions that must be asked about augmentative and alternative communication is Does it work? Answering this question requires examining answers to three other questions. First, has the student increased communication ability? Second, what, if any, effects are there on other areas of functioning? And third, how is the AAC user accepted by others? All of these questions could be used in determining the success or failure of an AAC system.

The first question is, without a doubt, the most important one. After all, the primary reason for using an AAC system is to improve the communication skills of the student. There is considerable evidence from both research and clinical practice that augmentative and alternative communication, when properly instituted, can enhance the communication skills of nonspeaking individuals (Mirenda & Mathy-Laikko, 1989). In our brief review of the literature on AAC, we have seen that even students with severe mental retardation can learn to use symbols (Romski, Sevcik, & Pate, 1988). We have also reviewed evidence that AAC users, given instruction in communication skills, can become more effective communicators (McGregor et al., 1992).

There is also some research evidence that when students with challenging behaviors learn an alternative means of communication, their behavior can improve (Doss & Reichle, 1989). Durand (1993) reported on three cases of students who each had significant behavior problems, in combination with mental retardation and the absence of spoken language. Their behavior problems included crying, hitting, tantrums, and hair pulling. The parents and teachers of these students attended a series of workshops at which they learned about using assistive devices for functional communication. Following implementation of these procedures, the students increased their spontaneous communication and significantly decreased their challenging behaviors—by as much as 95 percent. These data and results from other studies suggest that when students are helped to improve their communication, the results can extend to other behaviors, as well.

The third area of consideration in evaluating the AAC system is acceptance by peers. If students with disabilities are to be fully included in school settings, it is essential that they become accepted by their peers. If speaking peers have negative attitudes toward them, nonspeaking AAC users may shy away from interacting with peers. Although there is little research on this issue, there is evidence that improved ability to communicate is associated with improved peer acceptance (Guralnick, 1986). When Blockenberger, Armstrong, O'Connor, and Freeman (1993) compared the attitudes of fourth-grade children toward a child using an alphabet board, an electronic device, and signing, they found, interestingly, that there was little difference in the children's reactions. Their research suggests that children are not heavily influenced by the type of AAC system used by another child. While there is clearly a need for more research in this area, teachers often report that children are more accepting of peers with disabilities than adults would expect.

Summary

Every child can communicate. Physical and cognitive limitations are no longer impenetrable roadblocks to the development of communication skills. The rapid development of augmentative and alternative communication procedures means that there are now a variety of options available to help nonspeaking persons develop communication skills.

Despite the rapid proliferation of AAC techniques, there are still many nonspeaking persons who do not have access to communication aids. This may be due to factors such as lack of funding or lack of knowledge about augmentative and alternative communication on the part of teachers and clinicians. Whatever the reasons, to deny an individual access to effective means of communication is to deny that person the right to be part of the community. Therefore, it is incumbent upon teachers and clinicians to educate themselves about AAC and to advocate for the right of their students/clients to have access to AAC systems.

For those who need help getting started with augmentative and alternative communication, many states have an AAC resource center. If no center is listed for your state, you might try contacting a university medical center to see if they have someone with expertise in AAC systems.

Review Questions

1. What is the difference between alternative and augmentative communication? Why is this distinction sometimes not important?

2. List and briefly describe the three components of AAC systems.

3. Compare the advantages and limitations of aided and unaided communication devices.

4. What is scanning? How does it differ from direct selection?

5. Why have some researchers questioned the usefulness of sign-language approaches for students with autism and mental retardation?

6. What are some of the communication difficulties researchers have frequently described among AAC users?

7. Why has the candidacy model of AAC implementation been criticized?

8. List and briefly describe five learners' characteristics that should be considered in choosing an AAC system.

9. Define *guessability* and *learnability* as applied to symbol systems.

10. Find the story of Joshua in the chapter. How was instruction redesigned to help Joshua become a more effective communicator?

11. List the five steps in the selection of AAC systems.

12. What problems do you see that might inhibit the use of AAC systems?

Suggested Activities

1. Try interviewing a user of an AAC system. Find out about some of their experiences in using their system. What problems have they had? What are the reactions of other people? If the speaker has very limited communication skills, you might also have to interview a parent and/or staff member.

As you conduct the interview with the AAC user, note your own feelings. Do you find that you have any difficulty communicating with this person? What could be done to make the conversation flow more smoothly?

2. Try out an augmentative and alternative communication system yourself, an electronic device if possible. If you cannot get access to such a device, use a communication board or wallet. First, you will need to understand how the device works. Try it out. Then try to use it in a real environment (such as in a cafeteria or fast food restaurant).

How did you feel when you used the AAC system? How difficult was it to express yourself? How did others react to you? What could you have done to make the communicative exchanges work better?

3. Observe AAC users as they use their system. Note the following:

– Do they appear to be familiar with their device/procedure?
– With whom do they communicate?
– How frequently do they initiate interaction?
– How do others respond to them?

References

Barrera, R. D., Lobato-Barrera, D., & Sulzer-Azaroff, E. (1980). A simultaneous treatment comparison of three expressive language training programs with a mute autistic child. *Journal of Autism and Developmental Disorders, 10,* 21–37.

Blackstone, S. W., & Painter, M. J. (1985). Speech problems in multihandicapped children. In J. K. Darby (Ed.), *Speech and language evaluation in neurology: Childhood disorders* (pp. 219–242). New York: Grune & Stratton.

Bliss, C. (1965). *Semantography.* Sydney, Australia: Semantography Publications.

Blockenberger, S., Armstrong, R. W., O'Connor, A., & Freeman, R. (!993). Children's attitudes toward a nonspeaking child using various augmentative and alternative communication techniques. *Augmentative and Alternative Communication, 9,* 243–250.

Bryen, D. N., Goldman, A. S., & Quinlisk–Gill, S. (1988). Sign language with severe/profound mental retardation: How effective is it? *Education and Training in Mental Retardation, 23,* 129–137.

Bryen, D. N., & Joyce, D. G. (1985). Sign language and the severely handicapped. *Journal of Special Education, 20,* 183–194.

Calculator, S. N. (1988). Promoting the acquisition and generalization of conversational skills by individuals with severe disabilities.

Augmentative and Alternative Communication, 4, 94–103.

Calculator, S. N., & Dollaghan, C. (1982). The use of communication boards in a residential setting. *Journal of Speech and Hearing Disorders,* 14, 281–287.

Calculator, S. N., & Jorgensen, C. M. (1991). Integrating AAC instruction into regular education settings: Expounding on best practices. *Augmentative and Alternative Communication,* 7, 204–212.

Carlson, F. (1984). *Picsyms categorical dictionary.* Lawrence, KS: Baggeboda Press.

Carrier, J. (1974). Non-speech noun usage training with severely and profoundly retarded children. *Journal of Speech and Hearing Research,* 17, 510–512.

Carrier, J., & Peak, T. (1975). *Non-slip: Non-speech language initiation program.* Lawrence, KS: H & H Enterprises.

Clark, C. R. (1981). Learning words using traditional orthography and the symbols of Rebus, Bliss, and Carrier. *Journal of Speech and Hearing Disorders,* 46, 191–196.

Clark, C. R., Davies, C. D., & Woodcock, R. W. (1974). *Standard Rebus glossary.* Circle Pines, MN: American Guidance Service.

Crabtree, M., Mirenda, P., & Beukelman, D. R. (1990). Age and gender preferences for synthetic and natural speech. *Augmentative and Alternative Communication,* 6, 256–261.

Creagan, A. (1982). *Sigsymbol dictionary.* Hatfield, Hertsford, England: A. Creagan.

Dattilo, J., & Camarata, S. (1991). Facilitating conversation through self-initiated augmentative communication treatment. *Journal of Applied Behavior Analysis,* 24, 369–378.

Doherty, J. E. (1985). The effects of sign characteristics on sign acquisition and retention: An integrative review of the literature. *Augmentative and Alternative Communication,* 1, 108–121.

Doss, L. S., & Reichle, J. (1989). Establishing communicative alternatives to the emission of socially motivated excess behavior: A review. *Journal of the Association for Persons with Severe Handicaps,* 14, 101–112.

Durand, V. M. (1993). Functional communication training using assistive devices: Effects on challenging behavior and affect. *Augmentative and Alternative Communication,* 9, 168–176.

Guralnick, M. J. (1986). The peer relations of young handicapped and nonhandicapped children. In P. S. Strain, M. J. Guralnick, & H. M. Walker (Eds.), *Children's social behavior.* New York: Academic Press.

Hunt, P., Alwell, M., & Goetz, L. (1991). Interacting with peers through conversation turntaking with a communication book adaptation. *Augmentative and Alternative Communication,* 7, 117–126.

Hurlbut, B. I., Iwata, B. A., & Green, J. D. (1982). Nonvocal language acquisition in adolescents with severe physical disabilities: Blissymbol versus iconic stimulus formats. *Journal of Applied Behavior Analysis,* 15, 241–258.

Johnson, J. (1986). *Self-Talk: Communication boards for children and adults.* Tucson, AZ: Communication Skill Builders.

Johnson, R. (1981). *The picture communication symbols.* Salana Beach, CA: Mayer-Johnson.

Keogh, W. J., & Reichle, J. (1985). Communication intervention for the "difficult-to-teach" severely handicapped. In S. F. Warren & A. K. Rogers-Warren (Eds.), *Teaching functional language* (pp. 157–196). Austin, TX: Pro-Ed.

Kiernan, C. (1983). The use of nonvocal communication techniques with autistic individuals. *Journal of Child Psychology and Psychiatry,* 24, 339–375.

Light, J. (1988). Interaction involving individuals using augmentative and alternative communication systems: State of the art and future directions. *Augmentative and Alternative Communication,* 4, 66–82.

Light, J., Collier, B., & Parnes, P. (1985). Communication interaction between young nonspeaking physically disabled children and their primary caregivers: Part I: Discourse patterns. *Augmentative and Alternative Communication,* 1, 74–83.

Locke, P. A., & Mirenda, P. (1992). Roles and responsibilities of special education teachers serving on teams delivering AAC services. *Augmentative and Alternative Communication,* 8, 200–210.

Mayor-Johnson Co. (1986). *The picture communication symbols, books 1 and 2.* Solana Beach, CA: Mayer-Johnson.

McCormick, L., & Shane, H. (1990). Communication system options for students who are nonspeaking. In L. McCormick & R. Schiefelbusch (Eds.), *Early language intervention: An introduction* (pp. 427–472). Columbus, OH: Merrill.

McGregor, G., Young, J., Gerak, J., Thomas, B., & Vogelsberg, R. T. (1992). Increasing functional use of an assistive communication device by a student with severe disabilities. *Augmentative and Alternative Communication, 8,* 243–250.

Mirenda, P., & Beukelman, D. R. (1990). A comparison of intelligibility among natural speech and seven speech synthesizers with listeners from three age groups. *Augmentative and Alternative Communication, 6,* 61–68.

Mirenda, P., & Iacono, T. (1990). Communication options for persons with severe and profound disabilities: State of the art and future directions. *Journal of the Association for the Severely Handicapped, 15,* 3–21.

Mirenda, P., & Locke, P. A. (1989). A comparison of symbol transparency in nonspeaking persons with intellectual disabilities. *Journal of Speech and Hearing Disorders, 54,* 131–140.

Mirenda, P., & Mathy-Laikko, P. (1989). Augmentative and alternative communication applications for persons with severe congenital communication disorders: An introduction. *Augmentative and Alternative Communication, 7,* 3–21.

Musselwhite, C. R., & Ruscello, D. M. (1984). Transparency of three communication symbol systems. *Journal of Speech and Hearing Research, 27,* 436–443.

Mustonen, T., Locke, P., Reichle, J., Solbrack, M., & Lindgren, A. (1991). An overview of augmentative and alternative communication systems. In J. Reichle, J. York, & J. Sigafoos (Eds.), *Implementing augmentative and alternative communication: Strategies for learners with severe disabilities* (pp. 1–37). Baltimore: Paul H. Brooks.

Reichle, J. (1983). A survey of professional serving persons with severe handicaps. Unpublished manuscript, University of Minnesota, Minneapolis.

Reichle, J. (1991). Developing communicative exchanges. In J. Reichle, J. York, and J. Sigafoos (Eds.), *Implementing augmentative and alternative communication: Strategies for learners with severe disabilities* (pp. 133–156). Baltimore: Paul H. Brooks.

Reichle, J., Mirenda,. P., Locke, P., Piche, L., & Johnston, S. (1992). Beginning augmentative communication systems. In S. F. Warren and J. Reichle (Eds.), *Causes and effects in communication and language intervention* (pp. 131–156). Baltimore: Paul H. Brooks.

Reichle, J., & Yoder, D. E. (1985). Communication board use in severely handicapped learners. *Language, Speech, and Hearing Services in Schools, 16,* 146–167.

Romski, M. A., & Sevcik, R. A. (1988). Augmentative and alternative communication: Considerations for individuals with severe disabilities. *Augmentative and Alternative Communication, 4,* 83–93.

Romski, M. A., Sevcik, R. A., & Pate, J. L. (1988). Establishment of symbolic communication in persons with severe retardation. *Journal of Speech and Hearing Disorders, 53,* 94–107.

Romski, M. A., Sevcik, R. A., Pate, J. L., & Rumbaugh, D. M. (1985). Discrimination of lexigrams and traditional orthography by nonspeaking severely mentally retarded persons. *American Journal of Mental Deficiency, 90,* 185–189.

Romski, M. A., Sevcik, R. A., Robinson, B., & Bakeman, R.. (1994). Adult-directed communications of youth with mental retardation using the system for augmenting language. *Journal of Speech and Hearing Research, 37,* 617–628.

Romski, M. A., Sevcik, R. A., & Wilkinson, K. M. (1994). Peer-directed communicative interactions of augmented language learners with mental retardation. *American Journal on Mental Retardation, 98,* 527–538.

Rounsefell, S., Zucker, S. H., & Roberts, T.G. (1993). Effects of listener training on intelligibility of augmentative and alternative speech in the secondary classroom. *Educa-*

tion and Training in Mental Retardation, 28, 296–308.

Rumbaugh, D. M. (1977). *Language learning by a chimpanzee: The Lara project.* New York: Academic Press.

Scherz, J. W., & Beer, M. M. (1995). Factors affecting the intelligibility of synthesized speech. *Augmentative and Alternative Communication, 11,* 74–85.

Sevcik, R. A., & Romski, M. A. (1986). Representational matching skills for persons with severe retardation. *Augmentative and Alternative Communication, 2,* 160–164.

Shane, H. C., & Bashir, A. S. (1980). Election criteria for the adoption of an augmentative communication system: Preliminary considerations. *Journal of Speech and Hearing Disorders, 45,* 408–414.

Sigafoos, J., & York, J. (1991). Using ecological inventories to promote functional communication. In J. Reichle, J. York, and J. Sigafoos (Eds.), *Implementing augmentative and alternative communication: Strategies for learners with severe disabilities* (pp. 61–70). Baltimore: Paul H. Brooks.

Spiegel, B. B., Benjamin, B. J., & Spiegel, S. A. (1993). One method to increase spontaneous use of an assistive communication device: Case study. *Augmentative and Alternative Communication, 9,* 111–117.

Vanderheiden, G. C., & Lloyd, L. L. (1986). Communication systems and their components. In S. W. Blackstone (Ed.), *Augmentative communication: An introduction.* Rockville, MD: American Speech-Language-Hearing Association.

Zangari, C., Lloyd, L. L., & Vicker, B. (1994). Augmentative and alternative communication: An historic perspective. *Augmentative and Alternative Communication, 10,* 27–59.

Chapter 14

Language and Culture

In this chapter we will examine the special problems posed by children who speak differently from others—children with dialect and language differences. These children, in addition to speaking differently, also come from cultures that differ from the prevailing culture in the United States. Although most of these children do not have language disorders, many require help to achieve in school. We will consider the necessity of adjustments to assessment procedures in order to fairly and accurately assess this population, and we will also examine instructional approaches that can be used successfully with these children.

Some children with limited English proficiency (LEP) or dialect differences also have language disabilities. These children pose unique problems for educators. In this chapter, the special needs of this group of children are considered and recommendations for effective instructional practices are provided.

After completing this chapter, you should be able to:

1. Distinguish a *dialect* difference from a *language disorder.*
2. Understand the special instructional needs of bilingual students.
3. Select appropriate assessment procedures for children with language differences.
4. Describe effective programs for LEP children.
5. Understand the special problems of LEP children with disabilities.
6. Develop effective instructional practices for LEP children with disabilities.

_____ **Case Study: Jeanne** _____

Jeanne, a 10-year-old girl from Haiti, has been in the United States for less than a year. She is a student in a middle-class, suburban school district. Jeanne's first spoken language is Haitian Creole French. When she came to school, however, Jeanne was tested by a school psychologist who did not speak Haitian Creole and who determined Jeanne to have mental retardation. She was placed in a class for students with special needs. By January Jeanne's special education teacher realized that Jeanne had been inappropriately placed. She has acquired English quickly. Far from being mentally retarded, it is possible that

Jeanne is, in fact, gifted. She now assists the teacher in helping other students. The teacher has requested a change of placement for Jeanne, but this cannot be done until next year.

_____ **Case Study: Rosemary** _____

Rosemary was born in Mexico and came to California at age 2. She entered school for the first time at age 7½ and was placed in a multigrade classroom in which English was the primary instruction language. Her teacher began to notice that Rosemary had learning difficulties and referred her for help in the special education resource room, but Rosemary continued to make poor progress. A speech evaluation that included testing in Spanish indicated that Rosemary had a 4-year language delay and that her vocabulary was more developed in English than in Spanish. Rosemary was then placed in a special bilingual class for students with communication disabilities (adapted from Ruiz, 1989).

A new wave of immigration from Latin America and from Asia, coupled with high birth rates for minority groups, has changed the population of the United States to the point that before the end of the next century, the majority white population will become the minority. This has already happened in some parts of the country. According to Cole (1989), in California, in 25 cities and in many counties, minorities already total more than 50 percent of the population.

These immigrant groups from Mexico, Puerto Rico, and Southeast Asia bring with them cultural norms and languages that differ from those of the mainstream society. In addition, the culture and language of urban African Americans is different from that of the white middle class. How our society deals with these differences will, to a great extent, determine the future of the United States in the twenty-first century.

While changes in demographic patterns have an impact throughout society, they disproportionately affect schools. Younger people and people with families are more likely to emigrate to a new country, and higher birth rates for minority groups mean more children in the schools. So, in many parts of the United States, the schools have become the testing ground for our new society.

Cultural Diversity

As a nation of immigrants, the United States has been built on cultural diversity. Yet, there has always been a tension between the newer arrivals and those who were already here. Throughout most of this century, it was expected that immigrants would assimilate into the mainstream culture. In other words, they would give up their distinctive dress, food, and—most important—their language to become a part of "American" society. As a result, the myth of the "melting pot" developed. Many scholars now recognize that the United States is less a melting pot than a "tossed salad" of many different cultures living together (Emihovich, 1988; First, 1988). Terms such as *multicultural* and *cultural pluralism* have been coined to describe a society within which several subcultures exist. As Adler (1993) notes, these has been an ongoing debate between those who advocate assimilation of immigrant groups and those who urge the preservation of cultural diversity.

Whatever the outcome of the cultural diversity debate, educators have to deal with the reality of schoolchildren who hold varying cultural norms and speak many different languages. While this diversity can enrich our schools as well as our communities, it can also bring new problems. For example, a school district in New Jersey has struggled for years with how to celebrate holidays. Should it permit decorations for Christmas and Hanukkah? If so, what should it do about the Muslim, Hindu, and Buddhist children who have their own holidays? In this particular community (a midsized suburb) it is estimated that there are over a hundred languages spoken.

Language poses one of the biggest dilemmas for educators. We may acknowledge and accept the desire of persons from different cultural groups to maintain their cultural heritage. But what about their language? After all, the instruction language in U.S. schools is English. If children are to be successful in school, as well as in the larger community, won't they need to have good English-language skills? But what, then, do we do about their native language? Should we allow, or even encourage, students to use their first language? And what about children who speak English but in a different way? Should they be taught the "right" way to talk?

This is no mere theoretical issue. Some have responded to the increasing cultural and linguistic diversity in our society by calling for a declaration that English shall be the only language spoken in the United States. A number of states have adopted laws that make English the official language of the state; others are considering similar action. An organization called U.S. English has been lobbying Congress for an amendment to the Constitution to make English the official language of the United States. These developments indicate just how important language is to people and how strongly they feel about preserving their language.

These are a few of the problems posed by children from different cultural and language backgrounds. In addition, there is the issue of language disability. It is important to be able to distinguish children who talk *differently* from children with a language *disorder*. Yet, because of deficiencies in assessment materials and procedures, this is often difficult to do. As a result, some children are inappropriately referred to special education while others, who could use additional help, do not receive appropriate services (Gersten & Woodward, 1994).

Dialect Differences

A dialect is a variant of a particular language. Warren and McCloskey (1993) have defined *dialects* as "systematic subvariants of a particular language that are spoken by a sizable group" (p. 207). Dialects share most of the features of the main language but differ in pronunciation, vocabulary, and/or stylistic features. For example, in some parts of Boston, words that end with an *uh* sound, as *pizza*, are pronounced *er* (as in *pizzer*). President Kennedy, a Boston native, was faced with the challenge of the missile crisis in "Cuber." In some parts of the United States the words *Mary, merry,* and *marry* are each pronounced the same. In other regions they are differentiated from each other. In England, one works in a la-*bor*-a-tree, while in most regions of the United States, this word is pronounced *lab*-ra-tory. If you order a large sandwich on a roll, you get a *hoagie* in Philadelphia, a *torpedo* in some parts of the New York area, and a *grinder* in New England. People from the East and West coasts of the United States often feel that people from the South speak very slowly.

All of these are examples of regional dialect variations. Often these variations are minor; they may create brief moments of embarrassment or humor. However, some regional dialect differences are so great that it may be difficult for speakers and listeners to communicate easily. Some speakers from the Appalachian Mountains and those from isolated communities around the Chesapeake Bay area may use dialects that are very difficult to follow.

What we must keep in mind is that there is nothing "wrong" with these regional dialect differences. There is no one "right" way to talk, because the "right" way is different in different regions of the country. On the other hand, there is a widely held belief that there is (or should be) a standard dialect. A *standard dialect* is the one spoken by highly educated people in formal situations. Although this may be the standard used for broadcasting and in classrooms, there is nothing inherently superior about this dialect (Lindfors, 1987). It is simply a standard that certain elements of the society have set.

Social Dialects

In addition to regional dialects, there are social dialects. Social dialects are ways of speaking that are associated with a particular social group. The haughty, sometimes mumbled speech of the "aristocrat" and the dropped endings (*I'm goin'*) often heard in the speech of working-class persons are both examples of social dialects. Some social dialects carry with them the stigma of discrimination and the widespread belief that some are inferior versions of English. Nowhere is this more true than in the case of Black English.

Black English is a dialect of English that is associated with African American speakers. However, Black English is not used by all African Americans. In actuality, there is a great deal of variation in language use within the African American community (Terrell & Terrell, 1993). Some scholars (e.g., Labov, 1972) have attempted to draw a distinction between the general term *Black English* and the distinctive language used largely by inner-city, low-socioeconomic-status, young African Americans. Labov called the latter dialect *Black English Vernacular (BEV)*.

Black English Vernacular is the dialect that most people think of when they refer to Black English. BEV is characterized by differences in phonology, syntax, and pragmatics, as well as in aspects of conversational discourse (Cole & Taylor, 1990). Some of the unique features of BEV include: deletion or substitution of medial and final consonant sounds (*brother = brovah; walked = walk*), deletion of auxiliary verb (*The boy is running = The boy running*), deletion of the possessive

TABLE 14.1   Examples of Grammatical Features of Black English Vernacular

Grammatical Feature	Example
Deletion of past tense ending	cashed = cash
Variation in past tense of irregular verbs	saw = seen
	did = done
Use of double negatives	He didn't do nothing.
Use of *be* as a main verb	I be here in the evening.
Deletion of final *s* in third-person singular present tense	He walk.

Source: Adapted from S. L. Terrell and F. Terrell. (1993). African-American Cultures. In D. E. Battle (Ed.), *Communication disorders in multicultural populations* (pp. 3–37). Boston: Andover Medical Publishers.

suffix *(boy's = boy* as in *It is the boy ball)* (Walton, McCardle, Crowe, & Wilson, 1990; Terrell & Terrell, 1993) (see Table 14.1 for additional examples).

Even those African Americans who use Black English Vernacular do not do so at all times. They may use this type of language in some settings, with some people, but not in other situations. This phenomenon in which people switch from one language or one dialect to another is called **code switching.** It means that the individual is aware of environmental conditions that affect the choice of language.

Social dialects such as BEV are often considered inferior by speakers of a more standard form of a language. Not only do social dialects differ linguistically from the standard language, but when used by people of color or by lower socioeconomic groups, they carry the additional stigma of racism and discrimination. The idea that social dialects are inferior forms of a standard language was reinforced by research on the language of lower socioeconomic groups that was conducted during the 1950s, 1960s, and 1970s. One of the most prominent names associated with this research is that of Basil Bernstein. Bernstein's observation of language usage by working-class persons in England led him to conclude that their use of what he called *restricted* language resulted in more limited opportunities for language development. Restricted language is characterized by a narrower range of syntactic usage, greater reliance on nonverbal means of expression, and the use of slang (Bernstein, 1970).

Research conducted by Bernstein and others was applied to inner-city children in the United States. The result was the notion of *cultural deprivation*—the idea that, because of their environment, persons from lower socioeconomic strata (SES) are denied the opportunities for learning that are available to persons of higher SES. Labov (1969, 1970), however, demonstrated the fallacy of the deprivation argument. His research showed that children exposed to Black English Vernacular do not develop a deficient verbal system. In fact, these children engage in elaborate conversational interactions—at least under certain conditions. Labov (1970) presented examples that showed how the same African American child hardly talked to a white researcher, talked somewhat more to an African American adult, but engaged in a lengthy conversation with a friend from his neighborhood. Clearly, cultural deprivation is, at least partially, the result of how it is measured.

Today, most scholars agree that there is nothing inherently wrong with social dialects such as Black English. In fact, the American Speech-Language-Hearing Association (ASHA) issued a position statement in 1983 in which it stated that "no dialectal variety of English is a disorder or a pathological form of speech or language" (ASHA Committee on the Racial Status of Minorities, 1983). Despite a near unanimous consensus among researchers and clinicians that social dialects such as BEV are not inferior, concerns about what to do about speakers of these dialects continue to exist. Grossman (1995) notes three reasons for many educators' continued concerns about children who use nonstandard English dialects:

1. Although nonstandard English dialects are not substandard, they interfere with students' academic progress.
2. Competency in oral standard English is necessary for students to learn to write standard English.
3. Standard English is necessary for vocational success and in other areas in which nonstandard dialect speakers are branded as uneducated and ill prepared.

Although Grossman notes that there is little, if any, research that supports these concerns, some educators continue to hold these beliefs. Questions about whether to encourage or discourage students from using their particular dialect are haunted by issues of race and class. Later in this chapter we will examine the different approaches to teaching students with dialect differences.

Bilingualism and Limited English Proficiency

In the Preface to this book you were asked to think about how it feels to be in a situation in which you do not speak the language that others speak. Those of us who have been in such situations may recall feeling uneasy and embarrassed. Some may even have experienced physical discomfort. You may have felt confused, ignored, or ridiculed (whether this was true or not). For an increasing number of children who attend school in the United States, these feelings are a daily occurrence. They are students who speak a language other than English as their first language.

Like children with dialect differences, children who come to school speaking a language other than English as their first language pose significant challenges to teachers and other professionals. These children may be misunderstood as much for their cultural differences as their language differences. Sometimes these children are mislabeled as having disabilities and are inappropriately placed in special education. Often, they fail to achieve in school at anywhere near the rates that would be expected of them (Garcia, 1993). Our challenge as educators is to provide a program that will allow the child who speaks a language other than English to fully develop, both academically and socially.

There is not general agreement about what to call children who speak a language other than English. The terms *limited-English-proficient (LEP)* or *non-English-proficient (NEP)* are frequently used to describe these children in the research literature. But some researchers reject these terms, because they focus on apparent deficiencies (Genesee, 1994), favoring, instead, terms like *ESL (English-as-a-second-language)* students or *language-minority* students. Teachers and speech-language specialists should be aware that any of these terms might be applied to students who speak a language other than English.

Bilingualism refers to the ability to understand and use two languages. Bilingualism is not an all-or-nothing principle, but ranges from minimal ability to complete fluency in more than one language (Baca & Almanza, 1991).

Schiff-Myers (1992) distinguishes between three kinds of childhood bilinguality. One type is *infant* bilinguality. In this case, both languages are spoken to the child beginning in early infancy. When the child develops both languages simultaneously, that child's language competence in each language becomes similar to that of monolingual speakers. Most bilingual children learn to switch back and forth between their languages, depending on who they are talking to and what they are talking about. Schiff-Myers calls the other type of bilinguality *early childhood*. Early childhood bilingual children hear one language in their home but are later exposed to a second language in the larger community and in school. A third type of bilingual child acquires a second language only after beginning school. The first type of bilinguality is sometimes called *simultaneous* while the other two kinds are called *sequential* or *consecutive*.

For teachers and other education professionals, it is important to keep in mind that while generalizations can be made about bilingual students, they are still a heterogeneous group. They come to school with a variety of language and cultural experiences. Some are very familiar with the mainstream culture, while others are largely unfamiliar with any culture other than their native one. Some have good English language skills, while others have limited or nonexistent English language skills.

One of the major questions about bilingualism regards the effect of second-language acquisition on the child. Goodz (1994) notes that it is commonly believed that early exposure to two languages is detrimental to the child, and, therefore, it is assumed that learning two languages causes confusion and interference between the languages. In fact, however, research has found that children learning two languages do so at about the same rate as other children learning one language, although they may progress at different rates in each language (Goodz, 1994). Moreover, there is evidence that bilingual children actually have an advantage in metalinguistic development (Bialystok, 1991), and that they outperform their monolingual peers on tests of cognitive ability (Cummins, 1994). On the other hand, Schiff-Myers (1992) has noted that some children lose skills in their first language as they begin to acquire a second language. This seems to be especially true of children from minority cultures who begin to acquire their second language in school.

Compounding the problems of their differences in proficiency with English language skills and in familiarity with the mainstream culture is the fact that bilingual children and LEP children also differ from each other. Not only do their languages differ—the sounds, the words, and the grammatical rules—but their pragmatic and social rules—and worlds—vary as well. For example, in Asian cultures,

TABLE 14.2   Some Cultural and Conversational Differences

Cultural Group	Cultural Norms	Conversational Characteristics
African Americans	Touching of someone's hair may be seen as offensive. Verbal abuse is not necessarily precursor to violence. Asking personal questions of new acquaintances may be seen as improper.	Children may avoid eye contact with adults. Discourse may be loosely connected. Conversation may be emotionally intense.
Hispanics	Official or business conversations are preceded by lengthy greetings and pleasantries. Mexican-American children seldom ask for help. Students may deny responsibility for mistakes.	Respect is shown through use of formal language. Hissing to gain attention is proper. Avoidance of eye contact may be a sign of respect. Relative distance between speakers is close.
Asians	Touching or hand-holding between members of same sex is acceptable. A slap on the back is insulting.	Straightforward communication is impolite. Talk about sensitive or unacceptable topics is not proper.

Source: Adapted from: H. Grossman. (1995). *Special education in a diverse society.* Boston: Allyn and Bacon. L. Cole. (1989). E pluribus pluribus: Multicultural imperatives for the 1990s and beyond. *ASHA, 31,* 65–70.

children are expected to be seen and not heard. Since they are discouraged from interrupting teachers, Asian students may appear passive and be slow to participate in the classroom (Cheng, 1987). In the Hispanic culture, physical proximity and touching during conversations is not uncommon (Cole, 1989). Some African American children have been taught that making eye contact is disrespectful (Terrell & Terrell, 1993). Table 14.2 gives additional examples of cultural differences in communication style and nonverbal behavior.

Making generalizations about any culture is risky. There are often differences within cultures that are caused by country of origin, exposure to different cultures, and other factors. The important point for teachers is to be aware of the cultural differences that may exist in students from their community.

For educators, gaining an awareness of cultural differences and respect for different cultural values can be an important first step in building a functional classroom environment. In addition to their recognizing the obvious problems for students acquiring a second language, educators must also be concerned about the literacy skills and social skills of LEP students. Children with limited skills in English often do poorly in reading and writing English (Baca & Cervantes, 1989). Given these limitations, their performance is not surprising. Unfortunately, educational programs and instructional methods that try to teach children to read before they have mastered English only make the problem worse. Reyes (1992) has reported that when students with limited English proficiency are given the opportunity to read and write in their first language, their literacy skills improve significantly. Students who are linguistically and culturally different from other students also are at risk for problems in socialization. There are many reasons why this may be so. For example, there are different cultural norms for social interaction. Children from diverse cultures can be expected to have different patterns of eye gaze, speaker distance, and use of facial expressions. Other factors, such as prejudice and language differences themselves, can affect socialization (Damico & Damico, 1993).

Students with Limited English Proficiency and Special Needs

Some students with limited English proficiency have such significant problems in learning and/or socialization that they require special education services. The American Speech-Language-Hearing Association has estimated that approximately 3.5 million children who speak a language other than English have disabilities that have nothing directly to do with their use of a minority language (ASHA Committee on the Racial Status of Minorities, 1985). These children have needs that go beyond those of other LEP children because in addition to their learning or developmental disabilities, they also have language and cultural differences that may make it more difficult for them to learn. Rueda and Chan (1979) called children with disabilities and LEP "triple threat" students because they have three strikes against them before they even start school. Strike one is their behavioral and/or learning disability. Strike two is their limited English proficiency. Strike three is discrimination because of their race and/or social class.

One of the biggest challenges facing educators is appropriate identification of these students. Ironically, these students tend to be both overidentified and underidentified. Several researchers have found that children from language-minority groups are overrepresented in special education classes (Mercer, 1973; Ortiz & Yates, 1983). Use of identification practices that rely largely (or solely) on testing performed in English results in some children from language-minority groups being placed inappropriately into special education classes. At the same time, Gersten and Woodward (1994) claim that some school districts have become so concerned about the possibility of inappropriate placement of language-minority children that they may be allowing some children with real special education needs to "fall through the cracks." Other concerns relate to the ability of special educators, many of whom have received little or no training in working with culturally and linguistically diverse populations, to develop effective instructional programs for special needs students with limited English proficiency.

Appropriate Assessment

Assessment of children from culturally and linguistically diverse backgrounds serves two purposes. The first is to know about the child's skills in English. This will help in determining whether the child needs help in acquiring English. The second purpose is to identify those children who have significant learning and/or socialization problems. We need to know that the difficulties the child is experiencing are the result of a disability and not caused by the language and/or cultural difference itself. This is a difficult task. The goal is to avoid overidentifying children as in need of special education but not to deny services to children who really need them to reach their learning potential. What makes this identification task especially difficult are the inherent difficulties of testing children from diverse language and cultural backgrounds.

Public Law 101-476, the Individuals with Disabilities Education Act (IDEA), contains provisions that spell out the obligations of schools to conduct nonbiased assessments when evaluating children for special educational services. Among these provisions are the following:

- Testing and evaluation materials and procedures used for the purposes of evaluation and placement of handicapped children must be selected and administered so as not to be racially or culturally discriminatory.
- Testing and evaluation materials and procedures must be provided and administered in the language or other mode of communication in which the child is most proficient, unless it is clearly not feasible to do so.
- Tests must be administered to a child with a motor, speech, hearing, visual, or other communication disability, or to a bilingual child, so as to reflect accurately the child's ability in the area tested rather than the child's impaired communication skill or limited English language skill unless those are the factors the test purports to measure.

To summarize, IDEA requires that when students who are culturally or linguistically diverse are assessed for special education, testing must be culturally fair, conducted in the child's own language, and must be designed so that it examines the area tested rather than the child's communication skills in English.

These goals are supported by most educators who are interested in identifying those children from diverse backgrounds who need special education services. Unfortunately, these provisions of IDEA are often not followed (Figueroa, 1989). Among the reasons that testing regulations may not be followed are:

- Disagreement about what constitutes cultural bias in testing.
- A shortage of appropriate assessment materials for students from diverse cultural and linguistic backgrounds.
- A shortage of personnel trained in the assessment of children from diverse cultural and linguistic backgrounds.

Let's look at each of these problems in turn. First, although many educators are concerned about the possibility of bias in testing, the bias has often been difficult to prove. Court decisions have only added to the confusion. Throughout the 1970s, most court decisions supported the notion that there was bias inherent in standardized testing. But in *PASE* v. *Hannon* (1980) the court ruled that although black children were disproportionately represented in special education classes in the Chicago school system, there was little evidence that the tests used to determine placement were biased. The results of court decisions have caused continued disagreement about what constitutes fairness in testing. Even if the courts cannot agree on what constitutes bias in testing, many educators continue to have concerns about fairness in assessment procedures.

A second reason that the listed mandates of IDEA may not be carried out is that appropriate tests may not be available. For example, after an extensive review of the research literature, Figueroa (1989) concluded that psychological testing for children with varying levels of language proficiency and differing home backgrounds was inadequate. He criticized technical aspects of the tests, the knowledge base used for constructing psychological tests, and regulations regarding testing. Baca and Almanaza (1991) expressed similar concerns about educational testing. They noted that there is widespread concern about the content of test items, lack of cultural sensitivity by testers, and lack of test-taking strategies for students from diverse cultural and language backgrounds.

One solution to the problem of test fairness is to use a version of the test in the child's native language. Yet, even this is not always a totally satisfactory solution. Payan (1989) has pointed out that even if such tests are available, the test items may still be inappropriate for children from diverse cultural backgrounds. In addition, the tests are often translated into a standard dialect that may not be the one used by the child.

One of the main reasons that children from diverse language and cultural backgrounds are tested is to determine their skills in English. But serious concerns have been raised about the practice of using what are called *discrete-point* tests. John Carroll (1961) defined discrete-point tests as those that focus attention on one point of grammar at a time, such as phonology or syntax or vocabulary. While discrete-point tests certainly have their place in a comprehensive assessment of language, over-reliance on such tests can be a problem. The problem is especially serious when children with limited English proficiency are tested, because they tend to make more errors in the use of English rules (Damico, Oller, & Storey, 1983). Damico et al. (1983) explain that despite making errors on language tests, many children with limited English proficiency can be effective communicators. The researchers found that the examination of pragmatic language elements from language samples was a better measure of the language abilities of Spanish/English bilingual children than were standardized tests of language.

Cole and Taylor (1990) noted that researchers have often raised concerns about speech and language testing of African American children, claiming that few standardized tests of language contain items that are truly representative of the variety of dialects in use within the United States. When Cole and Taylor used three widely accepted tests of articulation in testing African American children, they found that the results varied considerably, depending on what norms were used. They suggest, then, that clinicians would get more reliable results by using language samples and other techniques that measure the *use* of language skills in communication rather than by using tests of specific language skills.

A third obstacle to the implementation of the IDEA testing requirements is a shortage of trained personnel. There are two problems related to personnel. One

TABLE 14.3   Principles for the Development of Appropriate Assessment of Children with Language Differences

1. Standardize existing tests on nonmainstream English speakers.
2. Include a small percentage of minorities in the standardization sample when developing a test.
3. Modify or revise existing tests in ways that will make them appropriate for nonmainstream speakers.
4. Utilize a language sample when assessing the language of nonmainstream speakers.
5. Use criterion-referenced measures when assessing the language of nonmainstream speakers.
6. Refrain from using all standardized tests that have not been corrected for test bias when assessing the language of nonmainstream speakers.
7. Develop a new test which can provide a more appropriate assessment of the language of nonmainstream English speakers.

Source: Adapted from F. B. Vaughn-Cooke. (1983). Improving language assessment in minority children. *ASHA, 25,* 29–33.

involves language abilities. It is often not possible to find a qualified test administrator who speaks a particular child's native language. Frequently, schools have to use a test administrator who is only familiar with standard English. The second problem involves possible bias. As Long (1994) pointed out, testers may misinterpret the child's limited responses as signs of uncooperative or resistant behavior when, in fact, the child may simply misunderstand or have difficulty completely expressing their thoughts in English. Testers may also hold inaccurate expectations for children from particular cultural and language backgrounds and may interpret the test results to confirm those expectations.

In response to the serious problem of test adequacy for children from diverse cultural and language backgrounds, Fay Boyd Vaughn-Cooke (1983) has suggested seven principles that should be used in developing more appropriate testing (see Table 14.3).

Recommendations for Assessment

Considering all of the potential problems in testing children from diverse cultural and language backgrounds, what can educators do to try to fairly and accurately assess these children? One suggestion is to carefully consider the abilities and background knowledge of the child being tested. Baca and Almanza (1991) recommend consideration of the following factors:

- **Experiential background:** Including school attendance history, quality of prior instruction, family history, and medical history.
- **Culture:** Including family goals and expectations, religion, extent to which child has become acculturated, and the child's ability to function in more than one culture.

- **Language proficiency:** Including identification of the child's dominant and preferred language, the child's extent of exposure to each language, and the child's level of proficiency in both languages.
- **Learning style:** Identification of the child's preferred learning styles and the extent to which these require instructional accommodations.
- **Motivational influences:** Including the child's self-concept and the family's attitude toward education.

With these factors in mind, educators can proceed to actually conducting the assessment. Payan (1989) has suggested a seven-step process for the assessment of LEP students. Although her recommendations were designed specifically for the identification of children with special needs, the steps are appropriate for any child with limited or different English.

Step 1 is the **referral.** Payan (1989) provides a rather lengthy form that includes information about who referred the student for assessment, a description of the student's present program, and the student's language and communication abilities. This information is useful for planning the assessment, as well as for discouraging inappropriate referrals.

Step 2 is the **parent interview.** This is an especially important step for children who speak a language other than English at home. In order to completely understand the child's language and cultural background, the interviewer must ascertain what languages are spoken at home, who speaks them, and any concerns the parents may have about their child's language development. A parent interview is also an opportunity to find out about the cultural norms and cultural background of the family.

Step 3 is an assessment of **language proficiency.** Several standardized tests have been developed for the purpose of assessing the language skills of children with limited English (see Table 14.4). However, most of these tests have been developed for use with Spanish-speaking persons.

Criterion-referenced tests and informal procedures such as language samples are alternative means for assessing language proficiency. Other alternatives include dictation tasks in which the examiner says words or phrases from normal discourse and the student writes down the word or phrase; cloze procedure in which the child fills in (either orally or in written form) missing words in a passage; and an oral interview to assess the child's language skills (Oller, 1988).

Step 4 is determining the **language for assessment.** The examiner should consider information from the parent interview and from assessment of the child's language in deciding in which language the assessment should be conducted.

Step 5 is an in-depth analysis of the child's **native language abilities,** including assessment of receptive and expressive skills in all areas of language.

Step 6 is a similar assessment of **English language skills.**

Finally, Payan (1989) recommends that in step 7, the clinician **summarizes the results and makes recommendations.**

Assessment of students with diverse cultural and language backgrounds is necessary to determine the appropriate instructional program for each individual child. Assessment can also be used to determine proficiency in the first language

TABLE 14.4   Standardized Tests of Language Proficiency

Name (Authors)	Ages or Grades	Language(s)	Oral Language Skills Assessed
Basic Inventory of Natural Language (Herbert, 1977, 1979, 1983)	Gr. K to 12	Spanish and 31 other languages	A language sample is scored for fluency, complexity, and average sentence length
Ber-Sil Elementary and Secondary Spanish Tests (Beringer, 1987, 19840	Ages 5 to 12 and 13 to 17	Spanish, Tagalog, Ilokano; Elementary also available in Cantonese, Mandarin, Korean, Persian	Receptive vocabulary
Bilingual Syntax Measure I and II (Burt, Dulay, & Hernándex-Chávez, 1978)	Gr. pre-K to 12	Spanish, English	Expressive syntax
Dos Amigos Verbal Language Scales (Critchlow, 1973)	Ages 5 to 13	Spanish, English	Expressive vocabulary
Language Assessment Scales-Oral (Duncan & DeAvila, 1990)	Gr. 1 to 12	Spanish, English	Phonemic, lexical, syntactical, and pragmatic aspects of language
Prueba de Desarrollo Inicial de Lenguaje (Hresko, Reid, & Hammill, 1982)	Ages 3 to 7	Spanish	Receptive and expressive syntax and semantics
Woodcock-Muños Language Survey, English and Spanish Forms (Woodcock Muños-Sandoval, 1993)	Ages 4 to 90	Spanish, English	Receptive and expressive semantics

Source: From *Assessing Special Students,* 4th ed., by McLoughlin, © 1994. Reprinted by permission of Prentice-Hall, Inc., Upper Saddle River, NJ.

and in English. In addition, the results can be used to decide if the child requires special education services. As we have seen, there are special challenges in assessing children with limited English proficiency or whose language differs from the prevailing standard. It is important that teachers and speech-language specialists be aware of these challenges and of the procedures found effective for assessing such children.

Instructional Programs

In the previous section, we noted that children with language and cultural differences are a diverse group. They come to school with different degrees of skill in their first language and in English; they differ in their exposure to the mainstream culture; and they differ in their learning and social skills. Therefore, there is no one program that will suit everybody. The task for educators is to find the most effective program for each individual.

Although each individual's program of study may differ, there are certain broad goals that are appropriate for all learners with language and/or dialect differences. One goal is to develop *competence* in English. But what is competence? Cummins (1980; 1984) describes two types of language skills: basic interpersonal communicative skills (BICS) and cognitive/academic language proficiency (CALP). Cummins cautions that children may develop BICS fairly quickly (1–2 years) but that CALP takes much longer to develop (5–7 years). Thus, when we say that a child is competent in English, we should clarify whether we mean that the child is able to engage in interpersonal interaction or the more advanced skill of applying English language skills to academic tasks. There is a danger that some children will be transferred out of programs that help them develop their English skills because they are able to demonstrate basic communication skills. But many of these children will not be prepared to use their language for the complex learning tasks posed in the classroom. Handscombe (1994) has suggested that in addition to the development of skills in English, programs for children with language and/or cultural differences should also help students enhance their academic achievement and social integration.

Cummins (1994) reminds us that a number of factors are working against the development of effective programs for children who speak a language (or a dialect) other than standard English. These include government policies that ignore the research on second language learning, curriculum that is skewed toward white, middle-class values and experiences, and a shortage of professionals who share the language and/or cultural background of many of the students in today's schools. Despite these obstacles, effective programs have been developed. In subsequent sections of this chapter we will examine programs for children with limited English proficiency, students with dialect differences, and students with special needs and language differences.

Instruction for Children with Limited English Proficiency

Students who come to school with competence in both their native language and English (bilingual) will usually not need any type of special program. But many children whose first language is other than English have limited skills in English, or limited English proficiency (LEP), and do need some type of instruction that helps them acquire the English skills they need for success in school. Gersten and Woodward (1994) described two issues that underlie decisions about what types of programs LEP children should have. The first issue involves how quickly students should be placed in classrooms where English is the only means of communication. The second is whether to use the child's native language merely as a bridge to help the child acquire English or whether the goal is to help the child become academically competent in both languages.

Instructional programs for LEP children range from those that require children to use English right from the beginning to those that emphasize the use of the child's native language. According to Garcia (1993) some of the prevailing program models include:

- **Submersion:** Language-minority children are placed in regular classrooms where English is the only language spoken. The children with limited English proficiency receive no special help with English.
- **English as a second language (ESL):** Students with limited English proficiency spend most of their day in a submersion classroom but do receive some help with English. Most instruction takes place in English. The teacher may or may not speak the child's native language.
- **Traditional bilingual education:** Academic instruction is conducted in the students' native language until they have learned enough English to succeed in English-only classrooms. Children learn to read first in their native language and then in English. There are two types of bilingual education models: *early exit,* which emphasizes transition to English, and *late exit,* which places more emphasis on the development of literacy in the child's first language.
- **Structured English immersion strategy (SEIS):** Developed in Canada, SEIS programs teach students through use of English, with the instruction language carefully controlled to match the student's ability to comprehend. Students may use their first language to talk to each other and to the teacher (who is competent in both English and the students' native language).

Which type of program is most successful? Unfortunately, there is no simple answer to this question. Research on the outcomes of bilingual education programs is limited by factors such as individual differences between students and variations in the ways that school districts choose to implement the basic models described above. Despite these limitations, there are some trends that have emerged.

Reviews of research on the outcomes of bilingual education programs—programs that combined instruction in a first language with instruction in a second language—have generally found that such programs can work (Baca & Cervantes, 1989; Gersten & Woodward, 1994). Most of the research has found that students in bilingual education programs perform as well as or better than their monolingual peers in assessments of academic, cognitive, and social functioning. This research has been conducted throughout the world, with speakers of a wide variety of languages.

One relatively recent study, conducted for the United States Department of Education, compared the effectiveness of three types of bilingual education programs: structured immersion, early exit and late exit (Ramirez, Yuen, & Ramey, 1991). The academic progress of some 500 students from language-minority groups was followed from kindergarten through fourth grade. Results of this comprehensive study indicated that immersion programs gave young children tested in English an initial advantage. However, by third grade this advantage had disappeared. By the end of the study, children in the three programs achieved comparable scores in academic and language skills.

If, in fact, there is little difference in long-term outcomes between programs that emphasize English compared to programs that emphasize the child's native language, which program is better? Cummins (1989) suggests that programs that emphasize the child's first language are preferable, arguing that "in programs in which minority students' first-language (L1) skills are strongly reinforced, their school success appears to reflect both the more solid cognitive and academic foundation developed through intensive L1 instruction and also the reinforcement of their cultural identity" (p. 113). As Cummins and others have reminded us, there is more that goes into bilingual education than language instruction. Since many speakers of minority languages face discrimination combined with language differences, bilingual education programs also serve to help such children develop a stronger cultural identity and self-concept.

Despite strong evidence for the effectiveness of bilingual education programs that incorporate the child's minority language into instruction, many school districts choose other kinds of programs for these children. The reasons for such decisions often have more to do with politics than with educational outcomes. Teachers and speech-language specialists should advocate for decisions based on the individual child's needs and program effectiveness rather than on factors such as prejudice, fear, and cost.

An important component of most instructional programs for children with a first language other than English is the development of literacy skills (reading, writing, and spoken language). Hudelson (1994) has suggested several strategies for literacy development for second-language learners (see Table 14.5).

Hudelson's suggestions are based on a whole-language theory of instruction. While this approach can work for LEP students (Gersten & Woodward, 1994), Reyes (1992) cautions that this approach should be used with care. She suggests that literature-based programs must include literature from the cultural traditions of *all* of the students in the class. Furthermore, teachers should not be afraid to correct syntax and spelling when necessary. Reyes observed that modeling was not always adequate to teach English grammar rules to LEP students. In addition, Reyes suggests that second language learners be given the opportunity to use their native language for both academic and nonacademic purposes.

Gersten and Jimenez (1994) described the art of teaching LEP students as a "balancing act." The teacher must challenge the students but not frustrate them and help those who need it but also include all students in instruction. The researchers suggested that the following constructs be included in instructional programs for language-minority students:

1. **Challenge:** Including implicit challenges (such as the use of higher-order questions) and explicit challenges (high but reasonable expectations).
2. **Involvement:** All learners should be actively involved in instruction.
3. **Success:** Activities and tasks provided should be within students' abilities. Students should know when they are successful.

TABLE 14.5 Strategies for Literacy Development of Second-Language Learners

- **Create a literate classroom environment:** The classroom should be a language-rich environment. Charts for attendance, favorite songs, and academic tasks; a classroom library; a writing center; and displays of children's written work can be used to enhance the classroom environment.
- **Encourage collaborative learning:** A collaborative learning environment has been found to be an important factor in the success of classrooms for linguistically diverse learners (Reyes & Laliberty, 1992). Children should be encouraged to work together, to rely on each other, and to support each other.
- **Utilize oral and written personal narratives:** Although second-language learners may take longer to feel comfortable producing personal narratives, this can be an effective procedure. Reyes (1992) notes that many second language learners will need help with some of the mechanics of writing in order to be successful.
- **Utilize dialogic writing:** Dialogue journals enable students and teachers to communicate with each other in a nonjudgmental way. Second language learners get the opportunity to see examples of standard written English.
- **Utilize predictable books:** Such books reinforce the idea that reading is a process of prediction. Students can be asked to predict what is likely to happen and to fill in missing words.
- **Include opportunities for self-selected reading:** Students need opportunities to select and read books of their own choice.
- **Include literacy development as a part of content study:** Content area study provides many opportunities for reading, researching, and writing. When students with limited English proficiency are grouped in classrooms with native English speakers, heterogeneous grouping can be used to give the LEP students an opportunity to be successful.

Source: Adapted from S. Hudelson. (1994). Literacy development of second language children. In F. Genessee (Ed.), *Educating second language children* (pp. 129–158). New York: Cambridge University Press.

4. **Scaffolding/cognitive strategies:** The teacher uses instructional methods such as story maps, visual organizers, and think alouds to assist students in developing cognitive strategies for learning.
5. **Mediation/feedback:** Feedback should be frequent and understandable to the student.
6. **Collaborative/cooperative learning.**
7. **Techniques for second-language acquisition/sheltered English:** Including the incorporation of the students' primary language into instruction and the use of extended discourse.
8. **Respect for cultural diversity:** Teachers should be knowledgeable about the culture of their students and respectful toward cultural differences.

Instruction for Students with Dialect Differences

The question of how and what to teach children with dialect differences continues to be a very sensitive one. The issue clearly involves more than what is best in terms of language development or educational practice. It is closely related to our society's struggles with the issues of race, poverty, and equity.

In 1979, a United States district court judge ruled in favor of a group of African American children who had brought suit against the Ann Arbor, Michigan, school district. The suit claimed that these children were being denied an equal education because their school did not take into account their use of Black English. The judge noted that there was evidence that teachers had unconsciously indicated to the children that Black English is wrong. As a result, the judge argued, the children had been made to feel inferior and became disenchanted with school. The court ruled that teachers had to attend in-service education programs about nonstandard dialects and that a child's dialect had to be considered when the child was being taught to read and write (*Martin Luther King Jr. Elementary School* v. *Ann Arbor School District Board*, 1978).

This case caused many educators to rethink their attitudes toward dialect differences. In addition, it prompted debate (that continues even today) about the relationship between dialect differences and the development of literacy skills. Grossman (1995) described the debate as between those who argue for **bidialectalism** and those who argue for the **appreciation** of dialect differences.

Those who argue for a bidialectical approach to instruction for children who speak nonstandard dialects of English (such as Black English Vernacular [BEV]) contend that although there is nothing wrong with such dialects, they interfere with the child's ability to achieve success in the mainstream society. As Sol Adler, one of the advocates for a bidialectical approach, put it, "So long as linguistic and cultural prejudices dominate the thinking of these establishment members of our society, nonstandard speakers will continue to need to learn the language of the mainstream culture if they wish to have an equal opportunity to enter into the mainstream" (1993, p. 21). Adler argues that bidialectal programs must be mandatory, not voluntary, since most children will not pick up standard English without formal instruction.

Proponents of bidialectal programs generally give three reasons for the need for such programs (Adler, 1993):

1. **Educational reasons:** They cite evidence that the reading skills of speakers of BEV lag behind those of other children, both white and black. Furthermore, since "standard" English is the language of instruction in classrooms, speakers of BEV and other nonstandard dialects are at a disadvantage.

2. **Employment reasons:** They cite evidence that use of standard English is an important factor in hiring decisions. They argue that it is unfair to speakers of nonstandard dialects *not* to teach them the language skills they will need for employment.

3. **Ethical and pragmatic reasons:** Ethically, it is wrong to deny children the use of their dialect. But, it is equally wrong to deny them the opportunity to learn standard English. The pragmatic argument is that, like it or not, standard English is required for success in the United States and children must be given the opportunity to acquire the standard dialect.

The objectives of a bidialectal program are to create in students an awareness of the need to adjust language for different purposes, to help them understand the importance of communication skills, and to provide them with opportunities to develop and practice standard English while continuing to use their dialect (Harris-Wright, 1987). Many bidialectal programs use an instructional technique called *contrastive analysis,* in which children are given examples of nonstandard and standard English forms for communicating and are taught to analyze and recognize the differences between the two dialects.

The appreciation approach to dialect differences urges respect for dialect differences and the development of language skills in whatever dialect the child speaks. Grossman (1995) has summarized the arguments in support of the appreciation position:

1. Efforts to teach students to speak standard English do not work.
2. Dialect speakers who are required to speak standard English become less fluent and have difficulty expressing themselves.
3. Teaching students standard English before they are completely fluent in their original dialects stunts their language development.
4. It is not possible to encourage students to learn a second dialect without also communicating that their way of speaking is less desirable.
5. Acceptance and appreciation of nonstandard dialects by schools and teachers improves students' self-esteem.
6. Teaching standard English to nonstandard-dialect speakers is a form of political and cultural subjugation.

While the research base in support of many of these arguments is limited, the arguments do represent points of view that should be considered. At one time in the late 1960s and 1970s, some linguists were urging the development of Black English texts so that children who used this dialect would be less disadvantaged as they began to read (e.g., Baratz, 1969). Today, however, most educators recognize the need for all children to develop reading and writing skills in standard English.

Clearly the debate about what to do about children who speak nonstandard dialects of English, especially BEV, is about more than education. Issues of race and class inject highly emotional feelings into the debate. While most can agree that nonstandard dialects are not inferior forms of English and that speakers of such dialects deserve respect, they differ on the extent to which standard English should be taught. In making decisions about what kind of program to adopt, educators should consider both the research base on nonstandard dialects and literacy, as well as the desires of parents, students, and the community as a whole.

Instruction for Students with Language Disorders and Language Differences

An earlier discussion in this chapter described a group of LEP children who also have disabilities affecting learning ability and/or social development. These students are sometimes referred to as **culturally and linguistically different excep-tional (CLDE) students** (Baca & Almanza, 1991). These students often need spe-cial programs of instruction that will help them both develop their language skills and address their particular learning problems.

Baca and Almanza (1991) describe three types of instructional models for CLDE students:

> **The bilingual support model:** Monolingual English special education teach-ers are teamed with native language tutors/paraprofessionals to provide spe-cial education services. The special education teacher provides ESL instruc-tion.
>
> **The coordinated service model:** A monolingual special education teacher is teamed with a bilingual teacher. The special education teacher is responsible for providing ESL instruction and implementing IEP goals in English. The bilingual teacher provides academic instruction in the child's native lan-guage.
>
> **The integrated bilingual special education model:** A bilingual special edu-cator is responsible for the implementation of the IEP. Teachers are trained in both bilingual education and special education.

Just as there is disagreement about what constitutes the best instructional pro-gram for LEP students, there is also great disagreement within the special educa-tion field about the most effective instructional practices. Often, this disagreement comes down to an argument between those who advocate a direct instruction approach versus those who favor instruction addressing cognitive learning processes. This debate is especially relevant with regard to LEP students with dis-abilities. Many educators have expressed concerns about the use of direct instruc-tion techniques with CLDE students (Cummins, 1984; Yates & Ortiz, 1991). They are concerned that programs focusing on the acquisition of specific language skills (such as phonics and vocabulary acquisition) may actually interfere with the child's acquisition of English. As we have noted earlier in this chapter, many edu-cators have suggested that whole-language programs that emphasize more natu-ralistic approaches to language development are preferable for helping LEP stu-dents develop their skills in English. Similarly, instructional programs for CLDE students should emphasize the development of naturalistic language skills. At the same time, we cannot ignore the fact that many CLDE students will need extra help in identifying and correcting errors in language usage.

Cloud (1994) has suggested that educators consider the *whole* child when planning instruction for LEP students with special needs. She means that we should consider the child's *disability,* as well as the *language* and *cultural* differ-ences; each should be given equal importance. Instruction should be based on a reciprocal-interaction model, where the teacher's task is to facilitate learning through modeling and sharing successful strategies for learning. In her review of effective practices for teaching CLDE students, Ruiz (1989) recommended that instructional programs:

1. Take into account students' sociocultural backgrounds and their effects on oral language, reading and writing, and second-language learning.
2. Take into account students' possible learning handicaps and their effects on oral language, reading and writing, and second-language learning.
3. Follow developmental practices in literacy acquisition.
4. Locate curriculum in a meaningful context where the communicative purpose is clear and authentic.
5. Connect curriculum with the students' personal experiences.
6. Incorporate children's literature into reading, writing, and ESL lessons.
7. Involve parents as active partners in the instruction of their children.
8. Give students experience with whole texts in reading, writing, and ESL lessons.
9. Incorporate collaborative learning whenever possible.

Summary

In looking at the impact of language and cultural differences on schools and schooling, educators must have an awareness of the difference between a language *disability* and a language *difference*. Many children come to school speaking a dialect that differs from standard English or a language other than English. There is nothing "wrong" with most of these children, and most of them do not require special educational services. But many do need special programs that will allow them to retain their first language or dialect while learning standard English.

We have seen that most research favors a *holistic* approach that emphasizes the development of *literacy skills* through use of the child's *first language*—that students are then better able to make the transition to English. It is important that teachers show respect for the child's language and culture as they try to help the child make this transition.

Some children with language and cultural differences also have learning and/or behavior disabilities. These children not only need help in learning English but also need the intensive instructional support that can be provided through special education.

Teachers and other education professionals need to be aware of the special needs of children with language and cultural differences. They should also respect the contribution that cultural diversity makes to our society.

Review Questions

1. Is there a "right" way to talk? Give arguments for and against this notion.

2. Give three examples of ways in which Black English Vernacular differs from standard English.

3. What is the effect of bilingualism on cognitive and language development?

4. What are the three threats faced by LEP children with special needs?

5. List four ways that assessment can be modified to more fairly and accurately evaluate the abilities of LEP students.

6. Compare and contrast submersion programs with structured English immersion programs for LEP children, discussing both their instructional methods and their use of English and the child's first language.

7. Why do most educators who are interested in bilingual education support approaches emphasizing the development of competence in the child's first language?

8. What is the rationale for a bidialectical approach to teaching children with dialect differences?

Suggested Activities

1. Listen carefully to the language of teenagers. You will probably find dialect differences, the most apparent, in semantics. Often, different groups of students within a community can have different dialects. For example, African American students can use a different dialect from white students. Try making a list of five to ten words that seem unique to one group of teenagers. Then ask another group to tell you what these words mean. What did you find? What do the results indicate about the ability of students from different social or cultural groups to understand each other?

2. If you have the opportunity to observe students who speak a language other than English, try to observe some nonverbal aspects of their interaction (you do not have to speak the language). Watch closely as they interact with their teacher. Also, try to observe as they interact with peers. Do you notice any differences in

- distance between speakers
- facial expressions
- gestures
- lengths of conversation

3. To find out about cultural differences, try asking a group of children or adults to share one thing from their culture that they think other people may not know about. This is a good opportunity to discuss the word *culture,* and some interesting (and enlightening) responses often surface.

References

Adler, S. (1993). *Multicultural communication skills in the classroom.* Boston: Allyn and Bacon.

ASHA Committee on the Status of Racial Minorities. (1983). Social dialects position paper. *Asha, 25,* 23–24.

ASHA Committee on the Status of Racial Minorities (1985). Clinical management of communicatively handicapped minority language populations. *Asha, 27,* 29–32.

Baca, L. M., & Almanza, E. (1991). *Language minority students with disabilities.* Reston, VA: The Council for Exceptional Children. (ERIC Document Reproduction Services No. 339 171)

Baca, L. M., & Cervantes, H. T. (1989). *The bilingual special education interface.* New York: Merrill.

Baratz, J. C. (1969). Linguistic and cultural factors in teaching reading to ghetto children. *Elementary English, 46,* 199–203.

Bernstein, B. (1970). A sociolinguistic approach to socialization: With some reference to educability. In F. Williams (Ed.), *Language and Poverty.* Chicago: Markham Publishing.

Bialystok, E. (1991). Metalinguistic dimensions of bilingual language proficiency. In E. Bialystok (Ed.), *Language processing in bilingual children.* Cambridge, England: Cambridge University Press.

Carroll, J. (1961). Fundamental considerations in testing for English proficiency of foreign students. In *Testing the English proficiency of foreign students.* Washington, DC: Center for Applied Linguistics.

Cheng, L. L. (1987). Cross-cultural and linguistic considerations in working with Asian populations. *Asha, 29,* 33–36.

Cloud, N. (1994). Special education needs of second language students. In F. Genesee (Ed.), *Educating second language children.* New York: Cambridge University Press.

Cole, L. (1989). E pluribus pluribus: Multicultural imperatives for the 1990s and beyond. *Asha, 31,* 65–70.

Cole, P. A., & Taylor, O. L. (1990). Performance of working class African-American children on three tests of articulation. *Language, Speech, and Hearing Services in Schools, 21,* 171–176.

Cummins, J. (1980). The cross-lingual dimensions of language proficiency: Implications for bilingual education and the optimal age issue. *TESOL Quarterly, 4,* 171–174.

Cummins, J. (1984). *Bilingualism and special education: Issues in assessment and pedagogy.* San Diego: College-Hill Press.

Cummins, J. (1989). A theoretical framework for bilingual special education. *Exceptional Children, 56,* 111–120.

Cummins, J. (1994). Knowledge, power, and identity in teaching English as a second language. In F. Genesee (Ed.), *Educating second language children* (pp. 33–58). New York: Cambridge University Press.

Damico, J. S., & Damico, S. K. (1993). Language and social skills from a diversity perspective: Considerations for the speech-language pathologist. *Language, Speech, and Hearing Services in Schools, 24,* 236–243.

Damico, J. S., Oller, J. W., & Storey, M. E. (1983). The diagnosis of language disorders in bilingual children: Surface-oriented and pragmatic criteria. *Journal of Speech and Hearing Disorders, 48,* 385–394.

Emihovich, C. (1988). Toward cultural pluralism: Redefining integration in American society. *Urban Review, 20,* 3–7.

Figueroa, R. A. (1989). Psychological testing of linguistic-minority students: Knowledge gaps and regulations. *Exceptional Children, 56,* 145–153.

First, J. M. (1988). Immigrant students in U.S. public schools: Challenges with solutions. *Phi Delta Kappan, 70,* 205–207.

Garcia, E. E. (1993). Language, culture, and education. In L. Darling-Hammond (Ed.), *Review of research in education* (vol. 19) (pp. 51–98). Washington, DC: AERA.

Genesee, F. (1994). Introduction. In F. Genesee (Ed.), *Educating second language children* (pp. 1–12). New York: Cambridge University Press.

Gersten, R., & Jimenez, R. T. (1994). A delicate balance: Enhancing literature instruction for students of English as a second language. *The Reading Teacher, 47,* 438–448.

Gersten, R., & Woodward, J. (1994). The language-minority student and special education: Issues, trends, and paradoxes. *Exceptional Children, 60,* 310–322.

Goodz, N. S. (1994). Interactions between parents and children in bilingual families. In F. Genesee (Ed.), *Educating second language children* (pp. 61–81). New York: Cambridge University Press.

Grossman, H. (1995). *Special Education in a diverse society.* Boston: Allyn and Bacon.

Handscombe, J. (1994). Putting it all together. In F. Genesee (Ed.), *Educating second language children.* New York: Cambridge University Press.

Harris-Wright, K. (1987). The challenge of educational coalescence: Teaching nonmainstream English-speaking students. *Journal of Childhood Communication Disorders, 11,* 209–215.

Hudelson, S. (1994). Literacy development of second language children. In F. Genesee (Ed.), *Educating second language children* (pp. 129–158). New York: Cambridge University Press.

Labov, W. (1969). Contraction, deletion, and inherent variability of English copula. *Language, 45,* 715–762.

Labov, W. (1970). The logic of non-standard English. In F. Williams (Ed.), *Language and poverty.* Chicago: Markham Publishing.

Labov, W. (1972). *Sociolinguistic patterns.* Philadelphia: University of Pennsylvania Press.

Lindfors, J. W. (1987). *Children's language and learning.* Englewood Cliffs, NJ: Prentice-Hall.

Long, S. H. (1994). Language and bilingual-bicultural children. In V. A. Reed (Ed.), *An introduction to children with language disorders.* New York: Merrill.

Martin Luther King Junior Elementary School Children v. Ann Arbor School District Board, 1979. 473 F. Suppl 1371.

McLoughlin, J. A., & Lewis, R. B. (1994). *Assessing special students.* New York: Macmillan.

Mercer, J. R. (1973). *Labeling the mentally retarded.* Berkeley: University of California Press.

Oller, J. (1988). Discrete point, integrative, or pragmatic tests. In P. A. Richard-Amato (Ed.), *Making it happen: Interaction in the second language classroom.* New York: Longman.

Ortiz, A. A., & Yates, J. R. (1983). Incidence among Hispanic exceptionals: Implications for manpower planning. *Journal of the National Association for Bilingual Education, 7,* 41–53.

PASE v. Hannon, 1980. 506 F. Suppl. 831, N.D. Illinois.

Payan, R. M. (1989). Language assessment for the bilingual exceptional child. In L. M. Baca. & H. T. Cervantes, (Eds.), *The bilingual special education interface.* New York: Merrill.

Ramirez, J. D., Yuen, S. D., & Ramey, D. R. (1991). *Executive summary. Final report: Longitudinal study of structured English immersion strategy, early-exit, and late-exit transitional bilingual education programs for language-minority children.* Contract No. 300-87-0156. Submitted to the U.S. Department of Education. San Mateo: Aguirre International.

Reyes, M. de la Luz. (1992). Challenging venerable assumptions: Literacy instruction for linguistically different students. *Harvard Educational Review, 62,* 427–446.

Reyes, M. de la Luz., & Laliberty, E. (1992). A teacher's "Pied Piper" effect on young authors. *Education and Urban Society, 24,* 263–278.

Rueda, R., & Chan, K. (1979). Poverty and culture in special education: Separate but equal. *Exceptional Children, 45,* 422–431.

Ruiz, N. (1989). An optimal learning environment for Rosemary. *Exceptional Children, 56,* 130–144.

Schiff-Myers, N. B. (1992). Considering arrested language development and language loss in the assessment of second language learners. *Language, Speech, and Hearing Services in Schools, 23,* 28–33.

Terrell, S. L., & Terrell, F. (1993). African-American cultures. In D.E. Battle (Ed.), *Communication disorders in multicultural populations* (pp. 3–37). Boston: Andover Medical Publishers.

Vaughn-Cooke, F. B. (1983). Improving language assessment in minority children. *Asha, 25,* 29–33.

Walton, J. H., McCardle, P., Crowe, T. A., & Wilson, B. E. (1990). Black English in a Mississippi prison population. *Journal of Speech and Hearing Disorders, 55,* 206–216.

Warren, A. R., & McCloskey, L. A. (1993). Pragmatics: Language in social contexts. In J. B. Gleason (Ed.), *The development of language.* New York: Macmillan.

Yates, J. R., & Ortiz, A. A. (1991). Professional development needs of teachers who serve exceptional language minorities in today's schools. *Teacher Education and Special Education, 14,* 11–18.

Name Index

Abbeduto, L., 96, 97, 98, 174
Abraham, L., 244
Adler, S., 278, 294
Alamanza, E., 282, 286, 287, 296
Allen, J., 114, 120
Alpern, G., 114, 120
Alpert, C., 215, 219, 221
Alwell, M., 105, 267
Andersen, E., 166, 167, 171
Anderson, M., 122
Anderson, R., 169
Aram, D., 68, 78, 212, 235, 246
Armstrong, R., 270
Atkinson, R., 228

Baca, L., 282, 283, 286, 287, 291, 296
Bain, B., 212, 213
Bakeman, R., 258, 264
Baker, J., 240
Baker, L., 78, 116, 122, 127
Baker, P., 130
Ball, E., 79
Baltaxe, C., 115, 123, 125
Bankson, N., 196
Baratz, J., 295
Baron-Cohen, S., 128
Barrera, R., 263
Bartak, L., 117, 119, 121, 122
Bartel, N., 228, 229
Bartolucci, G., 121, 122
Barton, S., 114, 120
Bashir, A., 78, 234, 235, 261
Bates, E., 41, 47

Baumberger, T., 122
Bear, G., 240
Bedrosian, J., 97, 199
Beer, M., 255
Belanger, A., 68, 78
Bellugi, V., 149
Belmont, J., 100
Benaroya, S., 117
Benjamin, B., 267
Bentler, R., 148, 150, 151
Berard, G., 131
Berko, J., 205
Berko Gleason, J., 21, 58
Bernard-Opitz, V., 125
Bernstein, B., 280
Bernstein, D., 51, 75
Best, S., 171
Bettelheim, B., 116, 119
Beukelman, D., 255
Bialystok, E., 282
Biemer, C., 246
Bigelow, A., 166, 167
Bigge, J., 171, 174
Biklen, D., 131, 132
Billow, R., 57
Birch, J., 238, 240
Bishop, D., 173
Blachman, B., 69, 72, 79
Blackman, B., 59
Blackstone, S., 253
Bleck, E., 172, 173
Bliss, C., 258
Blockberger, S., 170, 270

Eberlin, M., 132
Edelson, S., 131
Edwards, R., 120
Eheart, B., 103
Eimas, P., 47
Eisenson, J., 144
Ekelman, B., 78, 212
Elfenbein, J., 148, 150, 151
Ellis, N., 100
Eppel, P., 121, 122
Epstein, M., 93
Erin, J., 166, 169, 170
Eskes, G., 123
Evans, J., 200
Ewing-Cobbs, L., 178
Ezell, H., 95

Fay, W., 121
Fein, D., 120, 122
Feldman, H., 149
Fewell, R., 93
Fey, S., 75
Fifer, W., 47
Fillmore, C., 40
Finitzo, T., 158
Fischer, F., 70
Fish, B., 124
Fletcher, J., 178
Flood, J., 78
Flowers, C., 177, 178
Fodor, J., 19
Foley, R., 93
Folks, J., 58
Folstein, S., 120, 127
Footo, M., 158
Fors, S., 103
Foster, S., 225
Fouts, R., 130
Fowles, B., 57, 75
Fox, B., 70
Fox, S., 205
Fraiberg, S., 169
Freeman, R., 170
Friel-Patti, S., 158
Fristoe, M., 197
Frith, U., 128
Fromkin, V., 16
Fuchs, D., 67
Fuchs, L., 67
Fujiki, M., 205
Fulwiler, R., 130

Furman, L., 96, 98
Furth, H., 144

Gaines, B., 127
Galbraith, G., 99
Gardner, B., 6
Gardner, H., 31
Gardner, R.., 6
Gee, K., 105
Geers, A., 148, 149, 150
Gentile, A., 150
Gerstman, L., 93
Gibbs, D., 68, 72
Glanz, M., 57, 75
Gleason, J., 13, 15, 20, 54
Gleitman, A., 41, 47, 48
Gleitman, L., 41, 47, 48, 169
Goetz, L., 105, 220
Goldfarb, N., 127
Goldfarb, W., 121, 127
Golding, B., 97, 103
Goldin-Meadow, S., 149
Goldman, R., 197
Goldsmith, S., 73
Goldstein, H., 95, 212
Golinkoff, P., 173
Gordon, L., 173
Gorga, M., 148, 150, 151
Gravel, J., 158
Grice, H., 21
Grievink, E., 158
Grossman, H., 89
Guthrie, J., 200

Hall, S., 125
Halliday, M., 41, 203, 204
Hammill, D., 195, 196, 228, 229
Hanlon, C., 37
Harrington, D., 178
Healey, W., 158
Henderson, F., 158
Hendy, J., 97, 103
Hermelin, B., 115
Hintgen, J., 120
Hirsh-Pasek, K., 173
Hissock, M., 177
Horton, K., 145
House, B., 99
Howard, M., 26, 27, 32
Howell, K., 205
Howlin, P., 116

Subject Index

Negation, 53
Neologisms, 124
Nonliteral language, 57–58
  and learning disabilities, 75
Non-SLIP, 258
Normalization, 91
Northwestern Syntax Screening Test, 197
Noun phrase, 53

Otitis media, 158
  and mental retardation, 93

Parallel talk, 242–243
Parent-child interaction
  and autism, 127
  and mental retardation, 102–103
  and visually impaired, 167–168
Parentese, 47–48
Peabody Language Development Kits, 229
Peabody Picture Vocabulary Test—R, 197
Peripheral nervous system, 28
Perlocutionary state of early communication
    development, 47–48
Phonation, 26
Phoneme, 14
Phonological awareness
  assessment of, 70–71
  and auditory perception, 69–70
  defined, 59
  intervention for, 79
  and learning disabilities, 69–72
  and reading, 59, 69–72, 79
Phonology
  assessment of, 191, 204
  and autism, 121
  defined, 14–15
  and hearing impairment, 145–146
  intervention for, 227
  and learning disabilities, 69–72
  and mental retardation, 93–94
Piagetian theory, 32–33
Picsyms, 258–259
Picture Communication Symbols (PICS), 258–259
Plasticity, 177
Pragmatic-interactionist model of language
    acquisition, 41–42
  and intervention, 224
Pragmatics
  assessment of, 192, 203–204, 206
  and autism, 124–126

conversational rules, 21
defined, 20
and hearing impairment, 148
indirect speech acts, 21
intervention for, 229
and learning disabilities, 76–77
and mental retardation, 96–98
speech acts, 21
and visual impairment, 169–170
Preschool classrooms, 243–244
Preschool language development, 50–56
  complex sentences in, 53
  grammatical morphemes in, 51–52
  semantic development in, 54–56
  sentence types in, 53
  stages of, 50–56
Protodeclarative, 47
Protoimperative, 47
Prototype hypothesis, 55
Protowords, 49
Proverbs, 57
  and learning disabilities, 75
Psycholinguistic model of language acquisition,
    38–39
  and intervention, 223
Psycholinguistics, 39

Regular education initiative, 238
Reading
  and hearing impairment, 150–151
  and language, 68–72
  and metalinguistic abilities, 78
  phonological awareness and, 59, 79, 69–72
Rebus symbols, 258, 259
Remedial approach to language intervention,
    217–218
Remediation of Common Phonological Processes, 227
Requests, 58, 229
Respiration, 26
Restating and rewording intervention strategy,
    243
Retardation (*see* Mental retardation)
Ritualistic behavior in autism, 114
Rules
  conversational, 21
  morphological, 15
  phonological, 14–15
  phrase structure, 17
  semantic, 19
  syntactic, 17

language and, 168–170
mother-child interaction, 167–168
pragmatics and, 169–170
semantics and, 169
syntax and, 169–170
Vocabulary, 56–57
and augmentative and alternative communication, 256, 265
assessment of, 192, 203
and hearing impairment, 148
and learning disabilities, 74, 81
and mental retardation, 95
and visual impairment, 169

Vocal folds, 26
Vygotsky's theory and language, 33

Wepman Auditory Discrimination Test, 197
Wernicke's area, 30
Whole-language approach to instruction, 244–245, 293
Whorfian theory and language, 32
Withdrawal from interpersonal contact, 114
Writing, and hearing impairment, 151–152

Zone of proximal development, 224